HOMES FOR THE MAD

Ellen Dwyer

HOMES FOR THE MAD

LIFE INSIDE TWO NINETEENTH-CENTURY ASYLUMS

Rutgers University Press
New Brunswick and London

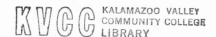

Library of Congress Cataloging-in-Publication Data

Dwyer, Ellen.
   Homes for the mad.

      Bibliography: p.
      Includes index.
   1. Willard Asylum for the Insane (N.Y.)—
History—19th century.   2. New York (State) State
Lunatic Asylum—History—19th century.
3. Psychiatric hospitals—New York (State)——History—
19th century.   I. Title. [DNLM: 1. Willard Asylum
for the Insane (N.Y.)   2. New York (State) State
Lunatic Asylum.   3. Hospitals, Psychiatric—history—
New York.   4. Mental Disorders—history—New York.
WM 27 AN6 D97h]

   RC445.N7N583   1987   362.2'1'09747   86–4355
   ISBN 0–8135–1182–8

British Cataloging-in-Publication information available

In Memoriam:

Gareth Paul Dwyer Huntsman

December 20, 1982–March 13, 1983

Contents

List of Figures and Table   *ix*

Preface   *xi*

Introduction   *1*

1. Life within the Asylum Walls   7

2. The Economics of Compassion   29

3. Medical Men and Medical Power   55

4. A Distanced Relative   85

5. Destiny in a Name   *117*

6. Attendants and Their World of Work   *163*

7. The Politics of Maintenance   *186*

8. An Unresolved Conclusion   *213*

Abbreviations   *219*

Notes   *221*

Bibliography   *275*

Index   *305*

List of Figures and Table

Table 2.1   Per Capita Expenditures in Dollars at the
Utica and Willard Asylums, 1869–1889   52

Figure 4.1   Utica Cases "Caused" by Emotional Stress   99

Figure 4.2   Utica Cases "Caused" by Economic Stress   99

Figure 4.3   Utica Cases "Caused" by Heredity   100

Figure 4.4   Utica Cases "Caused" by Epilepsy   100

Figure 4.5   Utica Cases "Caused" by Paresis   101

Figure 4.6   Utica Cases "Caused" by Senility   101

Figure 4.7   Utica Cases "Caused" by Physical Problems   102

Figure 5.1   "Recovered" as a Percentage of Admissions
(Five-Year Running Averages)   151

Figure 5.2   "Recovered" as a Percentage of Those Treated
(Five-Year Running Averages)   151

Preface

Discussions of what constitutes mental illness and how best to treat it evoke intense, and often contradictory, emotions. In the mid-nineteenth century, Americans, disturbed by what seemed to be an increasing number of the insane in their midst, began to build large state-funded asylums intended to cure as well as confine the mentally ill. One hundred years later, the initial promise of such institutions had been forgotten. During the late 1960s and early 1970s, radical psychiatrists such as Thomas Szasz and R. D. Laing suggested that our notion of "mental illness" was just that: a social construct. Others, even if they accepted a medical model of mental illness, attacked the therapeutic efficacy of mental hospitals. Such institutions, they claimed, more closely resembled prisons than hospitals, and behind their locked doors patients often served longer sentences than did convicted felons. How could the mentally ill learn to cope with the stresses of daily life within the artificial environment of such "total institutions," they asked. Out of their critiques emerged what has come to be known as a policy of "deinstitutionalization." Massive state mental hospitals discharged their chronic patients to a variety of community care programs. More recently, we seem to have come almost full cycle. The limitations of community care (at least in its present form) are all too painfully clear. Furthermore, the continued and highly visible presence of what seem to be chronic mentally ill men and women challenges Szasz's assertion that only a small percentage of those labeled "mentally ill" deserve that designation. Discouraged by stories of the plight of the so-called homeless mentally ill, some have begun to reconsider the potential of state mental hospitals to offer what their original appellation promised: asylum.[1]

This continuing debate about mental health care policies greatly interests me. Primarily a historian of nineteenth-century America, in the early 1970s I first discovered the writings of a diverse group of social critics of madness, ranging from Thomas Szasz and Erving Goffman to Michel Foucault and David Rothman.[2] More recently, I have read with concern the critiques of deinstitutionalization offered by Andrew Scull, Leona Bachrach, and others.[3] While I do not think that these contemporary writers predetermined my view of the past, they certainly influenced my choice of topic and research questions. For example, initially I most wanted to pursue the line of inquiry suggested by Szasz and Foucault and to find out how social definitions of madness (and its appropriate treatment) changed over time. I focused on nineteenth-century New York for several reasons. Not only did its state insane asylum system serve as a national model, but the medical doctors employed at its institutions also wrote extensively and well about their theories of insanity and how to treat it. Finally the extant manuscript sources for New York's first two state insane asylums, at Utica and Willard, are rich and accessible. I particularly looked forward to extracting from patient case histories clues to how nineteenth-century Americans defined mental illness.

In the course of my research, however, I slowly had to modify my goals. Most reluctantly abandoned was my ambition to measure changes over time in public perceptions of what constituted deviant behavior. Because families and communities rather than asylum doctors largely determined the boundaries of socially acceptable behavior, commitment records and patient casebook histories offer only a biased glimpse of that decision-making process. Yet, in combination with other manuscript and printed sources, they paint a rich picture of the complex internal dynamics of nineteenth-century asylums and their multiple social functions. While such institutions clearly were intended to modify the behavior of the men and women committed to them, they also provided a refuge for exhausted mothers, a respite for beleaguered families, a hospital for those with debilitated bodies as well as disturbed minds. By the time I began to write this manuscript, growing public concern about the difficulties of caring for the chronic mentally ill reinforced my interest in the asylums that were an earlier generation's solution to medical and social problems which continue to perplex us.

As in much historical research, finding relevant sources required time and ingenuity. Most of the extant manuscript materials related to the nineteenth-century Utica and Willard asylums remain at the Utica and Willard psychiatric centers. At Utica, Barbara and Lyle Engells have collected and preserved large numbers of nineteenth-century materials. Although I refer to a "Willard Archive" as well in my footnote references, there is no formal archive at the Willard Psychiatric Center. On my first visit there, I rescued the nineteenth-century casebooks from the basement of the abandoned Chapin building. Subsequently, extant nineteenth-century materials were stored in a former patient building. Primary sources related to Utica and Willard also can be found at the New York State Library Archives, the American Antiquarian Society, the Countway and Houghton libraries at Harvard University, and the Pennsylvania Hospital Medical Archives.

After locating the bulk of the Utica and Willard patient casebook records, I began to transcribe, code, and analyze them. During this lengthy gestation period, many friends offered personal support and professional encouragement. I am particularly grateful to colleagues at Indiana University in criminal justice, history, and women's studies. Once I began to look for manuscript records, I received much help from directors and staff at Utica and Willard. Deserving special mention are Lyle and Barbara Engells, whose creation of an extraordinary historical archive at Utica Psychiatric Center was done for love of the past. In addition, my conversations with them and others who work today at Utica and Willard greatly increased my appreciation of the complexity of life within large state mental institutions, whatever the century.

When I started this project, I had little background in the history of medicine and even less awareness of the difficulties of statistical analysis of nineteenth-century psychiatric records. Although I remain primarily a social historian, I have found my new acquaintances in the history of medicine to be extraordinarily generous and helpful. In particular, I want to thank Ann Carmichael, Gerald Grob, Dirk Hartog, Harvey Graff, Charles Rosenberg, Barbara Rosenkrantz, Andrew Scull, and Nancy Tomes for their useful comments on various parts and versions of this manuscript, although full response to their suggestions awaits a second book. I also appreciate the encouragement and assistance I received from Jim Beal, John Burnham, Joanne Fortune, Richard Jensen, Rick Jones, Eric Monkkonen, Irene Neu, Janet Rabinowich, Mike Sherry, Jan Shipps, and Peter Tyor. Barbara Hanawalt gave me the initial idea for this study, and Marlie Wasserman, my editor at Rutgers University Press, with great patience has helped it move to completion. Although he had little direct input into this particular project, I much appreciate David Brion Davis's support of my Ph.D. dissertation and his continued encouragement. Fellowship and research money from the Newberry Library's Monticello College Foundation; the National Endowment for the Humanities' State, Local, and Regional History Program; the American Historical Association; the Office of Research and Graduate Development at Indiana University; and the Indiana University Women's Studies Program gave me invaluable free time for writing. It also paid for the student assistants who helped to code patient casebook records and, in the case of David Lewis and Emil Pocock, shape my thinking as well.

My deepest debts are to my family. Paul and Marianne Dwyer, my parents, have long supported my work. My father, during his years at the New York State Department of Mental Hygiene, showed me that state officials' public pronouncements of concern for the mentally ill are, for some, much more than rhetoric. He further communicated his distress at the ease with which institutional realities move away from programmatic ideals. Jeffrey Huntsman helped in ways too numerous to list. Without his encouragement and support, I never would have tackled, let alone completed, this project. No one is happier about that completion than Elliott and Sara Huntsman, who, with varying degrees of patience, let their evenings, weekends, and vacations be disrupted for my research.

HOMES FOR THE MAD

Introduction

During the nineteenth century, insane asylums were simultaneously scourged as "tombs of the living dead" and praised as loving places of refuge to which troubled Americans could retreat for comfort and care. Such controversy over the functions of these institutions, and the meaning of their history, has persisted into the twentieth century, reviving with particular intensity in the 1960s and 1970s. The disputants, whatever their positions, often express concerns about contemporary policy toward mental illness and its treatment while reinterpreting the past. Although at times the debate bogs down in bitter arguments about the social control function of asylums, out of this dissension has emerged a growing awareness of the complexity of both the internal and external histories of nineteenth-century asylums, and a generally more positive evaluation of their therapeutic ambitions.[1] This book is part of that new perspective.

As the opening sentence suggests, Americans throughout the nineteenth century searched unsuccessfully for a single metaphor which would capture the essence of asylum life during this period when psychiatry was struggling to make treatment of the insane an increasingly medical procedure. But, while antebellum doctors pictured their institutions as the family home writ large, unhappy patients more often compared them to prisons, where superintendents endeavored to impose the order and discipline of the military or the industrial plant on their unwieldly populations. Ultimately, no one metaphor evoking either cell or sanctuary prevailed, for each truthfully illuminated a different facet of the asylum experience. Similarly, this book presents the complex interplay of a num-

1

ber of themes, concluding in part that nineteenth-century asylums sometimes differed dramatically from one another, that even state asylums served a range of social classes, and that the social and medical functions of such institutions cannot be separated from one another. While pursuing these arguments, the book also traces changes and continuities in definitions of the kinds of insane behavior that required asylum treatment.

The book presents a close look at the nineteenth-century development of New York's first two state insane asylums: the New York State Lunatic Asylum at Utica and the Willard Asylum for the Chronic Insane. They form a useful contrast to each other, for, while they shared some of the same administrative and medical concerns, they had different therapeutic goals. State legislators established the Utica Asylum in 1843 to care exclusively for the acutely ill; during its first several decades, asylum administrators attempted to restrict admissions to the recently afflicted and to discharge patients not cured within the first two years of treatment. In contrast, the Willard Asylum, which opened in 1869, accepted only chronically insane paupers whose therapeutic prognosis was grim. Many of its patients had already spent years in county asylums or other state institutions before their arrival at Willard.

Such official segregation of the acute from the chronic mentally ill was relatively rare in nineteenth-century America, although many asylums developed dual systems of care within a single institution. In New York State, the establishment of Willard had both the positive results desired by its supporters and the negative ones feared by its critics. For relatively small sums of money, Willard's doctors offered good medical care to its often physically enfeebled patients. They also protected patients from the abuse and neglect which the chronically insane so often suffered at both county poorhouses and acute care asylums. For Willard's staff, care of the chronic mentally ill was their first priority. The opening of Willard thus helped solve a pernicious problem at Utica: the relegation of the chronic mentally ill to "back wards" where they received neither the medical attention nor the therapeutic programs reserved for more promising patients. On the other hand, most Willard patients, no matter how serious their symptoms at admission, were discharged only by death. Despite doctors' acknowledgment that cases of chronic mental illness were sometimes cured, Willard's annual discharge rates seldom exceeded .005 percent. Within a few years of its opening, Willard became a permanent "home" for many nineteenth-century New Yorkers with few social resources: unskilled foreigners, female domestics, the senile old. In combination with Utica's, its history raises troubling questions, which have yet to be answered, about how best to care for those with recurrent or long-term mental illness.

Whatever the policy lessons of the Utica and Willard experiences, their histories make clear that nineteenth-century insane asylums performed a wide variety of social and medical functions. For most families, lunatic asylums were places of last, not first, resort. They institutionalized spouses, siblings, and children only after months of home care. When physically, emotionally, and often financially exhausted families could no longer control violent and unpredictable behavior or provide for the physical needs of individuals unwilling or unable to care for themselves, they looked to state lunatic asylums for affordable assistance. Although some historians picture these institutions as dumping grounds for the most marginal members of society, in fact they served a wide range of individuals, families, and communities. As the asylum doctors noted frequently in their annual reports, many inmates' poverty was a recent product of their illness, not a life-long condition. In addition, the Utica Asylum accepted a large number of private patients, who either could not afford or find room in New York's few private asylums. For some of the insane, such as women exhausted by childbirth, illness, and poverty, the Utica asylum lived up to its name and truly provided a refuge where they could rest and regain their health. For others it was a hated prison in which they had been trapped by machinations of exasperated families or scheming business acquaintances. In contrast, the Willard Asylum more closely resembled the conventional view of nineteenth-century social welfare institutions. Its patients were generally poor and often immigrants, who lacked familial and community supports.

In the eyes of both nineteenth- and twentieth-century commentators on these asylums, the diverse social functions of Utica and Willard often interfered with the institutions' medical mission. Asylum superintendents struggled with multiple burdens: the need to treat psychological symptoms, to cure physical disease, and to maintain institutional order. Too often, critics complained, the last goal became all-important. In response, asylum superintendents argued that only within a quiet, predictable environment could disturbed men and women begin to recover inter-

3

nal stability. They also fought, albeit unsuccessfully, the propensity of politicians concerned about costs and of medical professionals concerned about scientific progress to dichotomize treatment and care. Doctors, searching for ways to cure their troubled charges, naturally favored more promising patients over their fellows whose best hope was for stasis; politicians often looked chiefly for ways to insulate the general public from the mad, and at the lowest cost. Nevertheless, although Utica had a much higher cure rate than did Willard, both took great pride in their high standards of physical care, particularly as measured by their low death rates. As the records show, asylum superintendents had to fight fiercely for sufficient funding to maintain their physical plants, but much of their seeming obsession with such issues as ventilation and plumbing grew out of their concern for patients' health. At both Utica and Willard, polluted water supplies and contagious diseases several times threatened the lives of the entire institutional population, and although it sometimes troubled them to do so, superintendents often gave such concerns precedence over innovative psychiatric treatment.

After 1855, medical research at Utica turned in another direction. Convinced that insanity was a physical disease like tuberculosis or cholera, asylum doctors increasingly used laboratory tests and autopsies to explore the somatic bases of insanity. They hoped that such strategies would increase the general prestige of asylum medicine as well as unlock the mysteries of mental illness, but unfortunately they did neither. Utica's doctors replaced experiments in moral therapy with a reliance on chemical and mechanical restraints to quiet individuals and to ensure general institutional order. At Willard, where doctors had fewer research resources and less promising patient populations, members of the medical staff did much less pathological work. They also lacked the funds to use sedative drugs freely and therefore emphasized the soothing effects of physical labor.

Even while Utica's doctors tried to emulate research scientists in their work, they continued to refer to their patient populations as family members rather than as laboratory subjects. Superintendents at both Utica and Willard liked to consider themselves kindly fathers, although their institutional families had few of the qualities of the Victorian bourgeois ideal. Not only were asylum families much larger and more heterogeneous, but particularly at Utica by midcentury, internal conflicts on all levels frequently disrupted daily life. Several assistant physicians quit in anger and remained the superintendent's enemies for the remainder of their professional lives. According to the testimony offered at state legislative investigations and in patient memoirs, tension and even physical violence frequently characterized staff–patient relations. Patients also frequently fought among themselves. The family metaphor, even when grossly distended to apply to a community of two thousand, worked somewhat better at Willard, perhaps because its chronically ill patients were less likely to fight their assigned role as children. And Willard's physicians, who considered their patients incurable, did not have to emulate their Utica counterparts' efforts to maintain obedience to official rules while encouraging independence in their convalescing patients.

The family metaphor was inadequate for another reason; it conveyed little about asylums' therapeutic work. At both Utica and Willard, several factors influenced diagnosis and treatment of patients: actual patient behavior, the intellectual biases of the medical staff, particularly the superintendents, and the sociodemographic characteristics of patients. Most institutional diagnoses were based on fairly obvious behavior cues: melancholia on withdrawal, depression, or threats of suicide; mania on extreme mental or physical excitement; and dementia on evidence of temporary or permanent intellectual debility. More frequently these diagnoses confirmed judgments already made by the families and friends of patients than offered a new interpretation of aberrant behavior. Yet, there remained a substantial minority of cases in which the behavioral cues to diagnosis were ambiguous, particularly at Willard. It is these cases where nonmedical factors seemed most strongly to have affected doctors' responses to individual men and women. In particular, sex and ethnicity heavily influenced diagnoses and subsequent treatment, in combination with other variables such as age, civil condition, and occupational skills.

As this summary suggests, the book primarily offers an internal history of the two asylums during the nineteenth century. I rely heavily on manuscript records: patient casebooks, letters, scrapbooks, and so forth, as well as on published annual reports and journal articles. The richest and most difficult to interpret of these sources are the patient casebooks. They offer tantalizing glimpses of patients' preinstitutional lives as well as details about their institutional behavior and treatment, and they entice the twentieth-century reader into conjectures about the relationship between asylums and the communities they served. In the case of state asy-

lums, that relationship was particularly complex, for asylum superintendents had to respond to the expectations of many groups: state legislators,
who controlled part of their budgets; county officials, who controlled the
rest of their funds; newspaper reporters, who followed stories of abuse
and involuntary commitment with avidity; and the families, communities,
and employers of patients.

Understandably, it is this larger picture that most intrigues twentieth-
century analysts of the asylum, although few have managed to capture
fully the dynamic interaction of outside forces with internal developments. While insane asylums more often reinforced than provoked the
ethnic, class, and sexual biases of nineteenth-century New York, their
very existence and the force of their therapeutic ideologies certainly
affected the ways in which such biases were expressed. Asylum doctors
frequently failed to deliver the cures they promised, but they hardly were
to blame for the injuries with which their patients arrived or the unwillingness of many communities to reintegrate discharged patients. Such
examples suggest that, while doctors' policies and the growth of their institutions may well have been an important expression of nascent capitalism and industrialization in nineteenth-century America, it is not easy
to uncover the connections between macro-level economic change and internal institutional developments. The challenges to do so, issued by
scholars as diverse as Gerald Grob, Michael Katz, and Andrew Scull,[2]
cannot be ignored, and while none of us struggling to unravel the mysteries of the asylum have yet fully met them, I hope this book will bring us
some small way closer.

1

Life within
the Asylum Walls

However mundane the daily routines of closed institutions, those outside frequently suspect that dark secrets lurk behind their high walls and barred windows. Such certainly was a common attitude toward nineteenth-century insane asylums, an attitude encouraged but not sated by the revelations of attendants' brutality and doctors' incompetence which periodically appeared in contemporary newspapers. At the same time, there was relatively little public interest in readily available but mundane information about asylum budgets, diets, classification systems, and patient work programs. For a variety of reasons, such an imbalance in popular impressions of nineteenth-century asylum life has persisted to the present.[1] The work of social scientists such as Erving Goffman suggests that, in order to evaluate the therapeutic and social functions of such institutions, we need first to look at their workings as a whole.[2] While the rhythms of daily life varied somewhat from one institution to the next and also changed in tempo over the course of the nineteenth century, certain aspects of the asylum experience were sufficiently persistent to make possible a snapshot portrayal of it. This chapter attempts to catch the nineteenth-century doctors, patients, and staff at New York's first two state asylums in their typical activities. Subsequent ones explain how, against this background of continuity, specific actors and events were able to change the ways in which the nineteenth-century mentally ill were perceived and treated.

Homes for the Mad

The Physical Setting

When curious nineteenth-century taxpayers came to inspect the New York State Lunatic Asylum at Utica, they stood awestruck in front of its imposing classical facade. Built in 1843, the Utica Asylum was one of the first large state-funded mental hospitals in the United States. The facade made it resemble universities and statehouses built during the same period. Like Worcester State Hospital and the Pennsylvania Hospital for the Insane, the Utica Asylum embodied the architectural ideals of the first generation of asylum superintendents. These men felt that massive formal buildings signified the importance of their therapeutic mission. In New York, such a construct also satisfied the wishes of politicians for an institution in which the "Empire State" could take pride. They hoped that the Utica Asylum's lofty pillars and gracious halls would arouse sentiments of "grandeur" in its patients and thus drive away feelings of degradation.[3] As late as 1888, the state commissioner in lunacy, gazing at its well-cared-for grounds, saw in the luxuriant green lawns, bright flower beds, and cheerful swings evidence of the peaceful nature of life within "this cheerful and quiet retreat."[4]

Although intended to be a refuge from the stresses of industrializing America, the Utica Asylum was built on the outskirts of a bustling city which rapidly expanded to encompass it. Its founders did not anticipate the rapidity with which Utica grew before the Civil War, but they had no desire to remove patients entirely from a world to which they were expected to return. Locating the first state asylum near but not in a city would, they believed, permit convalescing patients to participate in social and religious activities. It also would make it easier for public authorities to oversee asylum activities and thus check abuse. On the grounds that patients needed protection from the curious, however, they built high wooden fences around the institution's perimeter.[5]

The Willard Asylum for the Chronic Insane presented a very different picture. During Willard's construction in the mid-1860s, New York State was struggling to cope with the economic impact of the Civil War. Furthermore, by that point, both legislators and doctors had lost confidence in the ability of medical science to unlock the mysteries of mental illness. For them, Willard's construction was an admission that some of the institutionalized insane could never be returned to society. Set up to house the incurable mentally ill who had begun to overflow county poorhouses and the Utica Asylum, Willard consisted of a central administrative unit and a large number of three-story detached "cottages." Its buildings were plain in style and their furnishings simple. Located on the east shore of Seneca Lake miles from any substantial settlement, Willard did not need fences to isolate its patients from the curious.[6]

Because of its geographical isolation, especially in the winter, Willard's administrators tried to make the institution as self-sufficient as possible. While the Utica Asylum relied upon goods and services from the city surrounding it, Willard could not. Over the course of the nineteenth century, in addition to basic housing and medical facilities, Willard's superintendents supervised construction of a fire station, a hotel, a cemetery, and even a small local train system. One visitor likened the resulting complex to "some thrifty and prosperous New England settlement." A newspaper reporter visiting the asylum in 1886 described it as a rural paradise, with buildings scattered across more than five hundred acres of rich, rolling farmland. Equally positive were those summer visitors from New York City who made a visit to Willard's sunny grounds part of their vacation plans. Unpacking their picnic lunches on its grassy slopes, they found amusement in both the beauties of Seneca Lake and the eccentricities of the asylum's patients.[7]

Not everyone responded to these two lunatic asylums so favorably. Many found Utica's high wooden fences and barred windows suggestive of ominous mysteries within. To a critic, the Utica asylum most closely resembled "the castle of an enchanter, whose dread power can only be dissipated by tearing down its walls." Ex-patients characterized it more bluntly as a prison and commented bitterly on the contrast between the asylum's beautiful facade and its internal realities. One noted that visitors, awed by the beautiful symmetrical architecture of the main building, failed to see the invisible inscription written over its main door in inmates' blood: "Who enters here must leave all hope behind."[8] While county officials who visited Willard were pleased by its scenic location and the sight of the chronic mentally ill working quietly in the fields, a New York City reporter who wandered through the halls characterized it as a "mammoth tomb" for its almost two thousand demented patients.[9]

Arrival

Many patients' first sight of Utica and Willard was further colored by the experience of having been dragged there in restraints. Those brought on public transport found themselves exposed to the jibes of young boys and the curious stares of their elders. One ex-patient, William Hotchkiss, years later vividly recalled the horrors of his transfer from a private home in Rochester to Utica in the 1840s. Hands and feet tied together, he had been thrown onto the floor of a wagon for the lengthy trip. Already delusional, he alternately regarded his friends as "the Thugs of India" and thought that he was returning to Yale College, where he had been an undergraduate. Asylum doctors argued, to no avail, that such harsh treatment not only led to bruises and even broken bones but also exacerbated patients' mental instability.[10] Furthermore, they claimed, most of the allegedly violent patients caused no problems once their restraints were removed. Typical was the case of the middle-aged Willard patient, an "unknown foreigner with mark of former respectability and intelligence," who arrived in 1874 wearing the chains he had endured for nineteen years. Once released from his bonds, he showed not the slightest proclivity to violence.[11] Asylum doctors also strongly opposed the use of trickery to persuade insane men and women to come to the asylum. Too often patients were told that their trip to the city of Utica was part of a vacation outing or that they could try the asylum for a few days and then leave if they did not like it. When such claims proved false, patients turned against the institution as well as their families. Better to bring such patients against their will, Utica's doctors advised, than to suggest that the asylum approved of such deception.[12]

Yet no matter how often they repeated them, asylum doctors' arguments and stories had little impact on public practice. Even late in the century, patients (including transfers from other state institutions) continued to arrive at both Willard and Utica in handcuffs, straitjackets, and chains. When Utica's doctors berated one overweight county official for manacling a ninety-five pound girl, he merely laughed.[13] Despite reformers' efforts to change attitudes toward the mentally ill, public fear of and contempt for excited or violent insane persons remained strong. And, for

New York's nineteenth-century mentally ill, the reality of their trip to the asylum was sometimes worse than their most lurid private nightmares.

Of course, some patients were too demented to notice the circumstances of their transportation to the asylum or their new surroundings. Others, particularly abused women with alcoholic husbands and many children, saw the Utica asylum as a refuge, a place to escape unbearable personal pressures. Yet, no matter what the circumstances of commitment, most patients experienced an initial shock at the contrast between the family scenes left behind and life within a large state institution. Conditions on asylum wards varied, but even the "quiet" halls had little of the homelike about them (despite institutional rhetoric to the contrary). When one female patient first glimpsed her fellow inmates, their "vacant faces and disconnected conversation" led her to fear for her life. Another woman assigned to the first female ward was initially pleased with its "gracious halls with happy women busy at work." In this ward reserved for the quiet and convalescent, each patient had a private room, which attendants could enter only after knocking. Yet, once she realized she could not leave, she began to feel like a "captive," trapped in a whirlwind of empty activities. Although she eventually became reconciled to her lot, she never again lost sight of the significant difference between domestic and asylum life.[14]

Occasionally doctors tried to ease the transition from private to ward life, but their gestures tended to be superficial. For example, Superintendent Amariah Brigham of Utica greeted new patient William Hotchkiss at the asylum door with great warmth and kindness and personally collected his case history. If Brigham had then led him by hand to a good bed, Hotchkiss later commented, he might well have begun to rest and regain his strength. But Brigham had too many patients in his charge to offer such individualized attention. Instead an attendant hurried Hotchkiss from Brigham's sympathetic presence to a basement cell with barred windows and no furniture. When the door clanged shut, Hotchkiss fell prostrate on the floor, tormented by delusions worthy of Edgar Allen Poe. The demented faces of his fellow inmates, peering from adjacent rooms, only fueled his feverish imagination. When they scrambled madly for a discarded crust of bread, Hotchkiss saw them as vampires "just risen from the dead." When he managed to shout a feverish plea for help from his window, two attendants, "beings bearing the form of men," entered the cell and threw him roughly to the floor. There he lay unconscious until morning. Thus went William Hotchkiss's first day.[15] Not surprisingly, he subsequently viewed the Utica Asylum as hell on earth.

No records remain to describe how patients felt when they arrived at Willard. Many already had spent years in other institutions; those in advanced stages of syphilis or dementia presumably paid little attention to their new surroundings. Hints of how Willard might have appeared to new patients can, however, be found in visitors' comments. Some praised the beautiful grounds, the busy farms, the bustling workshops. Others expressed shock at the contrast between Willard's pastoral exterior and the dark interior wards set aside for the "filthy and excited." When he entered a ward for male dements, one visitor reeled before the repugnant smells and unearthly screams. Even state officials, more accustomed to such sights, sometimes recoiled from them. One characterized the care of disturbed men and women as "trying and repulsive."[16] Both visitors and staff were so convinced of the superiority of state-level care, however, that they tended to assume patients would not share their perceptions. For the chronically insane, the doctors argued, even the worst wards at Willard represented an improvement over conditions in county poorhouses and families' attics. Whether patients agreed is not known. Few ever left Willard, and their correspondence with families has not been saved.

Life Inside

Patients

Just as the circumstances of arrival differed, so too did patients' experiences within the institutions. Most obviously, manic patients related to the asylum differently than did the seriously depressed; first-time patients interacted with their fellows and the staff more intensely than those who had been institutionalized for years. In addition, patients' living conditions and daily activities varied a great deal from ward to ward as well as from institution to institution. Both Utica and Willard classified patients on the basis of their self-control rather than their disease. For the quiet and industrious, life could be pleasant, if monotonous. One of Utica's more privileged patients, a middle-aged woman living on the first ward, praised her keepers in a poem entitled "Asylum Life; or, The Advantages of a Disadvantage." She lauded the carefree asylum environment where

> I have walks to take, and news to read;
> With chit-chat and work the hours to spend;
> Good company, sages, as good as the great
> Who have charge of the "Empire State."[17]

Even Willard, which specialized in cheap care for large numbers, provided the "convalescent and industrious" with pleasant observation halls whose walls were covered with pictures and floors with cheerful rugs. Caged birds sang while patients sewed, read, or talked with each other. In sharp contrast were conditions in the infirmary wards. Here, seriously demented men and women sat unmoving for hours and even years. Patients debilitated by syphilis or consumption tossed on straw-stuffed beds covered with rubber sheets. In addition to these two sorts of units within its central administration building, Willard assigned patients to sex-segregated three-story "cottages." Here, too, the details of daily life varied from building to building. One kept only "mentally enfeebled but not filthy" male patients, who went out daily to shovel and do gardening work. Another held those with "the better grade of harmless chronic mania and the lighter forms of dementia." At the latter, live-in attendants supervised farm work during the summer and mat making during the winter. Two detached buildings for women also contained a "better grade" of patient, capable of sewing and domestic work under the supervision of attendants. Although some patients complained about the length of their hours of work, many found in employment both physical release and an increased intimacy with fellow workers. As Stephen Smith noted with surprise on his first visit to Willard, he could not easily distinguish hired farm laborers from the insane patients working alongside them. His response was not unusual; visitors frequently commented on the air of contented productivity which characterized Willard's better patients.[18]

At Utica, patients and staff lived together in a single central administration building for most of the century. Wards closest to administrative offices and medical staff departments were the best; those farthest away held the "furious and filthy." Such an arrangement shielded both the medical staff and convalescent patients from the disturbing howls of the seriously deranged. One patient compared the Utica Asylum to a hotel whose accommodations varied sharply from hall to hall. State inspectors found the description only too accurate. An official visitor in 1884 noted that the first ward, which held twenty-nine convalescent patients and two attendants, was cheerful and orderly. On the second ward, where sixteen mixed-class patients lived with two attendants, the water closet smelled. The fourth ward, with four attendants for thirty demented and filthy patients, reeked of feces and had several patients confined in covered beds (the infamous "Utica cribs"). On the fifth ward, reserved for twenty-one seriously demented patients, many were filthy, and attendants relied heavily on restraints to maintain order. Even the sitting room was dirty.[19]

Patient memoirs make clear that, although the classification schemes were intended to facilitate recovery by grouping similar patients together, they could easily be used to threaten and punish. Although first and second hall patients were allowed to play cards, put on theatricals, go sleigh riding, and attend church services and entertainments in the city of Utica, little but their fellows' screams and the card playing of attendants broke the monotony of back-ward life.[20] Several of Utica's ex-patients alleged that those who exhibited the slightest insubordination were transferred quickly to a more restricted ward. Doctors somewhat unconvincingly denied such charges. As one assistant physician explained his practice, he did not "threaten" one of his difficult patients with removal but merely urged her to "exercise more control, or I should have to move her off." Whatever the individual circumstances, patients frequently were shifted from ward to ward, and in a number of cases, such transfers constituted their primary "treatment." As a result, a given patient might live on as many as five or six different wards in a single year. Asylum administrators claimed that such transfers permitted them to individualize treatment, even for the chronic mentally ill.[21]

In theory, the ward classification scheme exemplified insane asylums' commitment to individualized care for their deranged charges. But the rigid daily routines of both Utica and Willard limited the extent to which treatment could in practice be individualized. Asylum heads were convinced that only if every person in the institution followed a prearranged schedule could they cope with the large numbers assigned to their care.

At Utica, the board of managers worked out the institution's detailed daily schedule well before it actually opened its doors, and these preliminary guidelines remained in place for most of the nineteenth century. Nonmedical employees rose between half past four and half past five, depending on the time of the year, first to the sound of a bell and then, late in the century, to a bugle call. Attendants then awoke their charges, helped the feeble dress, and began to clean the wards with the assistance of able-bodied patients. At seven, attendants and patients sat down to breakfast together. Until the 1888 construction of a large communal dining hall, they ate in small rooms next to the sleeping areas. After breakfast, patients and attendants washed dishes and finished cleaning the wards. About ten o'clock, a young assistant physician walked quickly through the wards, usually at the side of a head attendant who pointed out particularly sick and troublesome patients. Then some patients were taken off to work on the farm, in the wards, or at the industrial shops, while others read, played ball, or walked in sex-segregated outdoor courtyards.

After dinner was served at half past twelve, patients continued to work for the institution or to amuse themselves. Tea at six was the last meal of the day. Except during Utica's first decade, few events were arranged for the evening. Patients once again were left to their own devices, under the surveillance of attendants, until bedtime. Only on Sunday did this schedule change. Then, all unnecessary labor and "frivolous" diversions ceased, while some patients and the entire staff attended religious services. Those patients too disturbed to be welcome into the asylum chapel sat on the wards or walked the grounds.[22]

The routine prescribed by Utica's first managers changed remarkably little between 1843 and 1890, except for a gradual decline in the number of "amusements" available to patients. For almost half a century, at least in its superficial aspects, daily life proceeded with a clockwork regularity managers found reassuring and doctors therapeutic. For patients, on the other hand, the days were so unchanging that the passage of time often lost all meaning. Some also complained that attendants used the official regulations to harass as well as control their charges. For example, they allowed only the seriously ill to return to their bedrooms during the day. When disturbed patients failed to help with ward housekeeping, they often were punished. Patients also suffered if they violated the unwritten rules of hall life. As one commented, he easily (although reluctantly) learned to conform to such institutional regulations as fixed rising and sleeping times, but he still found himself in trouble for inadvertently offending his keepers.[23]

A similar schedule dictated the rhythms of daily life at Willard, despite its very different patient population. For example, in 1882, Willard's attendants were still working the same hours as had Utica's first employees in 1844. The lives of attendants and patients were closely intertwined. They rose together at half past five. Attendants and the more competent patients then bathed, clothed, and prepared the "excited and filthy patients" for breakfast. Not surprisingly, attendants often delegated the worst of these shared tasks to patients, so that, for example, one E. M., "so much soiled an attendant could not touch her," was washed each morning by a fellow patient. At half past seven, all breakfasted together, except for those too destructive to be tolerated in the communal dining halls, who ate in their rooms. Housecleaning tasks absorbed the rest of the early morning. After medical rounds, attendants took some patients out to walk and assigned others sewing work. Dinner was served at noon, followed by still another round of housecleaning, sewing, and yard work. After supper at six, the dishes were washed, the silverware counted, night medicine and clean clothes distributed, and by 10 o'clock all had retired for the night. Since attendants slept in small rooms off patient wards, those with the energy to respond rose several times each night to quiet the disturbed and to assist the sick.[24]

Doctors at both Utica and Willard argued that rigid daily schedules would teach patients the valuable habits of self-discipline and regularity. Clearly, they also were reluctant to loosen their control of even the most trivial aspects of their many patients' lives. For example, when Willard's doctors reluctantly gave a few convalescent patients "parole" (permission to walk the grounds without the company of attendants), they defined the parameters of this limited personal freedom with great care. One woman was allowed to stroll through the south grove and up the flagstone path, but only as far as the vegetable cellar. Another could exercise south of the ravine, provided she did not go near the detached buildings. Patients who wandered outside their prescribed bounds promptly lost parole privileges, although offenders with skills vital to asylum workshops, whatever their offense, were punished least. For example, a patient accused of paying small girls to expose themselves lost his parole privileges for only nine days because he was needed to work in the tailor's shop. Others had their paroles permanently revoked when their mental health (and, therefore, their dependability) deteriorated. Although parole privileges enabled a small number of patients to experiment with limited freedom as a prelude to release, parole for the most part simply permitted patients to come and go freely from their places of work. By August 14, 1886, one such male patient had been paroled for seventeen years to work in the engine room, but he still was not allowed to go out alone between meals.[25]

In part, parole privileges were so restricted because attendants had difficulty keeping track of patients on Willard's sprawling grounds. Asylum authorities also feared the anger of local citizens should paroled patients leave the institution's premises. Although several did so, their wanderings seemingly upset asylum doctors more than the people of Seneca County. One such patient lost his parole rights when he returned intoxicated from the nearby town of Ovid, another when he hired himself out as a day laborer to local farmers. Only when attendants could not locate the latter patient at mealtime was his absence noted (a telling example of the gulf between asylum surveillance rhetoric and the much looser realities of daily life). Far from being upset when they learned that their worker was a Willard patient, his temporary extrainstitutional employers lauded the agricultural skills he had honed on the asylum's farm.[26]

Attendants

However constricted their liberties, Willard's parolees considered themselves privileged. Walks alone or with a designated companion, even to the edge of the vegetable garden, offered a welcome escape from the claustrophobic intimacy of ward life. Not only patients needed relief from the relentless routines of institutional life. Attendants also required, but too seldom received, breaks from their demanding jobs. At Utica, attendants worked fourteen to sixteen hours a day. For most of the nineteenth century, their leaves, whether for personal, medical, or business reasons, were limited to a half day once a month, two evenings a week, and every third Sunday. Not surprisingly, they took full advantage of their short breaks; Utica's patients complained that young attendants overindulged, returning to the wards drunk and noisy. Long hours of dealing with troubled and even violent charges wore out even the most devoted, and attendants seldom stayed at Utica for more than two years. Willard's retention rate was better, partly because of the lack of alternative employment possibilities in rural southwestern New York.[27]

Despite their concern that the medical staff not be overworked, Utica's superintendents had little sympathy for their attendants' stressful work lives. When a head supervisor assigned to a suicide ward had a nervous breakdown after eighteen months of day-and-night responsibility for her self-destructive patients, the superintendent, John Gray, criticized her lack of stamina. Eventually even the Utica board of managers recommended that attendants' work hours be limited, but Gray refused. "They are the companions and constant associates of the patients," he argued, "and they must be with them day and night . . . as a person is in a family." Although in his published writings Gray sharply criticized the impact of excessive family duties upon nineteenth-century women, he refused to acknowledge the extent to which he was replicating that situation within his institutional family.[28]

At Willard, the asylum's geographical isolation further limited attendants' outlets for release. To the regret of its officers, many of its approximately three hundred young male and female employees turned to drink and sexual flirtation for relaxation in their few free hours. To provide more wholesome outlets for his staff, Superintendent John Chapin requested legislative funding for a recreation hall where both attendants and the quieter patients might find "properly innocent amusements and diversions." While construction of such a facility did not eliminate alcoholism among attendants, it made possible the staging of numerous concerts and dramatic plays by staff and patients. By the end of the nineteenth century, a number of reforms finally broke the exhausting twenty-four hours a day, twelve months a year bond between attendants and patients. In 1888, Willard added a night shift and built a separate staff residence.[29] About the same time (shortly after Gray's death), Utica's attendants gained a two-week annual paid vacation.[30] While such relatively modest improvements did not eliminate tensions between patients and staff, they helped to reduce them.

The Medical Staff

Just as patients and attendants marched through each day to a prearranged beat, so doctors too followed a daily routine prescribed by early asylum trustees. For the superintendent, this meant an endless round of meetings: with the steward and matron, farmers and workshop heads, assistant physicians and visiting trustees. Quickly abandoned in the press of administrative demands was Superintendent Amariah Brigham's early habit of greeting new patients at the asylum door and of taking daily walks through the halls. Instead assistant physicians had responsibility for almost all direct interactions with patients, sometimes seeing as many as three hundred in a day. Not only did they supervise patient treatment and care—from the ventilation and heating of the wards to exercise and amusement programs—but they also corresponded with families, helped put together annual reports, and kept an eye on attendants. In addition, at all times, no matter how tired such duties left them, they were supposed always to exert a positive "moral force" on all whom they met.[31]

By the end of the century, four assistant physicians cared for 690 patients at Utica and seven for almost 2,000 patients at Willard. One asylum critic calculated that, in order to visit each patient twice a day, Willard's doctors would have to see a patient a minute for twelve straight hours.[32] Given the impossibility of such a task, most doctors focused their attention on three groups: the physically ill, patients with unusual problems, and those with the best prospects for recovery. Their relations with the remaining 60–70 percent of the patients tended to be perfunctory, and they relied on ward supervisors to keep them informed, a practice resented by many patients. As one complained, doctors' habit of asking attendants how well patients had slept the preceding night was absurd, since attendants themselves had been asleep. Another jibed that the doctors entered the halls "in rather a dignified, cool, forbidding manner, as though they had something of great importance to say that had never been said before." When a Utica patient dared to suggest a change in his medication, his doctor purportedly replied, "I am the boss of this shanty" and denied the request. During Utica's early years, patients also were allowed to approach doctors at weekly open meetings. The result was not an increase in individualized treatment, however, but pandemonium, with patients shrieking and gesticulating to attract doctors' attention.[33]

All doctor–patient relationships at the Utica and Willard asylums were not so negative, but satisfied ex-patients seldom published accounts of their asylum experiences. Those panegyrics to the medical staff which occasionally appeared in the Utica patient magazine, the *Opal*, were so formulaic as to reveal little about ward dynamics. For example, one poem compared Utica Superintendent Benedict favorably to the president of the United States and mentioned "the patients / Who smile at your coming." Another offered a rare picture of the young John Gray as a compassionate assistant physician, who "charms away the dismal mood / With precepts ever wise and good / His face benevolent and kind, / Bespeaks the feelings of his mind." Much later, Gray's successor as superintendent, Blumer, was praised by a patient for having transformed the institution "from a harsh and dreary prison for patients to a comfortable and pleasant dwelling place."[34]

Whatever their individual strength and weaknesses, asylum doctors worked long hours. They spent most of their time with the most difficult patients, those whose illnesses (both mental and physical) refused to respond to treatment. Yet, despite, such burdens, the medical staff also enjoyed the most freedom in the institution. Like all employees, doctors lived on the asylum grounds and found most of their social life within the confines of the institution. At Willard in particular, doctors took an active role in local entertainments and dramatics, working together with staff members and patients. Unlike attendants and their charges, however, doctors lived in private apartments and for the most part dined only with each other. Several married into prominent local families, and they clearly enjoyed high social standing inside and outside the asylum community. They also had many opportunities to leave the institution and, with the permission of the trustees, frequently went off for days and even weeks to give lectures, attend scholarly meetings, and take leisurely trips abroad.[35]

In a legislative request for an additional assistant physician, John Gray dramatically portrayed asylum doctors as so broken in health by middle age that few lived long enough to pass on their accumulated wisdom.[36] That he was here exaggerating for the sake of political impact is suggested by the readiness with which several of Utica's assistant physicians took on extra duties, ranging from the supervision of new construction to editing of the powerful, Utica-based *American Journal of Insanity* (*AJI*). They thus gained practical training for superintendencies elsewhere, to which several aspired, as well as special bonuses from the board of managers. When Gray took charge of the Utica Asylum, he immediately relieved his assistant physicians of their more menial responsibilities, such as giving tours, keeping patients' clothing accounts, and supervising patient baths, so that they might pursue research interests. At Willard, assistant doctors had heavier and less rewarding case loads. Yet, as late as 1886, they found time to meet regularly for discussion of both general medical topics and particularly interesting clinical cases.[37]

The Limits of Institutional Order

Doctors constituted the only group within the Utica and Willard asylums formally granted much freedom. Yet, even within the confines of their militarylike daily regimens, both patients and attendants frequently managed to bend, and even to break through, institutional constraints. Although not supposed to leave their halls while on duty, attendants often found excuses to visit other parts of the asylum. Patients could be forced to retire by midevening, but not to sleep. Screams, noisy songs, and loud obscenities filled the night air, despite vocal complaints from quieter patients. The most disruptive settled down only when heavily sedated. Equally ineffective were the measures taken to ensure peaceful meals. For example, attendants tried to prevent injuries by keeping forks and knives away from patients known to be violent and collecting the eating utensils of all after meals. Yet, at Willard one day, in the middle of lunch, a patient who did not want to eat threw his knife at an attendant. Fortunately, it missed him and embedded itself in a coffee pot.[38]

Such incidents, even when their consequences were serious, seldom reached public attention, for asylum administrators were unwilling to let what they viewed as isolated events tarnish their already flawed public image. Sometimes such cover-up policies backfired and, when revealed, further fueled the public's suspicion that horrors were being hidden behind asylum walls. For example, in 1882 a discharged attendant revealed that, a full month earlier, one Utica patient had crushed the skull of another with a broken table leg. (The murderer, a convicted criminal, had mistaken his victim for an attendant. He had planned to steal the attendant's keys and liberate the other patients.) Although few blamed the institution for the murder, reporters sharply attacked John Gray's attempt to keep the death quiet. Newspaper headlines blared, "Shocking Tragedy at the State Asylum" and "An Awful Crime Kept from the Public Four Weeks."[39]

In response to this hostile newspaper publicity, Superintendent Gray pointed out that such incidents were surprisingly rare, given the asylum's volatile patient population. Particularly impressive were Utica's low annual suicide and homicide rates, despite the admission of large numbers of such patients. Gray also complained about local judges' policy of sending insane criminals to the Utica Asylum. Such a practice disrupted already volatile wards by increasing the number of inmates with histories of serious antisocial behavior. Eventually, the state commissioner in lunacy, as well as several representatives of the state board of charities, investigated the 1882 Utica homicide. While they never issued a formal report, only one member of the board of charities agreed with the press that the matter should have been revealed to the public. The commissioner in lunacy argued that such events were frequent occurrences at asylums and hospitals. Like Gray, he felt that to reveal their details fully to the public would only frighten unnecessarily those in need of the asylum's services.[40]

Attempts by bureaucrats and administrators to explain the complex social realities of asylum life had little impact on the popular press. It preferred to focus on those terrifying random acts of violence most likely to titillate readers. For example, when two Utica patients suddenly assaulted a man waiting outside the asylum for a friend, the newspapers had a heyday. Even though the man was rescued almost immediately and not harmed, reporters commented that, had the patient been manacled, such an attack could not have taken place.[41] This position particularly infuriated asylum administrators, who complained that reporters one day warned the public that all lunatics were dangerous and needed to be confined more strictly and the next that many sane men and women were being unjustly kept in asylums.[42]

Systematic investigation of Utica's ward injury books in the 1880s also revealed that patients regularly suffered systematic (if seldom life-threatening) abuse at the hands of both attendants and fellow patients. On the witness stand at an 1884 legislative investigation, several ex-patients eloquently described their fear of fellow patients. One described his third-hall companions as continually "reckless, raving, and knocking each other down." Patient casebook comments suggest that his experience was not unusual. For example, when two well-known "fighters" were found hitting each other at Utica in 1879, doctors assigned the more maniacal to a different ward. They hoped that, once relocated, she would be unable to find another fighting partner. On the male side, a fourteen-year-old male patient also was transferred to another ward (and then sent to Willard) after he played tricks on and physically abused the old and feeble patients on his ward. His victims were those demented patients too incoherent to complain, let alone to protect themselves; such patients were also the most likely to be mistreated by short-tempered attendants. For one such victim, the nightmarish delusions generated by his insanity became so confused with the horrors of his asylum life that he could not separate the two.[43]

For attendants and fellow patients in the disturbed wards, the possibility of an unexpected physical attack was part of daily life. Doctors spent relatively few hours with potentially dangerous patients, but their social distance from such men and women seemed only to intensify their apprehensions. Under the editorship of John Gray of Utica, the *AJI* printed numerous reports of patient attacks on asylum doctors, both in the United States and abroad.[44] Yet in practice few patients seriously injured doctors at either the Utica or Willard asylums. The most serious nineteenth-century incident, the shooting of Superintendent John Gray in the head, was done by a Utica man who had never been institutionalized.

Newspapers, families, and the general public all paid less attention to incidents of patient abuse at Willard than at Utica. Most assumed that state-level care, even at its worst, was an improvement over that offered the paupered insane in county poorhouses. As a result, when Superintendent John Chapin reported to the state legislature that one patient had fatally battered another's head using a convenient chamber pot, not a single newspaper took notice. Perhaps because of their relative insulation from investigative reporters, Willard's administrators were relatively frank about the problem of patient violence. In 1883 they voluntarily sent to the commissioner in lunacy a detailed list of seventy-eight incidents which had taken place on a single day. They also noted that, during all of 1883, 263 patients, 5 attendants, and 1 physician had received skull contusions; 4 patients, bone fractures; 9, severe cuts; and 21 patients, 1 attendant, and a physician, a number of other injuries. These matter-of-fact injury reports reflected not a callous indifference, but rather the doctors' conviction that such rates of violence were low for an institution where almost two thousand disturbed men and women, together with more than three hundred keepers, lived together in close company.[45] The injury books at both Utica and Willard, like the descriptions of living conditions, also make clear that wards were not equally violent. Despite the monotony, both patients and staff preferred the predictability and quiet of life on convalescent halls to back wards' chaos and disorder.

Even the most ardent defenders of the use of restraints to control patients (a group which included most of the Utica medical staff) would not support their application to the entire patient population, as the reporters suggested. Furthermore, Utica's doctors had already been attacked, in the course of several legislative investigations in the 1870s and 1880s, for their overuse of restraints.[46] Yet, even at the end of the century, Utica's doctors and attendants did not hesitate to control violent patients by chemical and mechanical means. Such methods calmed wards at a heavy cost. Some patients died of drug overdoses; others sat on the floor all day in semicomatose states, moving only when pushed aside by attendants. Worst of all, noted critics, easy recourse to restraints encouraged attendants to treat patients like animals.[47]

In the 1880s, in response to harsh public criticism, doctors at both Utica and Willard finally began to look for alternatives to restraint for control of disturbed patients. They found that improving attendant–patient ratios, especially in combination with limits on overall ward size, was the most effective. As a result, at Utica in 1888, while three attendants looked after thirty-six patients in a convalescent ward, the same number were assigned to ten patients in a "refractory" ward. Initiation of more diversified patient employment programs also diminished ward tensions by providing outlets for bored and hostile patients.[48] Despite these experiments, however, underfunded asylums continued to find restraints, both chemical and mechanical, the cheapest way of dealing with disturbed patients.

The threat of overt physical violence was not the only source of tension on the asylum wards. Group living was difficult for both patients and their caretakers. Noisy patients kept quiet ones awake; profane patients bothered the religious; and middle-class patients objected to their forced intimacy with social inferiors, especially those who were Irish or black. One Utica patient declared of his associates, "Many are immoral, depraved, licentious, and therefore scarcely fit companions." Several female patients reported feeling great relief when they finally located other genteel female friends. That the medical profession shared many of these class biases did not ease tensions on the wards. As late as 1894, S. Weir Mitchell noted with dismay the indignities suffered by "refined and educated men and women" forced into public asylum wards. Most of their time was spent with cooks and maids, he noted in horror.[49] Class differences were not, however, the only source of friction. One young Irish alcoholic complained bitterly about being locked in "with old doating women and women who take fits . . . This is more like an assilam than an hoskital for their is a crazy girl in it and . . . I am afraid of my life of these old women."[50]

The squeamish were particularly likely to find their sensibilities offended. A common sort of dinner companion, declared one Utica patient, was the hungry man with "long, lean, lank lantern-jaws" who gobbled all the food in sight. After finishing, he blew his nose between "splashy digits strangers to pocket handkerchiefs" and then used his fork to pick his teeth. The same lecturer, however, described with compassion the sad spectacle of a quiet and dignified old man, tortured by delusions of persecution. In general, he praised his fellow inmates for their high quality, declaring that "in talents, in literature, in poetry, in oratory, in feminine beauty, intelligence and accomplishments, we shall compare with outside communities." At both Utica and Willard, patients often helped one another, especially in times of acute psychological stress. For example, three female epileptics at Willard frequently took their daily parole walks together, so that, if necessary, they could assist each other.[51]

Rigid sex segregation was probably the most striking difference between life within and without. Public lectures at the asylum, Sunday religious services, and art exhibits offered a small number of convalescing males and females the rare chance to gaze at, and even talk with, one another. Such patients described themselves as "rescued from the thralldom of observation and transferred to a class approximating to the enjoyments, interests, and duties of society and general life." Yet, one male patient found seeing women at chapel a mixed pleasure. "It seems," he observed, "rather too much like placing a dainty morsel within sight of a hungry man, without his being able to reach it."[52] Such an attitude was precisely what asylum authorities feared. They particularly wanted to guard against the sexual abuse of demented women which so plagued county poorhouses. At both Utica and Willard, not only were male patients housed in separate dormitories, but male employees could enter female portions of the insane asylums only with the express permission of the superintendent. For many years, female staff members also did not work on male wards, but for a different reason. Managers and doctors did not worry about them sexually abusing male patients, but they feared that female attendants lacked the physical strength required to control violent male patients. When, in 1888, a few older female nurses at Utica were sent to male wards for the first time, Superintendent Blumer discovered to his pleasure that their presence improved the behavior of both the patients and the male attendants.[53]

The Asylum and the Outside World

Although patients frequently complained of feeling cut off from the outside world, in one respect they felt they were not isolated enough. Although most did not see family members and friends for months and even years, patients at both Utica and Willard almost daily encountered hordes of touring citizens. Their doctors complained that such visitors disrupted daily routines and interfered with medical treatments, but they hesitated to limit them for fear of reviving speculations about the hidden horrors of asylum life. (Typically, visitors were shown only the front wards.) At best, such visitors as the forty schoolboys who chased deer around Utica's snow-drifted grounds and then went jingling and laughing away in their sleigh only reminded patients of their lack of personal freedom. At worst, patients experienced painful feelings of humiliation when they unexpectedly encountered former acquaintances among asylum visitors. Hiram Chase refused to move to Utica's first hall, despite its many amenities, because he did not want to become "a gazing stock for the multitude of visitors who daily flock to the asylum, take a walk through the first hall, gaze on the patients as they would look upon wild animals in a menagerie, and then depart."[54]

Visitors' insensitivity was a constant theme of writers for the Utica patient journal, the *Opal*. In bitter parodies, they described the thoughtlessness of those who came to the asylum for amusement. One essayist constructed a fictional composite of such visitors: a young New Yorker who decided to break the monotony of a long winter day by taking a sleigh full of friends to visit Utica. Arriving after visiting hours, she complained loudly until given permission to enter. Once inside, she protested angrily that "everything was very clean and all the patients looked and acted like other people." When she asked her guide to take the party to where they could "see *something*," he promptly bowed them back to their sleigh. Another such "nice young lady" allegedly asked of her apothecary guide to the asylum halls, "Where are the crazy people?" "O," the doctor replied, "we are all crazy." Despite the humorous notes in such satires, asylum patients resented visitors who seemed only to "derive a morbid satisfaction from looking on scenes of human misery" at the asylum. They also felt that those whose "sickly and vulgar anticipations" were disappointed by the sight of patients sitting quietly in the halls overlooked the real horrors of the asylum: men and women stricken by sorrows that could not be assuaged, weighted with fears that had withered the soul.[55]

During the latter part of the nineteenth century, doubts about the wisdom of open visitation finally began to outweigh fears of popular outrage at its discontinuation. During 1876 alone, John Gray reported, 11,794 men and women had toured the Utica asylum or visited with patients, in addition to uncounted numbers of county officers, clergymen, and physicians. By the 1870s, complained the commissioner in lunacy, even isolated Willard had become the well-advertised highlight of several holiday excursions. In 1889, a year before the New York State Asylum at Utica became the Utica State Hospital, its board of managers finally closed the wards to all visitors except officers of the law, scientists and other professionals, and patient's relatives.[56] Willard's administrators followed suit.

At the same time as Utica's administrators moved to exclude casual visitors, they also replaced with a short picket fence the high wooden walls which had surrounded the asylum for so many years. Now passersby could watch patients strolling the grounds and the staff scurrying from building to building. Yet the new physical openness of the institution did not eliminate public curiosity about and suspicion of those who lived within it. Despite the efforts of several generations of reformers to promote a scientific approach to insanity, most nineteenth-century Americans still feared the mad and envisioned those who controlled them as magicians with vital but fearsome powers.[57] They might have been surprised to read one Utica patient's letter to her sister, written in March of 1889. "Today," she scribbled, "I have folded sheets, towels and napkins at the laundry; attended school for two hours; talked with a new friend, a lawyer's wife; and eaten clam soup for supper."[58] Such a "domestication of madness," to use Andrew Scull's term, had its own potential for oppression, but the problems it involved were too subtle to make front-page headlines.[59] And patients as a group, particularly at the Willard Asylum, had few external advocates. Once families had made the painful decision to send disturbed members to a state asylum, they were reluctant to investigate the therapeutic and custodial deficiencies of their relatives' new homes. Newspaper reporters briefly played up sensational problems and then lost interest until the next scandal.

Over the course of the nineteenth century, the Utica and Willard asylums changed in a number of ways. Individual doctors and attendants came and went; their replacements occasionally brought new therapeutic philosophies. Patient–staff ratios changed, as did the kinds of men and women sent to the institutions. Funding levels shifted, especially in response to economic depressions and the Civil War. The state experimented with a variety of relationships between state supervisory agencies and state asylums, as well as between state insane asylums and county poorhouses. Yet, in a number of important ways, life within these institutions had a timeless quality. From 1843 to 1890, asylum bells summoned doctors, patients, and staff from one activity to the next with a monotonous regularity. Delusional men and women beat their heads on the walls built more to keep them within than overly critical eyes out. Depressed women strolled through Utica's greenhouses, and mad farmers ploughed up Willard's rich farmlands. While far from immune to the controversies swirling around them, New York's nineteenth-century state insane asylums remained as aloof as possible from the insanities of the public world which had driven so many of their charges to them.

2

The Economics of
Compassion

The massive institutional complexes that were the Utica and Willard asylums by the 1870s, along with the controversies which swirled around them, would have amazed the antebellum reformers who first had fought for state-level care of the insane in New York. Like most early nineteenth-century reformers, these New Yorkers felt glowing optimism about the potential benefits of insane asylums. Initially they found it difficult to sway fellow politicians and the general public to their position. Beginning in the 1820s, it took an alliance of politicians, physicians, and social reformers almost a decade to win approval for construction of a state-level facility for the insane. A number of factors contributed to their eventual victory: socioeconomic changes, improvements in medical care, and shifts in familial relationships. They also were helped by the emergence of an effective pro-asylum lobby in the legislature, which unified disparate local politicians under the banner of what might be called an economics of compassion. The component parts of this economics were neither complex nor novel, but their synthesis in the 1830s resulted in an emotional argument so powerful that it continued to appear in social welfare proposals well into the twentieth century (albeit in an increasingly formulaic fashion). Partly because of the intensity of political conflict in the antebellum legislature, its proponents made claims for the benefits of insane asylums so extravagant that they could never be realized. This tradition of rhetorical excess was both continued and deplored by reformers and asylum administrators for the rest of the century.

Sources of Support for Early Asylum Reform

New York legislators did not approve construction of a state insane asylum until 1836, but public concern about the best way to care for the mentally ill predated the American Revolution. During the seventeenth century, most were kept in private homes or local jails. When the New York (City) Hospital opened a separate building for "maniacs" in 1806, state legislators agreed to pay half of its construction costs and also to grant it an annual subsidy. Yet state aid covered only part of patient expenses at the Bloomingdale Asylum, as this branch of the New York Hospital became known. Since, for the most part, families had to make up the difference, most of the poor were excluded from institutional care. Even those with money did not always gain admission, for the Bloomingdale Asylum could accommodate only eighty patients at a time. A small private asylum in Hudson also accepted a few public patients, but it did so on the basis of contracts with local communities rather than with the state.[1]

As New York's population grew, the Bloomingdale and Hudson asylums became increasingly unable to care for the state's insane. An 1824 survey of the dependent poor in New York State intensified public awareness of this problem, for 446 of the 6,896 permanent poor were reported to be "lunatics." Out of this so-called Yates Report came the Poor Law of 1824, which ordered traditional settlement laws simplified and counties to assume more responsibilities for the dependent poor within their bounds. To their dismay, county officials found themselves required not only to maintain an almshouse for the dependent poor, many of whom needed only short-term shelter, but also for what looked to be a permanent population of insane paupers.[2] Struggling to meet their newly enlarged responsibilities for the poor, few of these inexperienced county administrators could cope with the additional burden of even small numbers of disruptive lunatics. Initially, they sent the most difficult to local jails, but that practice was outlawed in 1827. In desperation, some then locked the noisy insane into basements; others chained the destructive ones to walls. Not surprisingly, by the 1830s, many local overseers of the poor strongly supported the idea that the state should assume responsibility for its in-

30

sane citizens. State-level institutions for the insane, they hoped, would greatly lighten their own workload as well as save money.[3]

Joining the county officials in their campaign for state-level care of the insane were a number of New York's leading doctors. Among the most vocal were a group from the Oneida County Medical Society, led by C. B. Coventry of Utica. Like their compatriots in Massachusetts and Pennsylvania, these physicians were excited by reports of the new asylum-based treatments first developed in England which promised to cure (as well as to control) mental illness. They also were appalled by the sanitary conditions in local poorhouses. In the name of both progress and humanity, they called on the entire state medical community to rally behind the state asylum movement. They also worked closely with other social welfare reformers and several of New York's leading newspaper editors.[4]

Despite such diversity of support, it took New York legislators almost a decade to approve construction of a state institution for the insane. While some legislators opposed in principle such an extension of state powers, most of the delay was due to the rapidly changing social and economic conditions of antebellum New York. With their home counties' needs shifting from year to year, local politicians had difficulty developing consistent policy positions on such issues as poor relief and asylum reform. In addition, few served more than one term in the legislature. Turnover in the New York State Assembly increased steadily throughout the early nineteenth century until at its peak, in 1848, 89 percent of Assembly members were first-termers, and not a single legislator had served more than four years. Even the Speakers of the House lacked substantial state-level political experience. A similar volatility of membership characterized the Senate.[5] With so few legislators serving more than one term, the makeup of key legislative committees shifted frequently. For example, although the legislature produced six reports on asylum reform between 1830 and 1837, seldom did the same name appear on more than one report.[6] In such circumstances, legislators had difficulty formulating long-term policies of any sort, let alone in the new area of social welfare.

Although New York politicians began to discuss how best to care for insane paupers in the 1820s, the first formal state-level appeal for reform appeared in Governor Enos Throop's annual message of 1830. Throop called for legislators to consider establishing an asylum "for the gratuitous care and recovery of that most destitute class of the human family, who are suffering from a darkened understanding and the evils of poverty at the same time."[7] In response, legislators appointed a committee of three to investigate "the necessity of erecting new establishments for the insane." After visiting asylums in New York, Massachusetts, and Connecticut, that committee drew up a detailed report which argued for approval of a state insane asylum large enough to hold 350 of the insane poor. The committee even included engraved plans for several possible asylum designs, with estimates of the construction costs of each. But fellow legislators balked at the projected expense and did nothing.[8]

As a result, in 1831 and 1832, the governor had to renew his appeal. These later messages offered a somewhat different rationale. In 1830 he had warned of the social threat posed by the insane and described eloquently the financial and emotional burden so often assumed by their relatives. In 1831 he appealed less overtly to social fears and instead spoke loftily of the legislators' sense of public duty and Christian charity. Finally, in 1832, Throop offered a fully developed version of the economics of compassion. First he argued for sympathy "on behalf of a class of beings too powerless . . . to lay their griefs before you." Then he invoked his fellow politicians' pride in New York State's progressive image. Surely, he argued, New Yorkers deserved access to the best medical care available. Finally, he appealed to their pocketbooks, arguing that prompt institutional treatment of the pauper insane would save money.[9]

Throop's legislative allies presented similar petitions, both in 1831 and 1832. The second Assembly report offered a proposal almost identical to Throop's. Like the governor's message, that document divided neatly into three parts. The first described the nineteenth century's enlightened attitude toward lunacy. While in the past, Americans had relied upon physical force to restrain maniacal violence, they now had learned to pity, not to fear, those who had lost their reason. They also recognized that insanity, like other diseases, need not be a permanent affliction. With the curability of insanity now "an established fact," its authors argued, men of benevolence had an obligation to apply the new insights of medical science in such a way as to alleviate human misery.[10]

Despite such a progressive beginning, later sections of the 1832 report suggested that most New Yorkers, including reform-minded legislators, had not completely abandoned traditional notions of the insane. In the same document which boasted of their progressive attitudes, pro-asylum politicians described the insane as frighteningly unpredictable and prone to outbreaks of violence. The essence of insanity, these legislators claimed, was a giving way to "the basest propensities of human nature." Under its spell, the pious turned blasphemous and the gentle violent. The message was clear: while fitting objects of pity, the insane also properly evoked great fear.[11] Thus, the reformers implied, their fellow politicians could both gratify benevolent impulses and quiet deeply ingrained fears by agreeing to the establishment of a state insane asylum.

To this simultaneous appeal to benevolence and fear, pro-asylum legislators, like Throop, added a third persuasive element: the economic advantages of asylum treatment. If construction of a new asylum was approved, they claimed, the state's only expense would be the purchase of a site and the preliminary costs of construction. Surely, they argued, local county governments and families would gladly pay for patients' room, board, and medical treatment in exchange for getting rid of their most troublesome charges. Furthermore, economies of scale and efficiency of management promised to make state treatment less costly than local custodial care. Finally, since most pauper insane were not poor by choice but had been driven into poverty by their illness, medical doctors at a state asylum could restore not only their reason but their economic productivity.[12]

Neither Throop's messages nor the committee reports of 1830, 1831, and 1832 produced immediate results. They familiarized legislators with the arguments for asylum care, however, and subsequent legislative committees reprinted their reports. Such continuing pressure eventually helped persuade the powerful Albany Regency Governor William Marcy to call for action in his annual message of 1834. His call was again referred to a House committee, which reported a pro-asylum bill to the whole, but once more nothing was passed. As an 1835 Assembly committee noted, "enough and more than enough reports have been made on the subject," and the arguments so far presented were convincing. Feeling that further collection of evidence on the subject would only produce additional delays, the committee appended the 1830 report to their call for action.[13]

Once again, in 1835, a favorable committee recommendation was ignored. Still legislative lobbyists toiled on. They continued to benefit from the strong support of the medical profession. For example, the Oneida

County Medical Society sent to the legislature a petition and to the State Medical Society a memorial calling for state-sponsored construction of "a properly conducted asylum." Only such an institution could cure the recently stricken insane, rescue those languishing in local poorhouses, and protect the community from insane persons permitted to wander at large.[14] Whether or not this eloquent appeal turned the tide is impossible to determine, but finally, on March 30, 1836, the legislature passed "An Act to Authorize the Establishment of the New York State Lunatic Asylum."[15] It required the governor to appoint three commissioners to purchase a site for the new institution for not more than ten thousand dollars and three more to contract for its construction for the sum of fifty thousand dollars.

By that point, the pro-asylum argument was sufficiently broad-ranging to let politicians from all over the state win constituent support for the required increase in state expenditures. Some legislators found most useful the negative aspects of the appeal and emphasized the social threat posed by the increasingly visible insane people in their cities and towns. Those from areas burdened with large numbers of dependent paupers promised that a state asylum would lessen their counties' financial burdens. They also rejoiced in the prospect of turning social dependents into economically productive citizens. Whatever their individual motives, all also supported asylum reform in a spirit of self-congratulatory humanitarianism. Although later critics argued that the complex pro-asylum argument ultimately rationalized regimentation in the name of enhancing liberal democratic ideals, the early nineteenth-century reformers entertained no such misgivings about their activities. They firmly believed that there was no conflict between the rational self-interest of the state and its citizens and a wide range of humanitarian activities.[16]

Building the
New York State Lunatic Asylum

When they approved construction of a state asylum in 1836, New York's legislators moved into the forefront but not the lead of the national asylum movement. While they hoped to build an institution worthy of the

Empire State, they preferred not to spend much money doing it. From the perspective of those appointed to find a site, the initial ten-thousand-dollar allocation was "embarrassingly small." Legislators felt strongly, however, that an economics of compassion did not require budgetary extravagance. In practice, they often resorted to an impractical niggardliness. In 1838 the commissioners reported to the legislature that they had been unable to purchase a suitable site. They had located one in Watervliet (outside of Albany), but the owner finally refused to sell for the agreed upon price. Eventually, in the summer of 1837, they succeeded in buying a 130-acre site in Utica with the help of an additional six-thousand-dollar gift from the city. In part, the city's interest was due to the influence of a prominent local doctor, C. B. Coventry, who had long been active in the statewide asylum movement; it also hoped to benefit economically from the asylum's presence.[17] The Utica site filled most of the commissioners' requirements. Although somewhat smaller than they considered optimal, its grounds were "pleasant and attractive" and close enough to Utica so that patients could observe the bustle of daily life without being subjected to its stress. At least initially, the site also seemed to have sufficient supplies of water and farming acreage to support the proposed institution's population. Presumably the commissioners also hoped that Utica's location in the center of New York would permit the asylum to serve the entire state.[18]

As soon as the Utica property was purchased by the state, the governor appointed a second group of commissioners to superintend construction of an asylum there: William Clarke of Utica, Francis Spinner of Herkimer, and Elam Lynds. (Lynds had earlier been a controversial head of New York's first prison.) After visiting a number of other social welfare institutions in the Northeast, including almshouses and prisons, the commissioners developed plans for construction of the largest lunatic asylum in the United States, one suitable for a thousand patients. It was to consist of four buildings each 550 feet long, located at right angles to each other and connected by open verandahs. The completed complex would enclose more than thirteen acres. Legislators promptly approved the commissioners' plans but without increasing the initial $50,000 allocation for construction costs. Without hesitation, the commissioners proceeded with a design whose completion in brick, they estimated in advance, would cost $431,636. While they never provided a substitute estimate of the expense of the actual building material, native gray limestone, they spent almost $50,000 on the foundation alone.[19]

New York's governor at the time, William Seward (a man later to win national renown for his expansive dreams), supported the commissioners in their extravagance, eulogizing the projected asylum as "commensurate with the exigencies of the State, not unworthy of its growing wealth, and justly designed to endure as a monument of the taste and munificence of this age."[20] The commissioners' and Seward's bold plans won little legislative support, however. Most state politicians, worried about the depleted state of New York's treasury in the early 1840s, were horrified by the projected cost (as well as by the expenditures to date) of the asylum project.[21] They refused the commissioners' request for an immediate supplementary allocation of $100,000 and an additional appropriation of almost $432,000. Unswayed by Seward's argument that "nations are seldom impoverished by their charities," they eventually appropriated $75,000 to complete one of the proposed buildings and ordered the foundations of the other three covered over. They also replaced two of the commissioners, Lynds and Spinner, with W. H. Shearman and Anson Dart. The following year, Clarke and Dart were replaced by James Platt and Theodore Faxton. Despite legislative opposition, however, the cost of the Utica Asylum continued to rise. By the time the main building, with two additional wings, was finished in 1850, it had cost $435,100, more than eight times the initial legislative appropriation.[22]

These early cost overruns were to become typical of asylum building projects in New York State. With good reason, newspapers often accused those in charge of inefficiency or corruption, but problems caused by poor management were exacerbated by the legislature's insistence on underfunding new construction. The early commissioners' practice of ignoring what they felt were unrealistic fiscal restrictions was continued by the Utica Asylum's managers. When faced with inadequate appropriations for new construction projects, asylum managers often "borrowed" money for capital expenditures from other budgetary categories (such as furniture), then petitioned for additional appropriations to cover the resulting deficits. They also used county monies paid for patient maintenance to meet construction bills. Since the legislature always (if reluctantly) covered the resulting deficits, the cycle of underfunding, overspending, and the passing of supplementary appropriations became the customary mode of doing business.[23]

Asylum officials at Utica argued that both the late timing and the inadequacy of legislative appropriations put them at a competitive disadvantage in bidding for supplies and work. Yet their complaints had little effect on state politicians. Most of them held office for only a term or two, and they were unwilling to take full responsibility for mounting state social welfare costs. Yet the strategies developed by early asylum administrators to circumvent stingy appropriations, some of which led to higher costs for the taxpayers, did little to help them develop a sense of fiscal responsibility. Their budgetary ineptitude was further exacerbated by poor financial planning at the state level as well. For example, on several occasions, the Utica asylum's managers were denied access to already appropriated funds by the state comptroller because he had spent them elsewhere. This latter problem received little public attention, however, and by mid-century most critics laid total blame for the rising costs of state-level asylum care on Utica's managers and superintendent.[24]

In May of 1841 the legislature appointed five trustees for the new asylum, two of whom (C. B. Coventry and Nicholas Devereux) had long been supporters of social welfare reforms. Asked to prepare a plan of governance for the new institution, including regulations for the admission of patients, the trustees visited fourteen similar institutions in the Northeast and also read widely in the contemporary medical literature on insanity. As a result, their eventual statement of institutional goals and operating principles offered little original. It summarized the widely held notions of the day about the efficacy of kind, individualized treatment of the insane at institutions which isolated them from deranging social excitements and familial pressures.[25] It also emphasized that insanity was a treatable, physical disease. After receiving their report, the legislature passed an act to organize the asylum in April of 1842 and appointed nine managers, including Devereux and Coventry. It also appropriated twenty-six thousand dollars for purchasing furniture, fixtures, food, fuel, medicine, and enclosing the grounds.[26]

Almost immediately after their appointment, the new managers began to receive letters from desperate New Yorkers in search of help for insane family members and friends and relief for themselves.[27] To comply with such requests, the managers moved quickly to choose the asylum's principal officers: Amariah Brigham as superintendent, H. A. Butolph as assistant physician, E. A. Wetmore as treasurer, Cyrus Chatfield as steward, and Mrs. Chatfield as matron. On January 16, 1843, the new staff began to accept patients, even though the institution was still only partially furnished, its furnaces incomplete, and its water supply uncertain.[28]

Expansion of the Asylum System

As they grudgingly paid the high initial cost of building the Utica Asylum, most New Yorkers thought that they had met the needs of their insane poor for some time into the future. They were shocked to learn, almost immediately, that such was not the case. Hardly had the Utica Asylum opened its doors than some reformers began to talk about the need for additional facilities. Since Utica was intended only for those whose insanity was of less than two years' duration, local poorhouses continued to hold many chronic insane paupers. Perhaps the most vehement opponent of this practice was nationally known advocate for the insane Dorothea Dix. Dix arrived in New York in 1843, the year the Utica Asylum opened, to investigate the condition of pauper lunatics in local almshouses. Perhaps because the asylum movement was well underway in New York by the time she arrived, Dix received a less than enthusiastic welcome from her fellow reformers. In fact, the first superintendent of the New York State Lunatic Asylum, Amariah Brigham, regarded her investigation of county-level care of the insane as a hindrance to the state asylum movement. "By coloring and not accurately observing," he commented acerbically, "she was often mistaken and this has thrown a doubt over all her statements with many."[29]

Such criticisms little affected Dix, who was used to opposition and convinced that New Yorkers needed to hear her message. Despite the generous appropriations made for the acutely ill at Utica, she argued that many of the state's insane poor still lacked adequate care. Most desperate of all was the plight of a large group ineligible for Utica's therapeutic services: the chronic pauper insane.[30] In her efforts to broaden the mission of the fledgling New York asylum movement, Dix used familiar arguments. Like the reform-minded politicians of the 1830s, she complained about the frequency with which superintendents of the poor kept their violent insane in barred rooms. Keeping lunatics in "cages" or "cells" suggested that they were animals or criminals, Dix charged. She also claimed that a number of the county almshouses were cold and filthy, their insane inmates nude or only partially dressed, and the females vulnerable to sexual abuse. The histories of two such insane women, impregnated after their admission to the Oneida County House, were, she declared, "too shocking to relate." Although such "shameless immoralities" were rare, even the best of the county poorhouses frequently lacked "discipline, order, and method."[31] And Dix, like her fellow antebellum reformers, considered these qualities essential for the reformation of the dependent poor, whatever their physical or mental health.

While preferring to bombard her audience with such stories of individual barbarities and inhumanities, Dix occasionally admitted that the overall physical condition of the insane in New York's county poorhouses was better than she had expected. Her grudging commendation of the local reforms implemented in the 1820s and 1830s suggests that the legislature's 1836 approval of a state insane asylum had been but one manifestation of a general increase in popular concern for the insane. For the most part, Dix admitted, local social welfare appropriations in New York were surprisingly generous, although some taxpayers felt alarm at the rapidity with which county taxes were rising.[32] Yet, no matter how comfortable and humane it might be, Dix refused to admit that county-level care was appropriate for the insane. Even the best run local poorhouses lacked a professional medical staff, she argued, and the tenure of their heads, no matter how qualified, seldom was longer than that of their political patrons.

In her insistence on the absolute necessity of state-level care for the insane, Dix articulated a position which was to become orthodoxy among nineteenth-century mental health advocates. Like many committed reformers, she felt that only a dramatic, highly polarized presentation of the debate about county versus state care would increase state-level funding. Characteristic of her refusal to soften her position were her comments on the cheerful and comfortable Westchester county house, whose facilities rivaled those of the asylums at Utica and Bloomingdale: "If any thing could ever reconcile me to subordinate institutions, this certainly would do so; but nothing can."[33] Her attitude was shared by most other asylum reformers in New York. In 1844 one legislator proposed that, instead of enlarging the Utica Asylum, the state should direct its appropriations to the Bloomingdale and Hudson Lunatic asylums, both of which, he declared, could accommodate additional pauper patients for less than the interest on the sum requested for Utica's expansion. Despite the economic and geographical advantages of his proposal to diversify state funding, this politician was a minority of one on the Assembly Lunatic Asylum Committee.[34] Any relaxation of their insistence on the absolute necessity of state care, the reformers seemed to believe, would undercut the entire asylum movement. As a result, during this period, New Yorkers never seriously discussed the possibility of developing a complementary system of local and state care, such as that experimented with in the British Isles.

Although the New York State Legislature received Dix's report in 1844, it did not approve construction of a second state asylum for another two decades. In the meantime, the patient population grew at Utica to an average of 450 a year. Under the leadership of several powerful superintendents, such as Amariah Brigham and John Gray, the New York State Lunatic Asylum became well-known in the national campaign for asylum reform. Its heads became an important force in the campaign to expand state services, supporting those legislators concerned about the large numbers of the mentally ill still in county facilities and encouraging local superintendents of the poor to protest the heavy burdens involved in caring for chronically insane paupers. In both 1855 and 1856, those superintendents met in Utica to discuss their problems and possible political solutions. Out of these meetings came a petition to the legislature for additional funding. Noting the rapid increase in the absolute numbers of the insane and the inability of the Utica Asylum to take them all in, they suggested that the state immediately create two additional mental hospitals, one of which would care exclusively for chronically insane paupers. (Doctor John Chapin, then a Utica staff physician, was largely responsible for this second suggestion.)[35]

The political weight of this petition was substantial. Appended were the signatures of sixty-three local officials from across the state who had helped with its formulation, as well as of twenty-three superintendents and overseers of the poor. It thus suggested that support for "ample and suitable [state] provision for all the insane, not in a condition to reside in private families" extended beyond reformers.[36] Somewhat surprisingly, given the alarm in cities about increasing social discord, the strongest clamor for an additional asylum came from the small rural counties of northern and western New York. Presumably their more limited financial resources made it hard for them to construct separate buildings, or even apartments, for the insane poor. Despite its slightly higher maintenance costs, state care was a boon for communities unable to make the initial capital investment required for county asylums, no matter how primitive.

The asylum movement was just one of a number of antebellum reforms in New York State directed by a self-conscious, cost-effective humanitarianism. As L. Ray Gunn has suggested, in almost all of its policy decisions, the antebellum New York legislature emphasized "rational choices, cost–benefit analyses of proposed routes, and engineering expertise."[37] Very similar to the arguments used by superintendents of the poor were those offered the same year by a Senate committee to persuade the legislature to do more for the pauper insane. If treated promptly, pro-asylum politicians argued, 75 percent of those insane less than a year would recover; if left alone or sent to a county poorhouse, only 7 percent would regain their reason. Thus, they calculated, if there were 1,000 recently insane paupers in state poorhouses and only 7 percent could be expected to recover without treatment, 930 would be left to be supported by the public for an average life of eighteen years. At the low per capita maintenance cost of $1.50 per week, these 930 paupers would cost the counties $72,540 per year, and $1,235,720 for their lifetimes. Under a system of state care, 750 of these 1,000 insane paupers could be expected to recover within an average of ten months, for a total treatment expense of $90,000. The 250 incurables, even if provided for at the generous sum of $12 per month, would cost the state $648,000 over the course of their lifetimes. As a result, while the state system initially would cost taxpayers more, over a period of eighteen years it would save them $497,720 in support costs, as well as returning cured patients to the work force.[38]

Such fascination with economic calculations and statistics was not limited to antebellum reformers who thereby hoped to justify their particular version of the economics of compassion. As Patricia Cohen notes, numbers and statistical calculations fascinated many nineteenth-century

Americans. Reformers using appeals to economic self-interest benefited from the general prestige attached to quantitative data, as well as from politicians' desire to invest state funds wisely. Both reformers and politicians shared the new respect for facts and agreed with their fellows that "inventories of descriptive facts about society" would provide "an authentic, objective basis for ascertaining the common good."[39]

In practice, such descriptive information, when made part of the calculus of compassion, often proved more helpful in discriminating between groups than in locating a common good. For example, once reformers had collected masses of descriptive data on New York's dependent poor, they decided that the economics of compassion should be expressed in different ways, as well as at different times, for the various dependent populations. The first of the "dangerous and dependent classes" to be helped were those who showed the most economic and social potential: the able-bodied poor, juvenile delinquents, and criminals. Then, as medical science expanded its claims to be able to cure certain ills, or at least to modify their impact, asylums opened for treatment of the insane and schools for the education and vocational training of the deaf and blind. Last to be cared for in antebellum New York were that most discouraging group: the idiots and imbeciles.[40]

Once politicians became convinced of the need for asylum reform, they frequently tied support of the pauper insane to earlier successful antebellum humanitarian campaigns, especially those for prisons. While this strategy initially benefited the asylum movement by linking its funding requests to benevolent causes already well understood by citizens and taxpayers, its success tended to interfere with the general public's appreciation of the medical mission of asylums. Too often, early asylum superintendents complained, the public lumped together the rehabilitation of prisoners with the cure of the insane, an aggregation which was unfair to the law-abiding mentally ill and which fed public fears of the insane as social threats.[41]

Local and state medical societies also continued to lobby for the expansion of the state asylum system. Like Dix, the doctors saw three major problems in county care of pauper lunatics: lack of medical and moral treatment, "promiscuous" mixing of men and women, and unsanitary housing conditions. Construction of additional state facilities, they concluded, was the way to solve them.[42] An Assembly report submitted two months later made the same point. Quoting Edward Jarvis of Massachusetts on the tendency of insane asylums to serve localized populations, the Assembly committee argued for the construction of several smaller institutions around the state rather than the expansion of Utica.[43] Unfortunately, this sensible proposition was ignored by the legislature as a whole. Fiscal conservatives complained of the cost of such a comprehensive system; local politicians bickered about potential sites for new institutions. Finally the financial panic of 1857 ended the squabbling for a time, as expanded state expenditures for social welfare became impossible.

The Willard Idea

The financial panic of 1857 was followed quickly by the Civil War, an event which further strained New York's fiscal resources. Despite such obstacles, the fight to extend the benefits of state care to all of the insane poor continued. One of its most active leaders was John Chapin, a former physician at the Utica Asylum. Although he had left Utica in 1855 to join George Cook (another ex-Utica physician) at Brigham Hall, a small private institution for the wealthy insane, he did not forget the plight of the pauper insane. That same year he helped the superintendents of the poor draft their petition on behalf of the insane poor. Once they submitted it to the state legislature, he reiterated its arguments in an article published in the *AJI*.[44]

Chapin's 1856 *AJI* essay offers an early indication that the various strands of the economics-of-compassion argument had begun to unravel. The first part of the essay might well have been written twenty years earlier. In it Chapin praised the high cure rates of antebellum asylums and argued that, with the continued spread of prompt medical treatment, most of the social burden of chronic insanity eventually would disappear. Once that utopia arrived, the Utica Asylum would have more than adequately reimbursed the state for its generous capital investments. Such evidence of asylums' cost effectiveness, Chapin argued, should please both taxpayers and politicians, for, while Americans were seldom willing to act on the basis of benevolent impulse alone, they were always receptive to arguments based on a "humanitarian economics."

Chapin admitted, however, that insanity would not disappear immediately and that for several decades the state of New York would need to provide treatment and shelter for its most wounded victims: those whose insanity was of such long duration as to seem incurable. At this point, a fairly conventional presentation of the economics-of-compassion argument became more controversial. Needed immediately, Chapin argued, was a massive expansion of state fiscal responsibility for the dependent insane. New Yorkers must pay more attention to the almost two thousand of their fellow citizens who, impoverished and insane, could not speak for themselves. They should bring within the compassionate embrace of the state the chronic pauper insane as well as the curable insane. While taxpayers were unwilling to subsidize the kind of expensive therapeutic treatment offered at Utica for those with little hope of recovery, Chapin hoped they might be persuaded to underwrite cheaper custodial care. He turned out to be right.[45] Chapin's plea for state-level care of the chronically insane foreshadowed the substantial reformation of pro-asylum rhetoric which was to take place after the Civil War. An emphasis on the economics of maintenance began to replace earlier arguments for state-level care on the grounds that it would turn dependent victims of insanity into self-supporting citizens.

Chapin's article, along with a petition from the county superintendents of the poor, convinced many influential New Yorkers of the need to expand the state asylum system. Once again C. B. Coventry mobilized the State Medical Society to pressure the legislature. In turn, in 1864, the legislature asked Sylvester Willard, secretary of the State Medical Society, to collect information on the care of the insane in county poorhouses. Willard developed a lengthy survey to be administered in every county of the state by a judge-appointed local physician. Focusing on such issues as diet, housing, medical services, and sanitation, he made not even the slightest pretense to objectivity. The goal of his survey, he advised participating doctors, was to "discover the evils which exist in the management of the insane poor" so as to incite the legislature to immediate action.[46]

Although the county physicians tried to cooperate with Willard, they, like Dix before them, uncovered relatively few houses of horror. The most common problems found in county institutions plagued the Utica Asylum as well: use of restraints to control the violent; lack of adequate amusements and work, especially in the winter; and an inability to keep the filthy clean and dressed. In his 1865 report to the legislature, Willard ignored such evidence and concluded that a separate state institution for the incurable mentally ill was badly needed, a recommendation with which then-Governor Fenton concurred. Although Willard died almost immediately after submitting his report, the legislature that same year approved his recommendation, ordering construction of a new state asylum to be named "The Willard Asylum for the Chronic Insane." Once the Willard Asylum was completed, counties were to transfer their chronic pauper insane from local poorhouses and those discharged not recovered from the Utica Asylum were to be sent as well. The legislature also ordered local officials to send all recently insane indigents to the Utica Asylum for treatment at county expense. Under the provisions of its enabling legislation, per capita costs at the new asylum were not to exceed two dollars per week.[47]

The provisions of the Willard bill had been drawn up by the three physicians most intimately involved in the campaign for its passage: Sylvester Willard, George Cook, and John Chapin. Chapin subsequently was appointed a commissioner to oversee Willard's site selection and construction, as was John Gray, superintendent of the Utica Asylum, and a doctor from the State Medical Society. Soon after its organization, the commission decided the layout of the Willard Asylum would be markedly different from that of Utica. Instead of a single large building, Willard was to consist of a central administrative block with wings for the hospital care of the sick and excited and of groups of detached buildings for harmless, industrious, and tranquil patients. Having obtained title to the State Agricultural College in Ovid in December of 1865, the commissioners submitted their plans to Governor Fenton and the legislature in January of 1866. While some opposed the commissioners' choice of an isolated site on the eastern shores of Seneca Lake over another available in the growing city of Buffalo, the selection had definite political advantages. Perhaps most important was the desire of the prominent New York politician Ezra Cornell to move the agricultural college at Ovid, with its Morrill funds, to Ithaca. In addition, the state already had a fifty-thousand-dollar lien on the Ovid property. As a result, despite grumblings from an Erie County lobby which had fought for a Buffalo site, state legislators quickly approved the commissioners' choice.[48]

One of the three Willard commissioners, Superintendent John Gray of Utica, was not happy about the new direction in state policy represented by the decision to build Willard. Although he had complained in his annual reports about Utica's overcrowding, he opposed the idea of a separate institution for the chronically insane and resigned his commissionership in 1866. His opposition to what he began to call the "Willard idea" did not end with that resignation. He continued to attack the notion of distinct institutions for acute and chronic illness both in the pages of the *AJI*, which he edited, and on the floor of the national meetings of the Association of Medical Superintendents of American Institutions for the Insane (AMSAII). Gray's campaign was aggressive and vituperative. For example, when George Cook delivered a paper in defense of Willard at an 1866 AMSAII meeting, Gray mobilized almost the entire membership against him. Cook's fellow doctors attacked him on both philosophical and personal grounds. He cared only about saving tax dollars and nothing about the welfare of the insane, several charged. One of Gray's protégés suggested an even less worthy motive: that Cook's own private asylum in western New York would benefit financially from the location of Willard in the south central portion of the state rather than in Buffalo.[49]

At the same meeting, Gray himself attacked both Cook and the proposed Willard Asylum in a tirade which amounted to twenty-three pages when printed. Not only had the notion of a separate asylum for the chronically insane been thoroughly discredited by American and European authorities, he argued, but even the citizens of New York did not support it. The deformed brainchild of three men, Willard, Chapin, and Cook, it had been approved by a legislature distracted by the Civil War, the recent tragedy of Lincoln's assassination, and Willard's own unexpected death. Gray also repeated gossip about the Willard commissioners' extravagance. Instead of providing inexpensive care for the chronically insane, he charged, they were building what promised to be the most expensive asylum in the United States. Cook repudiated the last allegation from the floor, and once Gray's tirade drew to a close, Cook introduced a resolution calling for provision of special asylums for the chronically insane in all situations in which hospital accommodations could not be provided. Since Gray was one of the most powerful members of the AMSAII, Cook's motion failed. He won only a single vote for the motion: his own.[50]

Gray was not content with his AMSAII victory. He continued to attack both the Willard idea and Chapin's supervision of the asylum's construction. Frustrated and angry, Chapin responded by denying Gray's charges and complaining about Gray's generally obstructionist activities around the state.[51] He also went to the following year's AMSAII meeting in the hope of defending both himself and the notion of separate asylums for the chronically insane. Frustrated by Gray's dominations of the organization, Chapin took the offensive and attacked AMSAII members as conservatives unwilling to accept new social realities. They must give up their efforts to "fetter inquiry" into the growing problem of the chronically insane poor, he exhorted, or lose the respect of the rest of the medical profession. In the past, state asylum superintendents had too often used reports on the condition of the chronically insane poor in county poorhouses to win legislative support for acute care hospitals, he charged. Such misuse of "the most suffering, friendless, and helpless" must come to an end. Chapin also criticized asylum superintendents' adherence to an exaggerated "cult of curability" and demanded that they stop "gilding public reports with extravagant expectations" in order to win legislative support. More appropriate, he felt, was a modified version of the economics-of-compassion argument, which stressed the short-term benefits of cheap state custodial care rather than the long-term advantages of therapeutic treatment.[52]

Chapin's angry speech proved as initially ineffective as Cook's motion the year before, but John Gray paid a high price for his overwhelming AMSAII victories in 1866 and 1867. Although assured of his colleagues' support, he so slanted the published version of the AMSAII debates with Cook and Chapin that, for the 1868 meeting, the AMSAII hired a professional stenographer to replace Gray's reporter.[53] Furthermore, whatever his national victories, he was unable to stop, or even to modify, plans for the Willard Asylum in New York State. Completed in 1869, it immediately began to receive patients from county poorhouses. To Gray's additional dismay, the Willard trustees unanimously chose John Chapin as their first superintendent. By 1869, Chapin, once Gray's subordinate at the Utica Asylum, had become his political and social equal and, in Gray's eyes at least, an irritating professional rival.

Thus, while they did not persuade their colleagues in other states of the viability of separate institutions for the chronically insane, Cook and Chapin won the immediate local political battle. Others contributed to this victory, but the two doctors' articles and public speeches in defense of the Willard Asylum were models of political persuasion. Particularly effective was George Cook's 1866 "Provision for the Insane Poor in the State of New York." In it he grounded his defense of separate institutions for the chronically insane on carefully documented appeals to common sense, to the lessons of history, and to the medical profession's faith in progress. He characterized his opponents as impractical theorists, out of touch with the realities of New York State's fiscal situation and the miseries of poorhouse life for the insane. Rather than ignoring his opponents' arguments, he turned them on their head. In response to Gray's charge that establishment of a separate asylum for the chronically insane would stigmatize its patients and deprive them of all hope, Cook countered that the Utica doctors themselves had already stigmatized hundreds in a far more devastating fashion by sending them back to their local poorhouses "unimproved." When Gray argued that only the presence of the curable insane guaranteed continued public oversight of insane asylums and thus prevented patient abuse, Cook noted that, when relegated to the back wards of therapeutic institutions, the chronically insane received only the most minimal care.[54] Cook also emphasized that the Willard Asylum was not a utopian experiment. It promised to put into practice principles already well tested, particularly those relating to patient labor. If situated in a fertile agricultural district and run by competent managers, Willard's farms would both improve the health of their insane laborers and produce a substantial profit. Thus, despite his personal break with the first generation of asylum reformers, Cook ended his own political appeal with a slight reformulation of that tried and true argument, the economic advantages of compassionate care. While the Willard Asylum managers could not promise to restore most of their patients to economically productive lives, they could care for them in a humane, professional fashion, and at a very low weekly cost.[55]

In the long run, neither side was entirely victorious. Gray's charge that, once labeled incurable, few patients would ever leave Willard turned out to be disturbingly accurate. For a number of reasons, including the difficulty of distinguishing acute from chronic illness, few other states emulated the Willard experiment. On the other hand, many eventually adopted a modified version of it and constructed detached "cottages" for convalescent patients and quiet chronic ones next to their traditional hospital facility.[56] Committed to the notion of the superiority of state-level care, few states (except Wisconsin) thought to investigate another alternative: state-supervised county-level management of the insane.

Development of a
State Asylum System in New York

More significant than either Chapin's and Cook's local triumphs or Gray's national victories was the long-range impact of the Willard Act. It turned out to be a victory, not only for advocates of separate institutions for the chronically insane, but also for those who wanted to build ever larger social welfare institutions. The Willard Asylum eventually became the largest institution of its kind in the United States, caring for more than two thousand patients. Willard's opening in 1869 also marked official legislative recognition of the benefits of a specialized, comprehensive asylum system. Soon after Willard received its first patients, the state opened a second acute care facility in Poughkeepsie (1871), a homeopathic institution at Middletown (1874), the Binghamton Asylum for the Chronic Insane (1879), and the Buffalo State Asylum (1880). Although these institutions embodied a diversity of therapeutic philosophies, each held far more than the 250 patients the early AMSAII had considered an ideal limit. Before the Civil War, New York also had built a special asylum for insane criminals at the Auburn State Prison. Such growth suggested that much had changed since 1836, when Utica had been approved. Many New York State legislators, with the help of reformers increasingly well organized into groups like the State Board of Charities, now supported the notion of a unified approach to the treatment of mental illness. As a result, state care of the insane no longer could be characterized as fragmented and haphazard, the "accumulation of a number of highly individualized decisions."[57] Although still subject to local-interest lobbying pressures, it had begun to show signs of systematic social planning.

The growth of a statewide asylum system indicated that, despite their many differences, supporters and opponents of Willard agreed at least on one issue: their absolute opposition to any alternative to state-level institutions. Both Chapin and Gray, like their predecessors, consistently ignored evidence that certain county poorhouses managed to maintain their insane paupers in reasonable comfort. With their fellow superintendents, they refused to surrender the smallest part of their claim to monopolize care of the mentally ill. In increasing numbers after the Civil War, county superintendents of the poor expressed anger about the costs of state asylum care for the poor, which local governments had to absorb. Although they developed increasingly sophisticated noneconomic, as well as fiscal, rationales for local care, they ultimately failed to overcome the powerful pro-asylum lobby. Although the state legislature in the 1870s exempted a number of counties with their own asylums from the provisions of the Willard Act,[58] state asylum doctors and social reformers bitterly opposed every such exemption, no matter what its merits. They charged that the only motivation for the construction of local asylums was economic: exempted counties simply did not want to pay even the minimal costs of Willard care. Even though state insane asylums themselves were the target of much criticism and several legislative investigations in the years after the Civil War, social welfare reformers of all political persuasions continued to insist that there was only one appropriate response to mental illness: state-level care.[59]

Reformers' insistence on the need for state institutions was so adamant, so one-sided, that they almost totally obscured the social realities of local care of the insane. By midcentury in New York, highly repetitive, sensationalistic stories about the physical and sexual abuse of the pauper insane in county poorhouses had superseded time-worn diatribes against families keeping the insane locked up in chains. Thus, one sort of rhetorical excess succeeded another. Attacks on county poorhouses, whether written in 1843 or 1888, looked alike; they repeated the same themes and told the same horror stories, no matter who the authors or what the timing. With county care always available for rhetorical contrast, state asylum superintendents found it easy to ignore important problems shared by both county and state authorities. These included the poor quality of attendants (whether paid workers or paupers); the difficulty of providing consistently kind treatment for violent, abusive patients; the deadly monotony of institutional life, especially in the winter; and the difficulty of keeping self-destructive, filthy patients clean, well-clothed, and in good health. As a result, constructive discussion between local and state officials about how they coped with similar challenges never took place. By

Table 2.1. Per Capita Expenditures in Dollars at the Utica and Willard Asylums, 1869–1889

Year	Medicine		Patient expenses		Provisions		Utilities		Repairs		Furniture		Books and stationery		Consumables		Capital expense		Salary costs	
	Utica	Willard	Utica	Willard	Utica	Willard	Utica	Willard	Utica	Willard	Utica	Willard	Utica	Willard	Utica	Willard	Utica	Willard	Utica	Willard
1869	4.32		12.64		72.22		23.82		20.62		9.23		2.46		102.83		39.73		46.45	
1870	3.45		14.33		60.77		17.23		24.76		9.19		2.95		87.80		42.45		44.75	
1871	4.51		14.05		58.43		8.19	31.15	20.11	228.91	8.66	10.98	2.39	1.38	77.37	32.53	39.10	239.98	43.69	12.17
1872	4.74		13.37	9.94	64.07	52.30	18.22	21.29	22.89		6.81	4.31	4.47	.49	96.06	74.08	38.01	10.34	50.88	43.66
1873	5.39		11.91	13.01	65.15	57.12	16.44	20.60	43.42		8.37	7.04	3.99		95.36	77.72	61.34	14.44	55.33	50.60
1874	5.55	1.04	11.04	12.00	69.01	58.00	17.07	18.83	49.76		9.46	6.87	2.67		99.13	77.87	70.05	13.09	58.02	47.64
1875	6.33	1.08	10.55	8.80	63.15	53.25	17.68	19.38	27.00		9.00	11.34	2.98		97.01	73.71	45.63	18.01	57.24	45.93
1876	6.71	1.39	11.43	8.88	60.92	51.78	15.05	16.61	34.94	3.16	10.08	9.16	3.28		90.96	69.77	53.73	16.83	54.66	41.72
1877	4.59	1.57	11.43	9.54	58.05	59.05	13.05	15.22	47.38	3.43	6.96	8.92	2.01		82.40	75.85	62.52	16.94	55.48	41.74
1878	4.18	1.30	10.37	11.50	54.32	46.98	12.26	13.74	43.67	6.62	7.74	9.87	2.35		78.34	62.02	59.26	20.53	55.73	40.92
1879	4.46	1.00	9.07	9.34	37.10	35.66	10.88	10.90	29.93	2.27	8.90	13.94	1.61		57.28	47.56	45.03	18.69	44.60	34.75
1880	5.36	1.54	7.61	9.75	51.83	44.26	9.37	12.49	40.13	3.51	7.37	19.57	2.48		73.50	58.28	57.28	26.64	55.33	40.43
1881	5.36	1.70	9.77	12.32	56.71	47.07	14.10	14.82	30.57	2.85	10.05	13.77	3.35		82.94	63.59	54.54	19.67	52.86	42.11
1882	6.15	1.89	8.75	14.91	65.40	54.16	13.44	11.13	16.51	2.17	5.80	9.84	2.21		91.04	67.18	33.14	15.71	58.91	40.97
1883	5.33	1.59	8.15	10.12	58.44	50.89	14.79	13.88	8.05	1.67	3.44	10.19	3.04		85.59	66.35	24.06	15.68	60.17	43.01
1884	4.30	1.31	7.80		56.29	48.20	13.18	12.85	17.13	1.48	5.17	12.36	2.86		79.64	62.37	30.85	18.35	57.44	44.12
1885	4.09	1.34	8.47	11.70	50.59	39.73	12.04	11.63	40.10	1.45	8.26	12.23	3.11		73.67	52.70	58.72	18.01	62.26	42.60
1886	4.38	1.33	6.49	9.57	49.19	39.36	11.39	8.35	63.08	1.10	5.10	9.39	2.08		69.91	49.04	79.89	15.03	64.15	42.23
1887	2.80	1.45	6.47	10.56	43.13	38.39	12.21	9.49	48.94		7.49	9.90	1.86		63.01	49.34	61.81	13.72	65.64	43.50
1888	2.50	1.58	7.20	8.73	42.81	43.05	18.76	11.66	58.91	.72	8.60	10.95	2.47		69.77	56.29	74.58	15.67	61.76	44.51
1889	2.47	1.33	6.35	9.74	43.20	37.66	13.64	8.92	45.87	2.05	5.65	10.40	1.99		64.86	47.91	57.13	15.90	61.25	43.13

Data is taken from the Utica and Willard Asylum *Annual Reports*, 1869–1889.

diverting public attention to the horrors of county care, state asylum superintendents were able to sweep their own problems under their dusty rugs. Thus, as early as the 1870s, the new "comprehensive" system of state asylum care developed a self-imposed limitation: its proponents precluded any significant role for local communities within it.

Even while New York began to implement this state-level system of mental health care, its traditional ideological underpinnings began to show signs of strain. That appeal for asylum reform based on the economics of compassion which had seemed so simple and self-evident when articulated by Enos Throop in 1830 fit many fewer social welfare situations by the 1870s. The society's gradual loss of confidence in medicine's ability to cure mental illness was only one source of trouble. More serious was the increasing diversity of asylum's social functions, so that, although all of the insane were considered to deserve state care, certain groups were seen as meriting better care than others, at least as measured in monetary terms. One indicator of such an attitude was the difference in Utica's and Willard's budgets (Table 2.1). Consistently over the course of the nineteenth century, per capita expenditures on all sorts of items, ranging from food and medicine to utilities and library books, were two to three times higher for Utica's acutely ill patients than for Willard's chronic ones. The component parts of taxpayers' compassion differed sharply for the two groups: while Willard's patients were perhaps deserving of more sympathy, Utica's were more likely to benefit from additional funds.[60] The differential levels of expenditures for the two groups were too marked to be accidental, and an "economics of maintenance" argument slowly developed to rationalize the lower level of funding offered the so-called chronic cases.

The Limits of Benevolence

While early nineteenth-century reformers lauded the generosity of the New York State Legislature, its fiscal benevolence had clear limits. From 1843 on, the expensive therapeutic care of the Utica Asylum was reserved primarily for those most likely to benefit from it and, not incidentally, most likely to recompense the state for the costs of their treatment by returning to society as productive members. Conceptualized as an acute care facility, the Utica Asylum attempted (not always successfully) to limit its admissions to those whose insanity was of less than a year in duration, since these were considered to have the best chance of cure. It also was supposed to discharge all indigent patients after two years, whether cured or not.[61] As the number of chronically insane grew, both at Utica and in county institutions, state legislators eventually agreed to establish a separate asylum for them. Opened in 1869 in a beautiful, remote part of central New York, the Willard Asylum offered low-cost custodial care to its seemingly incurable patients.

To win even such conditional fiscal support for their proposals, antebellum reformers had had to stress, and often to exaggerate, four arguments: the curability of insanity, the abuse of the insane in local almshouses, the crucial importance of medical therapeutics, and the benefits of state care to the community (both in financial savings and feelings of benevolence). Over the course of the nineteenth century, the complexity of such multiple bases for their legislative support created many problems for state-funded asylums. Institutions such as Utica felt compelled to maintain high levels of cures, yet their superintendents also felt vulnerable to public resentment of the too-quick release of potentially threatening insane persons. Both Utica and Willard faced frequent scrutiny of their treatment programs from local and statewide reform groups, organizations often concerned simultaneously to keep costs low and cure rates high. The very decision to build Willard resulted from the despair of many doctors about the public's willingness to fund a second therapeutic institution in New York, so they settled instead for a largely custodial asylum where a heavy reliance on patient labor and high patient–doctor ratios helped minimize weekly maintenance costs.

By and large, social historians lack the accounting skills to dissect thoroughly the detailed budgets of nineteenth-century social welfare institutions. Evaluation of the merits and deficiencies of relative funding levels is not easy, for even the clearest indicators of quality of care lose their sharpness when considered in their social context. Yet, a comparison of the Utica and Willard budgets demonstrates that politicians', and even reformers', compassion had different limits for different groups. On the other hand, although Willard's per capita patient budget was small, its casebook records suggest that at least limited therapeutic benefits accrued from the decision to send "back ward" patients to an institution devoted to their special care. Once admitted to the Willard Asylum, few patients managed to regain their freedom, but almost all enjoyed lower mortality rates and a greater freedom from abuse than their peers in acute care facilities (Chapter 5). Willard's experience suggests that, at least in the nineteenth century, overt recognition of the chronicity of certain forms of mental illness and the construction of specialized facilities to deal with the chronic insane simultaneously produced devastatingly permanent labels and better patient care.

This is but one of the many paradoxes of asylum care with which social historians must struggle. The following chapters look at a number of additional aspects of nineteenth-century New York's asylum history which are equally complex and difficult to evaluate: relationships among families, asylums, and the state; the treatment philosophies of the asylums' medical staffs; their actual therapeutic practices; and the interactions on the wards of the attendants and patients. In many ways these aspects of life within New York's nineteenth-century asylums seemed far removed from life without. Yet, as the social and political forces which in the 1840s had produced an "economics of compassion" changed over time, even the most isolated and self-sufficient of New York State's insane asylums (like Willard) felt their ideological and fiscal impact. The reformist ideology which emerged after the Civil War might best be characterized as a "politics of maintenance." It expressed simultaneously the triumph of institutional approaches to madness and the increasing popular skepticism about the efficacy of such solutions.

3

Medical Men and Medical Power

Once the New York State Legislature approved funds for the construction of an insane asylum at Utica, the trustees of the new institution began to search for a doctor to head it. Their standards were high, some might have said impossibly so. In a letter to the New York State Senate, they described their ideal candidate in detail:

> An active, charitable, conscientious man, of good sense and mild manners, with perfect self-command, and a thorough knowledge of human nature; . . . a well educated physician, of tact, firmness and experience, familiar with the improved medical and moral treatment of insanity; . . . an energetic philanthropist, of calmness and decision, of moral and physical courage, who is never weary of *doing good*, whose benevolence can make the lunatic a companion and friend.[1]

Only a liberal salary, they added, could attract such a paragon.

The impossible challenge of fitting such a job description was to haunt New York's state asylum superintendents for most of the nineteenth century. And the resulting frustration was heightened by the onerous demands of their position. Frequently superintendents spent more time overseeing construction and ensuring that daily routines ran smoothly than in developing treatment programs (although they would not have seen such tasks as contradictory). As a result, opportunities to "make the lunatic a companion and friend" were few and far between. By the 1880s, Utica's patients complained that they saw then-superintendent John Gray only when he escorted important visitors around the wards. At Willard,

Superintendent John Chapin prided himself on the warm relations within his asylum "family" but could hardly know well his almost sixteen hundred "children." Late in the century, one New York observer criticized asylum superintendents for spending more time "raising turnips and striving to keep on the right side with the politicians" than in practicing medicine.[2] A more sympathetic commentator suggested that the management of insane asylums be rearranged so as to free their medical heads from routine business affairs. At the 1890 meeting of the AMSAII, Henry Hurd proclaimed that a superintendent "should not exhaust his energies in looking after the farm or a grade of calico to be purchased, or in seeing that the proper quality of flour is secured, or that the contract for coal is favorable, but he should occupy himself daily and only in becoming acquainted with recent cases."[3]

Because of the impossible breadth of the superintendent's prescribed duties, the choice of which duties to stress varied from superintendent to superintendent. The impact of individuals' personalities on the office of superintendent can be seen most easily at the New York State Lunatic Asylum at Utica. Between 1843 and 1890, the Utica Asylum had four superintendents: Amariah Brigham, Nathan Benedict, John Gray, and George Blumer. Between 1869 and 1889, Willard had two: John Chapin and P. M. Wise. Perhaps the most beloved was Brigham. When he died unexpectedly, his friends constructed a larger-than-life image of him as the ideal superintendent to whom all successors were compared.[4] Less well-loved but more powerful than Brigham was John Gray, who effectively controlled the Utica Asylum from 1852 until 1886. Gray's strong personality made him a controversial national figure within and without the world of asylum psychiatry. As a contemporary newspaper commented, Gray's accomplishments at Utica were considerable, but the very qualities of ambition and will which had pushed him to build such a system made him vulnerable to charges of autocracy and corruption.[5] In sharp contrast to Gray was John Chapin, superintendent of the Willard Asylum from its opening until 1884. Instead of establishing a personal fiefdom, Chapin worked hard to develop amiable relations with his staff and bragged of the "entire harmony" that prevailed within his household. While Gray prided himself on his national power and influence, Chapin most prized his skill at "holding affairs in the right groove, establishing good precedents, and adhering to them.[6] Neither Wise nor Blumer much resembled their towering predecessors, but like Chapin, they prided themselves on their moderation and openness to new therapeutic strategies.

Despite the variety of their administrative styles, all of New York's nineteenth-century asylum superintendents talked of their jobs in terms similar to those used by Amariah Brigham in the 1840s. Like many of his generation, Brigham thought of the asylum as the family writ large. Within it, the superintendent was the loving father. His power over patients and staff was absolute, albeit tempered with kindness and affection.[7] Aware of the strategic benefits of invoking Brigham's memory as well as of the power of such imagery in nineteenth-century America, his successors continued to use Brigham's rhetoric of domesticity. Yet, as their institutions grew, New York's superintendents came more closely to resemble remote biblical patriarchs than loving fathers. Furthermore, their authority, no matter how firmly exercised, proved often inadequate to control manic and demented patients who seldom resembled obedient, malleable children. The resulting social chaos created a topsy-turvy version of the Victorian family which little conformed to the clichés of domestic fiction. Nonetheless, these nineteenth-century superintendents continued to offer domestic conceptualizations of the asylum world. Gray, Chapin, Blumer, and Wise all clung to familial metaphors to rationalize an institutional expansion which gradually emptied those metaphors of significant meaning. Perhaps they also relied on patriarchal imagery to give them the authority so often withheld from nineteenth-century doctors and which their twentieth-century successors expect as a matter of course.

Amariah Brigham, 1843–1849

The first choice of the Utica trustees for their new superintendent was Samuel Woodward, then head of the Worcester Asylum. Woodward fit their job description as closely as any doctor of the day, but when they offered him a salary of two thousand dollars, Woodward turned them down for a more attractive counteroffer from his home institution.[8] The Utica managers then looked to Amariah Brigham, head of the Hartford Retreat, who accepted their offer eagerly. Since the managers' correspondence with Brigham has been lost, it is difficult to know why they chose the intense young doctor. Possibly the Utica managers had met Brigham during their information-gathering visits to leading northeastern asylums. His views on insanity, and in particular his emphasis on its physical origins, closely resembled their own.[9] While Brigham was not a highly original medical theorist, he had synthesized the major thinking of the day in a number of well-received books and articles.[10] He also possessed the requisite practical experience. After years in general practice and a term as professor of anatomy and surgery at the College of Physicians and Surgeons in New York City, Brigham had served several years as superintendent of the Retreat for the Insane in Hartford, Connecticut. In addition, he was somewhat familiar with New York State politics, having spent part of his young adulthood in Albany.

While most histories of the Utica Asylum do not rehearse the details of Amariah Brigham's life before 1843, the year he went to Utica, his early history prefigured in important ways his adult career. From childhood, Brigham had excelled at defining personal goals and achieving them, no matter what the obstacles. In order to fulfill his early ambition to become a doctor, after the death of his father the eleven-year-old Brigham left home for an apprenticeship with his uncle, a doctor. When the uncle died only ten months after Brigham had moved to his home, the young boy then proceeded alone to Albany, New York, where he became a bookstore clerk. In his free time, he read voraciously, trying to compensate for his lack of formal education. Eventually, he moved back to his mother's home in Marlboro, New Hampshire, where he studied, taught, and served an apprenticeship with a local doctor. After a second such apprenticeship and attendance at a medical lecture series in New York City, by the age of twenty he was ready to start his own practice. Once in practice, he continued his self-education, learning first French and then chemistry and saving his money for a European tour, so as to complete both his cultural and medical education.[11]

During his year abroad, Brigham visited cultural landmarks and a number of hospitals. While in Paris, he attended a course of lectures at the School of Medicine which profoundly influenced his future intellectual development. According to Eric Carlson, here he absorbed French notions about the importance of "clinical observation, localism as shown through lesions. . . , and medical statistics."[12] According to a Utica friend, when Brigham finally returned to the United States at the age of thirty-two, "His ambition had in no respect been cooled, nor his confidence in himself abated, by travel and a more extended acquaintance with the world."[13] Discontented with his career opportunities in Greenfield, Massachusetts, he moved to Hartford, Connecticut, in 1831. There, with the help of influential friends, he quickly developed a lucrative practice as both a surgeon and a physician.

During his Hartford years, Brigham continued the habits of hard work and intense intellectual activity which had characterized his life to that point. With the help of a large medical library, he began to reflect upon his professional experiences. In a number of books and articles, he developed the notions about mental illness and its care which were to shape his years at the Utica Asylum. The most influential of these publications, *Remarks on the Influence of Mental Cultivation and Mental Excitement upon Health,* which appeared first in 1832, went through three American editions by 1845 and appeared in Scotland as well. In both this book and his *Observations on the Influence of Religion upon the Health and Physical Welfare of Mankind* (1835), Brigham argued that, while insanity occasionally was caused by a blow to the head or a fever, more often it was produced by moral causes. Particularly dangerous were violent excitements of the mind which then generated morbid activities in certain parts of the brain. Like many of his contemporaries, he argued that those who lived in democracies with great social opportunity were at greatest risk of insanity.[14] Among the many dangerous trends in nineteenth-century America, he felt that the worst was the overstimulation of children's brains to the neglect of their bodies and to the detriment of their emotional stability.

Brigham also spoke out strongly against the unsettling impact of protracted religious revivals.[15] Excess of any sort, even of good qualities, was undesirable, he argued. To illustrate, he once recounted the story of a young man who, after a head wound, began to display an excess of benevolent feelings. Not only did he attempt to feed the poor and shelter the homeless, but whenever he saw cattle in a poor pasture, he moved them to a better one. His efforts to relieve suffering eventually created so many problems that he was put in an insane asylum.[16] (Whether Brigham, himself a man involved in a large number of reform efforts, saw the similarities between this man of excessive benevolence and himself is not recorded.) An ambitious self-made man who never let his uncertain health constrain his activities, Brigham criticized in his medical writings the many Americans who lived as he did. Stressing the need for balance and moderation, he celebrated Jeffersonian virtues while living a Jacksonian life. In a revealing quote, Brigham described his ideal person as "the agriculturalist, with a good farm and well-selected library." This mythical farmer, he argued, could maintain a valuable independence of others at work and spend his leisure improving his mind, thus assuring health of mind and body.[17]

In 1833 Brigham also arranged for the publication in the United States of a book by J. G. Spurzheim, a leading European phrenologist who had visited Hartford. In his 1833 edition of *Remarks on the Influence of Mental Cultivation,* Brigham defined the brain in terms borrowed from phrenology; it was, he asserted, "the material organ by which the mental faculties are manifested."[18] Similarly, in his 1840 book, *An Inquiry Concerning the Diseases and Functions of the Brain, the Spinal Cord, and the Nerves,* he argued for a close association between insanity and the dysfunction of specific parts of the brain.[19] Particularly attractive to Brigham after his introduction in Paris to clinical medicine was the phrenological notion that "the phenomena of mind could be studied objectively and explained in terms of natural causes."[20] Such a position accorded well with Brigham's own empiricist tendencies.

Initially, Brigham's support of phrenology, especially since he combined with it attacks on emotional excess in religion, won him many enemies. One pamphleteer accused him of denying the spiritual reality of the brain and the benefits to civilization of organized religion.[21] Enemies of phrenology also found offensive Brigham's insistence that a person able to distinguish right from wrong might still be unable to resist an impulse to evil. Here, they complained, he undercut the notion of responsibility for sin. Brigham was called an atheist and burned in effigy when he left Hartford. Yet Brigham consistently refused to disavow what he considered to be scientific truths. In this and similar situations, he responded that religious convictions worth holding on to did not need protection from science.[22] As a reformer, Brigham also found attractive the phrenologists' social optimism, their confidence that environmental changes could improve the lot of mankind.[23]

Over time, Brigham was to modify his views on phrenology but in response to empirical evidence, not public pressure. When he measured the heads of his Utica patients, he found their size and shape to be the same as those of the sane. After doing a number of postmortems on Utica patients, to his disappointment he found few indications of structural disease in those portions of the brain where, according to phrenologists, the organs that controlled these faculties were situated.[24] As a result, while continuing to believe that the brain was a "congeries of organs," he disavowed the phrenological position on craniology.[25] In the 1840s, Brigham's first assistant physician at Utica, H. A. Butolph, embraced phrenology with even more enthusiasm than his superintendent. Although by that point Brigham himself had moved away from phrenology, he commented gently on Butolph's notions at the fourth annual meeting of the AMSAII.[26]

In 1837 Brigham left his private practice in Hartford to become a professor of anatomy and surgery in the College of Physicians and Surgeons in New York City. Forced to resign after a year because of poor health, he returned once more to Hartford, where in 1838, he became assistant editor of the *American Journal of Medical Sciences*.[27] Having written an influential review of nineteenth-century insane asylums, as well as his study of the brain and its diseases, Brigham successfully applied to become superintendent of the Hartford Retreat in 1840. Opposed from the start by some of the Retreat's directors for his strong allegiance to the Jacksonian Democratic party, Brigham stayed at the Retreat for only two years. One historian has suggested that public dissatisfaction with his management of violent patients and his own unhappiness with the Retreat's board of managers prompted his resignation in 1842 and his move to Utica.[28]

While Brigham's early writings stressed the cultural roots of insanity, as an asylum superintendent he turned his attention primarily to ways of treating it. Despite his commitment to empiricism, most of his notions about treatment developed logically out of his theoretical writings. Insanity, he declared in an early annual report for the Utica Asylum, was a "chronic disease of the brain" which could attack any one of its several faculties. Some of the insane, he argued, suffered from impairment of the intellectual faculties alone and others of the emotional faculties, though most from both.[29] To explain why specific men and women fell ill, Brigham turned to the conventional wisdom of nineteenth-century medicine and divided the causes of insanity into two: the predisposing and the exciting.

Predisposing causes were the most important, he argued, for the physically and mentally stalwart managed to cope with even the most stressful events. While he regarded heredity as the most influential predisposing cause, he felt that even those "infected" at birth could protect themselves by a strong early education which taught them how to control their passions and to maintain good physical health. Furthermore, he argued, attacks of insanity were almost always preceded by sleep deprivation. Those thus weakened in body and mind became highly vulnerable to mental illness.[30]

Such ideas, according to Brigham's successors, made him a pioneer in the scientific treatment of mental illness. He was, they declared, one of the first superintendents to apply the laws of physiology to problems of brain disorders. By reducing insanity "to a simple problem of impaired nutrition," New York's first commissioner in lunacy declared in the 1870s, Brigham had eliminated "the black bat of superstition" which had so long clouded Americans' views of insanity.[31] Yet such a presentation of Brigham, however laudatory, misrepresented both his thinking and practice. In passages often overlooked by his successors, Brigham argued explicitly that so-called moral causes were more often at the root of insanity than physical ones. Indeed, he pointed out several times, many of the so-called physical causes, such as apoplexy, epilepsy, and dyspepsia, were actually the first symptoms of brain disorders produced by moral causes.[32] Furthermore, although concerned to replace popular superstitions about insanity with scientific notions, Brigham did not feel that medical treatments alone could cure diseased minds. In fact, he was bitterly opposed to the heroic medical strategies of the early nineteenth century and, like most of the first generation of asylum superintendents, felt that moral treatment was most likely to cure. He included under the aegis of moral treatment "everything related to the personal management of the insane, exclusive of medical treatments."[33] From a phrenological perspective, moral treatment led to the suppression of disturbed organs by calling other mental organs into greater action.[34]

The treatment programs Brigham developed for his Utica patients reflected his interest in both the moral and physical causes of mental illness. In his annual reports and published articles, Brigham described his theories about the best treatment strategies for dealing with the institutionalized mentally ill. He strongly attacked the lay tendency to rely on depletion strategies, whether bleeding, excess use of emetics, or harsh purgatives, was often leading to the weakening and death of the mentally ill.[35] To strengthen exhausted bodies, Brigham prescribed a variety of drugs, particularly opiates and tonics, but he also emphasized imaginative and diverse moral treatment programs. Most important, he declared, were the following: removal of the insane from their home and past associations, kind treatment, manual labor (in most cases), attendance at Sunday religious services, the inculcation of regular habits and self-control, and the diversion of the mind away from morbid turns of thoughts.[36] Brigham's advocacy of moral instead of medical treatments was so well-known, he ruefully noted to his friend Pliny Earle, that other superintendents felt he was "not practical."[37] An ex-patient, on the other hand, praised Brigham as one who poised "the weapons that his science gave / with wariest skill, as one who feared their power."[38] An American pioneer in the asylum treatment of the insane, Brigham remained always open to new ideas. In close contact with both national and international medical circles, Brigham eagerly greeted innovative treatment suggestions, even when they conflicted with his own practices. For example, upon hearing of the English doctor John Conolly's decision to abolish all physical restraint at his asylum, Brigham immediately resolved to try a similar experiment at Utica, despite doubts about its viability and the need to hire extra attendants to carry it out. Similarly, after reading a French doctor's comments on the therapeutic value of hashish, he acquired some for his own institution.[39]

As Utica's superintendent, Brigham also had to deal with a number of administrative problems little connected to direct psychiatric care. When he arrived at Utica in 1843, the asylum was far from finished, and construction continued for almost the entire term of his superintendency. Daily he had to cope with problems caused by an inadequate water supply, poor ventilation, and buildings which began to decay soon after their construction. In letters he often complained to friends of the fatigue attendant upon living with and having to supervise what amounted to constant chaos.[40] Yet he found excitement as well in solving such problems. "Eureka!" he began one letter describing his discovery that new principles of ventilation could be applied to Utica's wing.[41] Before coming to Utica, Brigham had characterized the ideal asylum as a small institution where men and women, living in gracious comfort, could receive kind, individualized attention. With more than four hundred patients, his situation in New York was far from that ideal. With what his chaplain described as "iron will and determination," Brigham handled the resulting political and therapeutic challenges with graceful competence, although at some cost to his health. At least, unlike some superintendents, he encountered few challenges to his authority from his board of managers.[42]

Despite demanding administrative responsibilities, Brigham continued to work to limit the spread of insanity as well as to cure it. Feeling that local asylum work by itself could not achieve these goals, in 1844 he started the United States' first professional psychiatric publication: the *AJI*. In addition to other asylum superintendents, it had two intended audiences: the general public and those professionals who dealt frequently with the insane, physicians and lawyers.[43] Starting such a new publication was not easy, and Brigham complained frequently of the need to beg for articles, scrabble for subscribers, and subsidize the *AJI* out of his own pocket. One letter to his good friend Pliny Earle started out, "I intend devoting part of the day to celebrating the advent of cheap postage and inflicting letters upon various persons and shall begin with yourself."[44] Brigham was never in strong health, and the demands of editing occasionally threatened to overwhelm him. He invariably signed his almost illegible letters "in haste."[45] Yet he obviously valued the intellectual contacts with peers in both the United States and Western Europe that the *AJI* provided. As he noted to Earle in a letter begging for news about the national asylum movement, "I am in the woods and hear but little that does not get into print. . . ."[46] Writing articles for and editing the *AJI* protected Brigham from being swamped by his multiple mundane institutional responsibilities. He also maintained contact with his professional peers through the AMSAII, of which he was a founding member.

For much of his life, Brigham's nervous energy and determination enabled him to cope with the daily demands of asylum administration, lobby for state funding, edit the *AJI*, and figure prominently in the fledgling AMSAII, despite his life-long poor health. When first his only son and then his mother died suddenly in 1847, however, the resulting depression weakened his always-feeble physique.[47] A subsequent attack of dysentery led to his death in 1849 at the age of 59. At his funeral, friends evoked both the man's achievements and his complexity. Obviously dearly loved by those who knew him well, he also had driven hard both himself and those around him. "Few men were less covetous of personal popularity, or more regardless of the opinions of those around him, so long as he was sustained by the approbation of his own conscience," noted one of the Utica managers.[48] Most often repeated in later years was the story that Brigham could distinguish a lunatic by his appearance alone, a feat he supposedly demonstrated by pointing out a seriously disturbed man sitting in the crowd in a courtroom to which Brigham had been called for psychiatric testimony.[49]

Nathan Benedict, 1849–1854

After Brigham's death, his first assistant physician, George Cook, served as acting superintendent while the board of managers searched for a worthy successor. Their choice, Nathan Benedict, had studied medicine at the University of Pennsylvania. Following graduation, he went into private practice until becoming medical superintendent of the Pennsylvania Almshouse in 1846. There he paid particular attention to the insane and developed innovative ways of heating and ventilating their quarters. Although he had written little before being chosen to become Utica's second superintendent, his practical experience appealed to the asylum's board.[50] Like Brigham, Superintendent Benedict was to spend much of his brief superintendency supervising repairs and overseeing new construction. His most noteworthy accomplishments were the completion of a new heating and ventilation system and the landscaping of the asylum grounds.[51] He continued most of Brigham's therapeutic programs, agreeing with him about the importance of moral treatment. Benedict too liked to describe himself as father to what he called "our great family," but unlike Brigham, he always took care to distinguish his institutional from his "private" family. The latter did not always appreciate the former. Benedict's wife, fatigued after childbirth, complained about their "public mode of living" and, in particular, about having to eat with patients and staff.[52] Like Brigham, Benedict disliked comparisons of asylums with prisons. When several patients escaped during his first year, Benedict received a letter from Dorothea Dix mentioning the harm such escapes were doing to Utica's na-

65

tional reputation. In reply, he declared that he felt that the institution
almost deserved special merit for allowing patients so much liberty as
would facilitate their escape, and he added that he found it more humane
to injure a patient by letting him escape than by too rigid confinement.[53]
Not surprisingly, such a position was not popular with Benedict's board of
managers or patients' families. A subsequent "epidemic" of suicides did
little to improve his relationship with his managers.[54]

Benedict's family had to endure the inconveniences of institutional life
for only a short time. Plagued by ill health, in 1853 he made the mistake
of temporarily turning over control of his institution to his first assistant,
one John Gray, while he took a trip south to convalesce. He was never to
resume charge of the Utica Asylum. The circumstances of his dismissal
were unclear at the time and remain so today. Late nineteenth-century
asylum histories most often described it as a "resignation" owing to ill
health,[55] but at the time, Benedict fought bitterly the request from the
board of managers that he resign. Seeds of his eventual conflict with them
can be seen as early as Benedict's first annual report, in which he wistfully
hoped in the future to "have the ability as well as the will" to improve his
somewhat unsatisfactory work.[56] His letters to friends express a similar
tentativeness, far different from the strong self-certainty which characterized most of the early leaders of the asylum movement. Benedict's failure
as a superintendent suggests that the successes of his contemporaries
were far from automatic, that early superintendents needed to exercise
vigorous, assertive leadership to satisfy their many constituencies.[57]

Yet Benedict's personality alone did not turn the Utica managers against
him. Extant correspondence suggests that his first assistant physician,
John Gray, left in charge of the institution while Benedict was on leave,
took an active role in the unseating of his superior. Gray consistently advised Benedict to extend his leave if he wanted to regain his health, even
while complaining to the managers about the problems it created. Eventually, as Benedict's leave dragged on, the board wrote asking him to resign. Shocked and bewildered, Benedict decided to return to Utica before making his decision.[58] Upon his return, he found Gray confident of
his managers' support, planning to marry the daughter of the powerful
asylum treasurer, and determined not to give up his new position of authority. Extant correspondence suggests that, in the ensuing battle, Benedict never had a chance against the powerful and manipulative Gray, but
he refused to resign for another six months.[59]

In June of 1854, Romelyn Beck, a prominent New York doctor long on the Utica board of managers, wrote to the head of that board suggesting a compromise course of action. Benedict, he reported, most objected to the suddenness with which he had been asked to resign and only wanted an extension on his superintendency until October. The managers consistently refused this and every other request of Benedict's. In a January letter, Charles Mann expressed to another board member the fear that Gray would leave if Benedict were granted an extension and that the rest of the staff would not get along with him. He offered a compromise: that Benedict be allowed to continue until September if he continued his leave and that Gray be given an extra supplement until then.[60] The ensuing controversy shook the fledgling AMSAII, whose members were shocked to see a fellow superintendent harassed out of office without serious cause. Yet, while some national asylum leaders expressed their displeasure with Gray to each other, they were unwilling to air AMSAII dirty linen in the public press.[61] After several months of negotiations with the trustees, the bewildered and defeated Benedict agreed to resign and left for Florida. Although he lived for another seventeen years, he never was able to find another position in the asylum movement.[62]

John Gray, 1854–1886

Even after his "resignation," Nathan Benedict continued to hope that his friends in Utica would succeed in exposing John Gray as a scheming politician. He was but the earliest of Gray's enemies to hope that somehow Gray's "true nature" would be exposed, and like his successors, Benedict's expectations were never realized. Although he frequently referred to himself as following in the beloved Brigham's footsteps, Gray was a very different kind of superintendent. By the 1860s, the board of managers largely had abandoned its supervisory role, and within the institution, John Gray's word was *the law* and (added a patient) all had to "bow to his sceptor."[63] Anyone who challenged Gray's power, even one of his handpicked assistant physicians, was quickly discharged. He fought so bitterly with three members of his medical staff—George Cook, John Chapin, and Louis Tourtellot—that the quarrels escaped the asylum walls to spread across the pages of the popular press. His disagreements with less influential employees, such as attendants, surfaced at several legislative investigations in the 1880s.[64]

The details of Gray's early life are too scant to explain how and why he developed into such a powerful figure, both within and without the Utica Asylum. Born in Pennsylvania in 1825, John Gray studied first at Dickinson College and then at the University of Pennsylvania. He never practiced privately but immediately after graduation became a resident physician at Blockley Hospital in Philadelphia under Nathan Benedict, who was chief of staff. After moving to Utica, Benedict brought Gray there too in 1851, as a third assistant. He moved up to become first assistant and then was named acting superintendent in 1853. That same year he was appointed medical superintendent of the Michigan State Lunatic Asylum and developed plans for new buildings at Kalamazoo. Although he visited Kalamazoo several times, he resigned from that position when made Utica's superintendent in 1854, at the age of twenty-nine. In 1855 Gray also took over the editorship of the *AJI*. He was to make it well-known (and, in some eyes, notorious) as a vehicle for his personal views, both in the United States and Western Europe. As his fame spread, so did his appointments and honors. In 1874 he was named professor of psychological medicine at Bellevue Hospital Medical College in New York City, and in 1876 he received a similar position at Albany Medical College. He was successively president of the Oneida County Medical Society, the New York State Medical Society, the New York State Medical Association, and the AMSAII. The British, French, and Italian medico-psychological associations elected him to honorary memberships. He also frequently served as an advisor to a range of charities, reformatories, and insane asylums.[65]

In the succeeding years, in large part through the *AJI* but also through public addresses and his annual reports, John Gray developed and publicized a strongly held position of insanity, its causes, and treatment that was quite different from Amariah Brigham's (a difference Gray did his best to obscure). To counteract those who viewed the insane as possessed or bestial, Brigham had emphasized that mental illness was a disease similar to all other diseases. Yet he felt that its roots could be found in moral or psychological as well as in physical causes. Gray, in contrast, argued that only physical causes could produce insanity and, in the late 1850s, he totally eliminated tables of moral causes (such as disappointment in love or religious excitement) from his annual reports. To counteract his medical colleagues' disapproval of what they considered an extremist position, Gray spelled out his views in every possible arena: annual reports, public lectures, the floor of AMSAII meetings, and the pages of the *AJI*. Essays such as "The Dependence of Insanity on Physical Disease" state the essence of Gray's argument: so-called moral causes affected the mind only if and when the body's physical condition was weakened, whether by a morbid condition, lack of sleep, or poor nutrition.[66]

Although Gray is often called an early somaticist, he developed a view of the mind–body relationship which owed as much to nineteenth-century religion as to medicine. He explained his position clearly in a lecture he delivered to students at the Bellevue Hospital Medical College in 1874. Some view insanity as a disease of both the brain and the mind, he explained to them. Others persist in holding onto the antiquated belief that insanity is essentially a disease of the mind. This perspective he dismissed as merely the latest version of the superstitious notion that insanity is a form of demoniacal possession. According to the third and "true" theory, insanity is a morbid physical state of the brain which disturbs manifestations of the mind but not its essence. Such a theory assumes that the mind is a soul or spirit independent of the body, as far as disease and death are concerned.[67] Consistent with his mind–body perspective, Gray strongly attacked those of his fellows who believed in affective rather than functional disorders of the mind. As one of his obituaries noted, for Gray, "moral insanity, dipsomaniacal and kleptomaniacal insanity were psychiatric myths and misnomers invented to shield depravity and crime."[68] Although he failed to persuade all of his psychiatric brethren, Gray's opinions were enormously popular with the general public, who applauded when he testified at the trial of Charles Guiteau, the man who assassinated President Garfield.[69] Gray was a frequent expert witness for the prosecution at a number of similar trials involving the insanity defense.

Gray's deep moralizing streak, which surfaced often in his comments at AMSAII meetings, contributed in other ways to a somewhat peculiar version of somaticism. Traditional religious values, as well as a commitment to scientific empiricism, influenced his thinking. Determined to protect the "immortal" mind from physical influences, he strongly attacked more thoroughgoing somaticists like Harvey Wilbur who refused to preserve what was for Gray an essential distinction between the mind and the brain. At the same time, through microscopic analyses of autopsy tissues, Gray attempted to plumb the full mysteries of the brain. When, like Brigham, he saw patients institutionalized after religious revivals, he insisted that true religion only strengthened resistance to mental illness. Unfortunately, he admitted, the lack of sleep and mental exhaustion which so often accompanied revivals could unsettle the most conventional of church members. He was harsh in his treatment of such "popular errors" as second adventism, spiritualism, and similar "morbid social phenomena"; they arose, he declared, in "selfish and depraving passions" and spread "by contagion through the erratic and morbid elements of society." Similarly complex was his attitude toward heredity and mental illness. While opposed to naive hereditarianism, he described many of the Utica patients as predisposed to insanity from childhood as a result of early neglect and immoral associations. Such "immoral associations" constituted physical, not moral, causes of insanity, he claimed.[70] While Gray himself refused to acknowledge the tensions within his psychiatric thought, his critics (of both the nineteenth and twentieth centuries) have not been so kind. When one contemporary historian tried to unravel Gray's thought, he decided that Gray saw insanity simultaneously as organic disease and as a lack of conscious ego.[71]

During the last sixteen of his thirty-four years at Utica, John Gray simultaneously reached the apogee of his power, locally and nationally, and became the target of relentless criticism. In many respects, the attacks were well justified. Several New York State legislative investigations made clear that Gray had grown accustomed to distributing asylum patronage to his friends rather than to the lowest bidders; that he spent more of his time testifying as an expert witness than walking the wards at Utica; that he frequently refused to print in the *AJI* articles which offered views on insanity and its treatment different from his own; and that he misrepresented events at AMSAII meetings when it benefited him to do so. Less attention has been paid to his achievements. For example, he encouraged his assistant physicians to continue to educate themselves on the subject of mental illness, relieving them of nonmedical duties whenever possible, approving educational trips to Europe, and publishing their analyses of particularly interesting cases in the *AJI*. However primitive the research done by the pathologists he hired to work at Utica, Gray's successors almost completely abandoned the research programs he fought so hard to set up.[72]

By 1886 Gray's empire showed signs of toppling, but his death that year prevented a final confrontation between him and his critics. The circumstances which led up to his final illness had a peculiar irony. The evening of his return from testifying at the Guiteau trial, while sitting in his office, Gray was shot in the face by a man named Henry Remshaw, a local masseur supposedly seized with a fit of temporary insanity. Although he lived for another four years, his health was never good. Thus, as historian Robert Waldinger notes, Gray "fell victim to the same unpredictability in human behavior which he both feared and denied in his dealings with men who were on trial for murder."[73]

John Chapin, 1869–1884

In sharp contrast to Gray was John Chapin, superintendent of the Willard Asylum from its opening until 1884. While newspapers attacked Gray for neglecting his asylum duties in order to build his national reputation, the commissioner in lunacy praised Chapin for his ability to supervise the management concerns of his vast asylum while simultaneously remembering in detail the mental state of his more than one thousand patients. However unlikely such an accomplishment, its attribution to Chapin suggests his reputation for hard work.[74] Nothing in Chapin's and Gray's similar educational backgrounds accounts for the substantial differences between the two men. Educated at Williams College, in 1850 Chapin began to study medicine with a physician who worked at the New York Hospital. Two years later he himself became a member of the house staff there, having graduated from the Jefferson Medical College in Philadelphia in 1853. He spent the next several years at the New York Hospital, gaining an expertise in the management of a wide range of illnesses, including cholera and typhus, which was to prove highly useful at Willard. Chapin also visited that department of the hospital reserved for the insane, the Bloomingdale Asylum, although he did not work there; and he attended an annual meeting of the AMSAII which took place in New York

City. In 1854 John Gray invited him to take a position at Utica. While Chapin had had no previous training in psychiatry, Gray felt that his broad medical background well qualified him for dealing with mental disease.[75]

As an assistant physician at Utica, Chapin not only cared for patients, but he also helped to edit the *AJI* and, at Gray's request, assisted the superintendents of the poor with their 1856 memorial to the state legislature asking for construction of more facilities to care for the chronically insane. Presumably this experience was a turning point in Chapin's life for, ever after, he had a profound interest in the fate of the chronic pauper insane. In 1857 he resigned from the Utica Asylum for reasons which remain obscure. Although he briefly headed a Kentucky institution for the blind, in 1860 he joined another former Utica assistant physician, George Cook, at Brigham Hall, a private insane asylum in Canandaigua, New York. From that position, he helped lead the fight in New York for the construction of a separate state facility for the chronically insane. Named one of the first commissioners to select a site and oversee construction of the new asylum, he subsequently became its first head. There he had the opportunity to put into practice his notions about how best (and most cheaply) to care for the chronically insane. Perhaps most important were his insistence on a segregate rather than congregate architectural style, so that the quietly insane could live in so-called detached buildings, with only the violent and seriously ill kept in the central administration building. He also developed an elaborate work program which cut the costs of patient care while winning much praise as a therapeutic strategy.[76]

Unlike John Gray, Chapin did not develop a distinctive theory of insanity; insofar as he was an innovator, his contributions lay in notions about treatment of chronic cases. When, in his annual reports, he offered observations on the causes of insanity, he clearly was describing his Willard experience. The insane, he felt, were increasing in number more quickly than the general population, and they tended to come from the lower and middle classes. Unlike Brigham, he did not feel that mental work produced mental illness. Most likely to unbalance those already troubled, whether mentally or physically, were poverty and deprivation. He refused to let himself be drawn into philosophical debates about insanity, noting that, whatever the best general theory, it was impossible to deny that "injudicious marriages, social vices, and the direct and indirect effects of intemperance" were among the most powerful factors predisposing the general population to mental derangement.[77]

End-of-the-Century Superintendents

The personality differences between Gray and Chapin are so striking that they easily obscure the two men's shared problems as asylum superintendents. Despite the fact that few ever questioned the efficacy of Chapin's administration of Willard, his annual reports, like Gray's, justified S. Weir Mitchell's criticism that asylum superintendents unrealistically expected themselves to be "farmers, stewards, caterers, business managers, and physicians."[78] By the end of the nineteenth century, even some of the superintendents themselves agreed that, if lay superintendents were appointed to take over all nonmedical supervisory responsibilities, the superintendents, as chief medical officers, could focus on the care and treatment of patients.[79] Neither Gray nor Chapin supported this notion, however, for both felt that only a single head could run an institution effectively. Typically, Gray was the one to articulate their shared position loudly and repeatedly. The superintendent, he argued, was supposed to act as a consulting medical director and not as an attending physician. No superintendent could personally direct a large staff and care for some six hundred patients (or, in the case of Willard, almost two thousand), especially at an institution which received four hundred new patients every year. While he might walk through the wards, he could not adequately supervise patient treatment himself. Only by cooperation among staff members could high-quality medical care be provided.[80] While this response did not answer the charge that Gray devoted too much time to extra-institutional activities, including medical school lectures and expert testimony at trials, he did pinpoint here what seemed to be an inevitable administrative trend at large state institutions. Critics' proposal for split authority at the top of the asylum administrative structure was never implemented in New York. Perhaps a number of state officials agreed with Gray and Commissioner of Lunacy John Ordronaux that the final authority at a large asylum had to rest in one person's hands and could not be divided effectively.[81] More likely, the legislature balked at the notion of adding another expensive administrative position to the asylum budgets.

Even though Gray won the first skirmishes over the extent of the superintendent's powers, the office lost much of its unrestricted authority after his death. Almost all of the reform proposals Gray had fought so bitterly were implemented eagerly by his successor, George Blumer. The careers of Blumer and of Chapin's successor, P. M. Wise, were very different from those of Brigham, Gray, and Chapin. Having slowly worked their way up the ranks of asylum medical staffs, they had less interest in theoretical problems, whether of psychiatry or administration, and more in practical issues of patient care. Understandably, they also were more open to reformers' criticisms of policies formulated by their predecessors. Yet they did not strike out in new directions, for they were conservators rather than explorers. Revealing is the Willard board of trustees' comment on Wise in 1884: "The change of supervision was not a change but the continuation of a fixed, settled, and successful policy."[82]

When Blumer discontinued many of Gray's policies, he did so in the name of a return to the past, to the practices of Amariah Brigham. After describing his abolition of the use of restraints at the Utica Asylum and his revitalization of moral treatment programs, Blumer worried lest he "furnish evidence of ruthless iconoclasm on the one hand, or unseemly haste for personal methods on the other."[83] Certainly John Gray never in his life made such an apologetic statement. Equally suggestive (and unlike Gray) was his statement of editorial policy for the *AJI*. In the future, he proclaimed, "we bind ourselves to no school of thought and to no asylum coterie. . . . New blood shall mingle with the old; reform and conservatism act as check and counter-check. . . ."[84]

While Blumer's geniality was a welcome relief to many, both within and without his institution, he lacked the vision and zeal for experimentation which had characterized both Brigham's and Gray's administrations. Certainly patients benefited from the reinstitution of moral therapy at Utica, but in many respects, Blumer's programs seemed somewhat superficial. Gray had lectured local audiences on the relationship between physical debility (especially among women) and mental illness; Blumer gave an address called "Music's Impressions on the Mind." Just before the Utica Asylum entered the twentieth century, Blumer reintroduced broom and braided-mat workshops for patients. Such, he claimed, would "make sick people well by the process of manufacturing."[85] He then left to become superintendent of Butler Hospital in Rhode Island, leaving his staff to cope with an overwhelming new challenge, one for which brooms and concerts were inadequate therapeutic tools: the swamping of all the state insane asylums with the chronically mentally ill as a result of what was called the State Care Act.[86]

The career of P. M. Wise was similar to that of Blumer, although Wise had a slightly longer list of publications to his credit. Most of these offered no theoretical perspectives on insanity or its treatment, however, but summarized careful clinical observations.[87] Initialed comments in Willard patient casebooks suggest that, as late as December of 1889, Superintendent Wise was making ward notes on patients, thus involving himself to an unprecedented extent in direct patient care. According to a local newspaper, his diagnostic skills were legendary in his upstate community; one reporter told of a sixteen-year-old boy whose eye problems were recognized only after his father brought him to Wise at Willard.[88] Such stories make clear the benefits of Wise's long years of training as an assistant physician at Willard, in which position he had learned to cope with a wide range of physical as well as mental problems.

When Wise and Blumer together attended the 1887 meeting of the AMSAII, a local newspaper reporter in Detroit observed them both. Wise, he declared, was about thirty-five; his sharp eye saw everything that happened in his vicinity. Known to be an authority on all forms of chronic insanity and a good disciplinarian, he obviously was capable of keeping Willard's many patients under his control. Blumer was somewhat quieter than Wise. The youngest member of the association (being barely thirty at the time) and yet the influential editor of the *AJI*, he had an intellectual face "brightened by a paid of kindly eyes," whose sparkle was somewhat hidden by his glasses. While his demeanor was mild, the reporter assured his readers that the shape of Blumer's head suggested great force of character. Such a comment was remarkably appropriate, given Blumer's desire to mold himself in the image of his phrenologist predecessor Brigham.[89]

Assistant Physicians

Although in the first few years of the New York State Lunatic Asylum, Amariah Brigham greeted incoming patients at the door and walked the halls, Brigham and his successors as superintendent quickly found themselves totally preoccupied with administrative details. As a result, by the 1860s, they allocated most direct patient medical care to assistant physicians, whose formal responsibilities had been outlined in detail by the asylum board of managers.[90] As with almost all asylum positions, the daily duties of the medical staff were clearly too overwhelming to be met in a single day. For example, when the New York State Lunatic Asylum first opened in 1843, its single assistant physician was ordered to serve as the institution's apothecary; to supervise all aspects of patient treatment and care, from ventilation and heating of the wards to exercise and amusement programs; to accompany the superintendent on morning rounds and himself to see every patient at least once a day; to report instances of abuse and neglect to the superintendent; and at all times, to exert a "moral influence" on those with whom he was in contact. In his free moments, he also was expected to maintain patient accounts, correspond with patients' families, and look after visitors whenever the steward was absent or engaged.[91] In 1847 the board revised and expanded these duties even further into a list that remained in effect until the end of the century. Still expected to oversee patient treatment, assistant physicians (by then there were two) also were ordered to ensure that "the attendants and assistants are faithful and kind, attentive to the wants of the patients, and vigilant in the discharge of their duties." (That this was a near impossible task for doctors who visited the wards at most twice a day did not deter the board from prescribing it.) They also had to keep the superintendent informed about patients through daily written reports on the general condition of their divisions, on sick and excited patients, and on the number of patients in restraint or seclusion, as well as through notes in casebook records. (Surviving casebooks make clear that this duty was often performed perfunctorily, for notes on a patient might be as infrequent as once a year, unless the patient's condition changed suddenly.) Finally, assistant physicians were ordered to "always be ready to perform whatever services may be required of them by the Superintendent."[92]

Surprisingly, such lengthy lists of duties and responsibilities did not deter well-qualified doctors from applying for these positions. When Edward Jarvis, later to become famous for his statistical report on the insane in Massachusetts, applied for a position at Utica in 1842, the board of managers claimed to be swamped with applications.[93] Although it was not until 1885 that the State Civil Service Board established uniform standards for staff medical positions in all state institutions,[94] the credentials of the Utica and Willard assistant physicians were impressive. When one nineteenth-century asylum critic complained about the poor quality of asylum doctors,[95] John Gray retorted that he considered only applicants with general hospital experience as well as medical degrees.[96] Even late in the century, with asylum pay growing less competitive, the New York institutions were able to attract well-qualified candidates. For example, one assistant physician graduated from Bellevue Hospital Medical College and then worked at a private insane asylum for two years before coming to Utica in 1876. Another, before accepting a position as fourth assistant physician at Utica in 1888, earned degrees from Cornell and the College of Physicians and Surgeons in New York City and worked at both the Blackwell's Island Asylum in New York City and Hudson River State Hospital.[97] At Willard, between 1869 and 1884, John Chapin advertised openings widely and also asked his friends to nominate particularly promising candidates. Letters of recommendation were solicited for all candidates, and personal interviews were scheduled for the most promising. The result was an impressive pool of applicants, most relatively young, from both New England and New York.[98]

While the medical staffs at Willard and Utica were not subject to the overt pressure to hire political favorites that plagued many midwestern asylums, their boards and superintendents sometimes responded to more subtle forms of influence. John Gray's advancement at Utica from assistant physician to superintendent obviously was helped by his marriage to the daughter of the powerful asylum treasurer; and in 1885 he did not hesitate to appoint his own son to a temporary staff vacancy.[99] Yet, when one of his assistant physicians adopted a similar strategy (and in so doing, challenged Gray's authority), he reacted with great hostility to the man's "pretensions."[100] Ties to the local community helped applicants for medical positions at Willard too. For example, one successful applicant, a graduate of the Medical and Surgical Department of the University of Michigan with

77

outstanding references from the faculty there, also offered recommendations from an uncle in Ovid, the closest village to Willard, and from two men who lived in the nearby village of Lodi.[101] Although Alexander Nellis had strong references from a medical school professor and his supervisor at the Albany County Insane Asylum, his letter of support from the powerful secretary of the State Board of Charities surely helped his application.[102] A somewhat different case was the application of G. B. Bristol, who deluged Chapin with obsequious letters of application for two years. (In one, he ineptly characterized Willard under Chapin as guided by "only one *will*, to which others must conform, repressing their own individuality.") Despite his self-proclaimed academic excellence, Bristol's references were mixed. One former employee said that, while he was "not prepared to give a wholesale unqualified recommendation," Bristol was above average and "as far as we know free from any possible objections." In a personal interview, Chapin continued to discourage Bristol, but he finally capitulated and hired him only a short time before leaving Willard for the Pennsylvania Hospital.[103]

One prerequisite for assistant physician not mentioned by the Utica or Willard superintendents was male sex; yet, when a bill to require state insane asylums to hire female physicians was first introduced into the New York State Legislature in the late 1870s, both Chapin and Gray responded with great hostility. With his usual political astuteness, Chapin immediately wrote to superintendents in other states who had been forced to hire female physicians. He then incorporated their negative responses in a twenty-one-page letter to the New York State Senate. He marshalled a wide range of arguments against the proposed legislation, including the inability of female physicians to protect physically the buildings to which they would be assigned, the absurdity of the notion that only female doctors should care for female patients, and the negative impact of the use of female doctors on the prestige of asylum medical service.[104] While Chapin's letter carefully avoided inflammatory rhetoric, the "for your eyes only" letters Chapin received from his fellow superintendents were less restrained. One doctor complained that his female assistant "disgusted everybody" by her desire to examine all of the patients and her obsession with work. "She was headstrong, arbitrary, uneven in her dealings with patients and a mischief maker generally," he asserted. While willing to admit the theoretical possibility of a female physician with common sense, executive ability, and good medical training, he felt sure that such a woman would not study medicine and would be spoiled if she did.[105] Another reported that he had voluntarily added a female physician to his staff in 1873 but quickly found that she had become too independent. Not only did she develop her own ideas about how to run the institution, but she had the temerity to repeat them to the superintendent. When she became interested in one of the young male physicians, she was fired. To his dismay, she almost immediately managed to get herself elected to the board of trustees, a position that gave her more power than she had had before. The disgruntled superintendent harrumphed that women managers were as useful as "the fifth wheel of a coach."[106]

Despite the defeat of this 1879 bill, Chapin began to get female candidates for Willard medical staff positions. In 1880 one Nellie Keith, an expert in female complaints, was recommended by a local minister on the grounds that her "peculiar ways and qualities of heart," as well as her devotion to hard work, well qualified her to take charge of a new building for female patients.[107] The subject of hiring female physicians also was discussed at both the 1880 and 1884 legislative investigations of asylum conditions. While most asylum witnesses testified against the idea (including the Utica matron), it was supported by the commissioner in lunacy and included in the recommendations made by the 1884 investigative committee. The senators noted that, although asylum officials felt that women lacked the mental power to control female patients, they could (and would) do more gynecologic examinations.[108] The State Board of Charities also supported the innovation, noting that provision of female physicians to supervise the bathing of patients would help check patient abuse.[109] Despite their endorsement, however, not until 1890 did the New York State Legislature mandate the appointment of female physicians to state asylums, and even then, they failed to appropriate the requisite funds.[110] Somewhat surprisingly, given Chapin's attitudes, his successor, P. M. Wise, appointed a female physician in his first year of office. Wise selected Theoda Wilkins after advertising in local newspapers a position paying six hundred dollars a year plus lodging, boarding, and washing; the position was open to female graduates of reputable medical schools who were unmarried and between the ages of twenty-two and forty. (At that time, he paid male assistant physicians two thousand dollars a year, plus room and board.)[111] The Willard Asylum thus moved to the forefront of the movement to employ female physicians in New York State. In contrast, the Buffalo State Hospital superintendent asserted that, if forced to hire a female physician, he would use her to supervise and train nurses and attendants, thus relieving the male medical officers of much work.[112] His attitude was not unusual. As a doctor at an annual meeting of the Conference of Charities and Corrections complained, so many hospitals gave their female doctors clerical rather than professional duties and consistently passed them over for promotions that it was not surprising that women were reluctant to enter asylum work.[113] At Willard, the name of the female physician was set off from those of her male counterparts on staff listings until 1893, and although the reason for the resignation of male doctors was always noted, female doctors simply disappeared from the rosters.[114]

Despite the alleged shortage of qualified female physicians, Willard's second one, Alice Farnham, produced research superior to that of many of her male colleagues. For example, in an innovative essay on uterine disease in female patients, she attacked the notion that female gynecologic diseases create insanity. Comparing twenty Willard females with a matched control group of noninstitutionalized women, she found more gynecologic abnormalities in the "sane" control group than in her Willard patients.[115] Farnham was not the only asylum doctor to engage actively in research, of course. Although in the 1870s and 1880s, the New York neurologists bitterly attacked the quality of the research being carried on at asylums in general (and Utica in particular), at least these young physicians were being encouraged to observe their patients' symptoms systematically. Especially prolific were several assistant physicians at Utica, perhaps because Gray's editorship of *AJI* made it relatively easy for them to get into print. Most asylum doctors wrote narrow comments on unusual cases and autopsy results, but a few continued the older tradition of general essays on patient management.[116] Despite the varying quality of such publications, that the Utica and Willard assistant physicians managed to write at all, given their grinding daily routine and the physical and cultural isolation of their institutions, is impressive.[117] Even those articles which just detailed patients' responses to specific drug therapies belied the neurologists' criticisms that asylum doctors failed to contribute to the advancement of psychiatry. On the other hand, many of the neurologists' complaints about asylum medical service were prophetic of future developments. Despite his recruitment successes, John Chapin himself warned the legislature in 1879 that the asylum should not be held responsible if the quality of its underpaid and overworked medical staff declined in the future.[118] E. C. Seguin's picture of the state institution in which experienced assistants were preoccupied with their own duties and the superintendent so immersed in business that he had not time for teaching increasingly described New York State's asylums as the nineteenth century drew to a close.[119] Certainly superintendents after Brigham did not lecture to their juniors, provide them with monographs, or show them how to analyze patient cases, as Seguin wanted. Yet, despite a ratio of 1 doctor for 350 patients, Willard physicians as late as 1896 met regularly with each other to discuss medical topics and especially interesting cases.[120]

Throughout the nineteenth century, a few of the assistant physicians at Utica and Willard (primarily those with ambitions to become superintendents) went aboard to study during their early years of asylum work. For example, P. M. Wise went to England for a four-month visit in 1880; George Blumer studied abroad for six months in 1884–1885; and Charles Pilgrim left for a year of special studies and institutional visits in 1885.[121] More rarely, they sought extra-asylum training at home; for example, in 1882 a young Willard doctor spent his vacation time to gain "special instruction in the obscure diseases of women" in New York City.[122] While they supported such trips for their favorites, New York's asylum superintendents felt that their medical officers most benefited from on-the-job experience. It was considered sufficient to prepare them for institutional advancement.[123] The ease with which ten of the seventeen Utica assistant physicians became superintendents suggests that the profession agreed.[124] Willard assistant physicians were equally mobile: William Goldsmith became superintendent of the Butler Hospital for the Insane; E. C. Carson, of the New York Institution for the Instruction of the Deaf and Dumb; and H. E. Allison, of the State Asylum for Insane Criminals at Auburn. Both Utica and Willard provided medical libraries for their staffs, and the critical neurologists were not the only doctors to see the potential of state asylums as research centers. In 1879 when Chapin petitioned the New York State Legislature for money to build a research laboratory he envisioned Willard as a center for the general study and investigation of nervous diseases, to which the most promising young doctors would come for training.[125] His dream of the state's largest (and most cheaply run) asylum also becoming a center of medical research was of no interest at all, however, to the legislators of the state of New York, who felt that they were doing quite enough in offering state-level care to chronically mentally ill paupers.

Since the Utica and Willard assistant physicians neither left diaries nor published memoirs, the details of their daily lives are difficult to reconstruct. According to John Pitts, the assistant physicians came the closest to being "genuine therapists" in the state asylums.[126] Yet contemporaries were critical of the quality of care proffered by doctors with responsibility for between one hundred and three hundred patients each.[127] According to testimony given at legislative investigations in the 1880s, the medical staff coped with such workloads by walking quickly through patient wards and halls, at the side of a supervisor or head attendant, who drew their attention to critical cases. By the end of the nineteenth century, when almost half of the patients were seriously ill at admission, the assistant physicians devoted most of their attention to the physical rather than the mental health of their patients.[128]

Like all asylum employees, assistant physicians were supposed to make the asylum their first priority, and John Gray fired at least one (Louis Tourtellot) for his seeming reluctance to do so. Scrapbooks kept at nineteenth-century Willard suggest that assistant physicians at this relatively isolated institution, like the rest of the staff, had little choice about making the institution their life. At both Utica and Willard, assistant physicians often had to spend their evenings keeping up with casebook records, correspondence with patients' families, and the maintenance of statistical data on patients.[129] Yet, a survey of the Utica Asylum's "Record and Daily Census Book" for the time from May of 1857 to December of 1859 reveals that the doctors there were absent from the institution an average of 15.1 person workdays a month. While the figure for this time period may have been inflated by the extended absences of Edwin Van Deusen, preparatory to his assuming a new position at a Michigan asylum, doctors were allowed many more breaks from asylum routine than were other members of the staff.

The Lives of Asylum Doctors

We know remarkably little about the daily lives of physicians who lived and worked in nineteenth-century asylums, in large part because we have been more interested in their theory than their practice. Perhaps best understood are the superintendents. Final authorities in every matter, subject only to the rare intervention of managers or trustees, New York's nineteenth-century superintendents attempted to conform their institutions to a rigidly hierarchical (albeit patriarchal) social model. Yet, the frequent failures of even such powerful personalities as Amariah Brigham and John Gray to control those under them, whether patients or staff, showed that asylum superintendents' authoritarian tendencies were severely constrained by the complex social structure within which they operated. As Nancy Tomes observes, most nineteenth-century asylum superintendents "shared the same concept of paternal absolutism in hospital management and the same difficulties in maintaining it."[130]

With varying degrees of grace, superintendents further limited their power by turning the medical care of patients over almost entirely to assistant physicians. Amariah Brigham described his assistant as "a friend and counselor, on whose discretion and devotedness to the welfare of the institution, I can confidently rely."[131] In contrast, neither Gray nor Chapin reported such close relations with subordinates, and Gray's habit of quarreling violently with his more independent assistant physicians was notorious. Signs of a shift back toward greater intimacy appeared in Blumer's first annual report; he claimed to have left the medical ranks too recently to have forgotten the vital contributions assistant physicians made toward the smooth running of the institution.[132] Yet, no matter how tyrannical their superiors, the Utica and Willard assistant physicians were located close to the top of the institutional social hierarchy. They often ate with the superintendent and his family and socialized with managers, trustees, and local politicians. Several married well; all who chose to stay within the asylum advanced steadily up its occupational ladder, a number reaching the top. Like that of the superintendents, the authority of assistant physicians was both enormous and circumscribed. They could order attendants and patients to perform certain tasks and to conform to a predictable schedule; sometimes they were obeyed, other times not. Hoping to become experts in psychiatry, they more often found themselves curing sick bodies than sick minds. Yet young doctors competed intensely to become assistant physicians. Within the precarious world of nineteenth-century medicine, they preferred walking the asylum wards to coping with the economic uncertainties of private practice.

4

A Distanced Relative

Even before 1843, when the New York State Lunatic Asylum at Utica officially began to accept patients, its newly appointed managers found themselves besieged with imploring letters. Sent by families and friends of the insane, they sought help not for insane paupers locked in prisons and poorhouses but for troubled New Yorkers of the "middling sort." One such, a young man "of brilliance, talent, and exacting education," had lost his reason as a result of "too close application to study." In repeated letters addressed to the asylum superintendent, a friend begged for the scholar's admission that he might "avail himself of the advantages of this valuable and humane institution." Another potential patient, a woman of "good reputation but no money" who had become deranged while studying spiritualism, needed shelter after having lived too long on the charity of friends.[1]

Such correspondence suggests that middle-class families expected to benefit from construction of a state insane asylum in New York at least as much as did the poor. They were permitted to do so by some curious twists in New York's early commitment laws. Some managed to get themselves declared "indigent"; others agreed to pay for that asylum treatment usually subsidized by counties. Early asylum superintendents encouraged the admission of such private patients on the grounds that mixed-class institutions better protected their patients from the double stigma of poverty and insanity. County superintendents of the poor, struggling to care for the poor and insane in the same almshouses, equally eagerly greeted the construction of the Utica Asylum. Almost as soon as the new institution opened its doors in 1843, it filled to capacity; the same happened upon completion of the Willard Asylum in 1869–1870. Families of all sorts sought in these institutions relief from and, in some cases, renewed hope for their mentally ill members.

The relationships among the insane, their families, asylum superintendents, and the state of New York were extraordinarily complex in the nineteenth century. Families looked to asylums for relief from unmanageable burdens of care; the asylums looked to families for the clients which justified their existence. In nineteenth-century New York, most often families initiated the commitment of members whom they alleged to be mentally ill. Yet, in the case of indigent and pauper patients, they could not do so arbitrarily; they had to follow legal procedures established by the state legislature. County officials also had to agree to assume the relatively expensive costs of state care. (By contrast, until 1874, private patients could be admitted without any formal papers beyond promises by families to pay for their care.)[2] Although asylum superintendents frequently complained about overcrowding in their institutions and the commitment of the inappropriate, they simultaneously led a campaign to bring all of the state's insane poor under their care. Over the course of the nineteenth century there emerged a complex and often tense symbiotic relationship among families, asylums, and the state. The first two made the major decisions, but the state defined the outer limits of their activities.

The Decision to Institutionalize

Patient Casebook Records

The opening of the New York State Lunatic Asylum in 1843 did not of itself change relationships within nineteenth-century New York families, but in combination with new commitment laws, it offered a way for beleaguered families, both rich and poor, struggling to care for difficult members, to transfer that burden of dependence to the state. Yet, while families turned to asylums for a wide range of reasons, few eagerly made the decision to institutionalize. Not only was asylum care relatively expensive (at least in comparison to such alternatives as county poorhouses), but families did not willingly surrender loved ones to the care of un-familiar medical doctors located at forbidding, geographically distant in-stitutions. Asylum doctors were well aware of their reluctance and fre-quently harangued against the shortsightedness of those who refused to admit that delays in institutionalization lessened the likelihood of cure.[3]

In contrast to the heads of private hospitals, state asylum doctors had little control over their patient populations, except through the limited influence of their writings. In almost all cases, the decision to commit someone to a state asylum in nineteenth-century New York was made by the patient's family. If that family was poor, it also had to persuade county officials to subsidize state care. Thus, the initiative to institutionalize came primarily not from the asylum but from families and local commu-nities (or in the case of insane criminals, the courts). Most often families took that step only after long struggles to confine that madness within fa-milial rather than asylum walls. They tolerated delusions, eccentricities, and threats of violence for months, even years, and sent disturbed rela-tives to Utica only if they became suddenly worse, "maniacal and raving," or if they threatened physical harm to persons or property. In general, the greater a family's (or community's) social resources, the longer it tended to postpone seeking institutional assistance.[4] On the other hand, New York State's asylums could neither turn away patients (unless they lacked legal commitment papers) nor forcibly institutionalize them.

For the entire period from 1843 to 1890, families continued to domi-nate the commitment process, although the uses to which they put New York's state asylums shifted somewhat over time. The kinds of familial situations which most often led to institutionalization were described in patient case histories collected by asylum doctors at admission. Of course, these histories did not offer complete accounts of patients' lives. They fre-quently failed to distinguish between real events and social responses to them. Most often, they recaptured only the most disastrous events of the immediately preceding days or weeks. Since many families felt guilty about their reluctant decisions to send insane members to Utica or Willard, some in self-justification exaggerated threatening or unusual behavior; others hid particularly embarrassing incidents of family conflict. Yet, de-spite their deficiencies, casebook histories vividly chronicle the daily stresses of nineteenth-century domestic and work lives and suggest the structural limits of certain families' abilities to cope with stress.

Inevitably, admitting doctors also shaped the information collected in casebook histories. On their surface, the earliest Utica records seemed to offer primarily shorthand versions of families' stories. For example, the description of one twenty-three-year-old man read: "talked of suicide but never attempted it; is violent; threatened to kill his friends and was thought to be dangerous." Another young woman, admitted in July of 1848, had lost much sleep in January and become "somewhat deranged" as a result but recovered quickly and seemed well until May. Then her health deteriorated, and she "suddenly became very crazy." "Her mind is full of fearful apprehensions," her worried mother reported, for "she thinks she swallows me when she drinks and that she is drowned."[5] Yet, although such early Utica case histories lack the standardized format and medical language characteristic of those collected during the second half of the nineteenth century, they were less haphazard than a first reading might suggest. Even the earliest generation of asylum superintendents tried to collect systematic information about four key items: behavior which might present management problems to the institution, such as noisiness, suicidal tendencies, destructiveness, physical violence, and personal filthiness; medical problems and their treatment; the immediate or "exciting" cause of insanity; and if known, its "predisposing" cause.[6] Concern for these issues unified such superficially disjointed notes as the following: "Talks of religion and philosophy; not much violent, but is if opposed—has struck and thrown a little—has talked of suicide but has made no attempt—has said he would kill himself. Had epileptic fits when a child, is costive—has taken laxatives. Doesn't sleep well—up and running about—broke through windows—eats poorly."[7]

The scholarly concerns of Utica's early record keepers reflected the conviction of the asylum's first head, Amariah Brigham, that public insane asylums should become "valuable schools of instruction for all medical men." Here Brigham expressed the widely held conviction of antebellum reformers that the systematic collection of information could solve social and medical problems.[8] Because of his commitment to gathering a broad variety of statistical data about the insane, Brigham and his assistant physicians asked families for details about physical as well as psychological problems, especially those relating to digestion and menstruation. If doctors had not taken the initiative, few families would have volunteered such information, for medical issues seldom seemed to have entered into a family's diagnosis of insanity. In part because they felt incapable of sort-

ing the relevant from the trivial, asylum doctors also conscientiously recorded even minor incidents recalled by patients' families. Doctors frequently complained that families too often confused precipitating events
with the causes of insanity, but their very disdain for such anecdotal data
limited their efforts to shape it. With exasperated sighs, they took down
highly elaborate accounts of domestic conflicts, work histories and financial transactions, friendships and enmities, just as family members presented them. Then, whenever possible, asylum doctors attempted to
probe deeper by asking about underlying physical and moral weaknesses
as well as about hereditary predispositions to insanity.[9]

Despite doctors' efforts to collect consistent sorts of information, patient records varied a great deal in both length and content. Some casebook histories covered an entire page or two; others (especially at Willard)
comprised only a few lines when the persons accompanying new admissions knew little, if anything, about patients' preinstitutional lives.[10] As a
result, for many of Utica's patients, the precipitating cause of institutionalization or of mental illness was relatively clear-cut; for others, it was
buried in a multiplicity of details. At Willard, most often it had long been
forgotten, and all that was known of new patients was their earlier institutional histories. Antebellum asylum doctors hoped to use information
about the epidemiology of mental illness embedded in such casebook histories to uncover its etiology, but this proved an impossible task. Patients'
preinstitutional histories revealed much about familial and community responses to mental illness, but they failed to explain why environmental
stress created mental illness in some and not others. Most clearly, case
histories showed the extent to which local communities, and not asylums,
defined insanity. In New York, as elsewhere in the nineteenth century,
committing families and local officials were most concerned with specific
problems created by alleged insane persons and the question of who, if
anyone, could cope with and control them.[11]

The Familial Perspective

In the nineteenth century as in the twentieth, not everyone who showed
symptoms of mental illness was sent to a state asylum. Some ended up in
local jails or state prisons; others stayed in the community, their eccentricities tolerated by family and friends. Without complete local records,

historians cannot pinpoint the social and behavioral factors which influenced communities to institutionalize certain of the insane and to keep others at home or deal with them through the criminal justice system. No doubt patterns of decision making varied from community to community, although those who lived close to asylums clearly used them the most heavily. In addition, patient casebook histories suggest that certain kinds of events were likely to overcome most families' inclination to ignore mental illness by "normalizing" aberrant behavior.[12] These included serious threats or actual harm to persons or property; the incapacitation of caretakers through illness or death; and the intensification of physical disabilities in men and women with epilepsy, paresis, and alcoholism to the point where families could no longer care for them. Families did not always initiate the institutionalization process, however; the Utica asylum in particular received at its door exhausted men and women who, after years of taking the major responsibility for the well-being of their families, sought rest and refuge within its walls.

Without doubt, families committed members most rapidly (albeit still with a great deal of pain) when they threatened or inflicted substantial physical damage on themselves, others, or property. Considered the most tragic cases in this category were those women who, while deeply depressed, killed or attempted to kill their children. Despite his general antipathy toward the use of the insanity plea in criminal trials, Utica's long-time superintendent John Gray felt great sympathy for such exhausted wives and mothers and castigated his fellow citizens for not supporting overworked women, particularly in the weeks immediately following childbirth. One such mother, admitted to Utica in 1848 at the age of thirty-two, first neglected her household duties, then attempted to give her four children away out of fear that they would come to a bad end, and finally drowned two of them. She also attempted to drown herself. According to the doctor who observed her at the asylum, she appeared to be "an excellent woman," who felt great remorse once she realized what she had done. A year after admission to the Utica Asylum, she left recovered, with her husband.[13]

A number of male patients at Utica also had turned violently against their families or neighbors shortly before admission, although many fewer actually had committed murder. (Perhaps homicidal males were more likely than their female counterparts to be sent to prison.) A middle-aged farmer, "long prone to spells," was not sent to Willard until he tried to shoot a local woman. Although they had not objected to his earlier eccentricities, the attempted homicide so alarmed his neighbors that they wrote to the Willard superintendent begging that the man not be released until all symptoms of madness were clearly gone.[14] Reports of such long community and familial tolerance for deviant behavior appear in many patient records. Some communities even expressed sympathy for homicidal patients, if such individuals previously had led blameless lives. For example, when a melancholic blacksmith well known for both his superior craftsmanship and love of family threatened his wife and children with an axe, he was handcuffed and taken to Willard. According to local newspapers, the community was "saddened" by his fate and filled with sympathy for his "heart-broken family."[15]

While most commitments were initiated by families, neighbors sometimes intervened when family members would not, as in the case of a sixteen-year-old pyromaniac. His mother was described as a "nervous, garrulous, and rather feeble-minded woman," and his father had deserted the family when the boy was two. Although mischievous, the boy had been well regarded until he began to set fires. Although he always helped to put them out and worked to repay the damage, neighbors eventually uncovered his responsibility for the blazes. His mother then sent him to live with relatives in Michigan. Later setting fire to several buildings there, he was sent home, certified insane by two physicians. At that point, fearful neighbors pressured local authorities to send the young pyromaniac to the asylum, where he impressed doctors as a "model patient" always eager to please.[16] What is most remarkable about his case is not the eventual intrusion of the community in the internal affairs of a troubled family but its lengthy patience.

Another common precipitant to institutionalization was the death of a long-disturbed insane person's family caretaker or the addition of new family members (including stepparents, in-laws, and siblings). For example, the doctors who signed the admission certificate of an unmarried thirty-seven-year-old female epileptic declared that she had suddenly become violent and abusive toward her friends. Her brother-in-law, however, clarified the circumstances leading up to institutionalization by reporting that the marriage of a sister about a year earlier had deprived the epileptic of her usual refuge when periodic behavioral problems surfaced. Although she had recovered from several previous attacks sufficiently well to support herself, upon admission to Utica she was labeled a chronic manic. She then spent the rest of her life in New York State mental hospitals. Sadly, although her hospital records note that she usually was "troublesome and incoherent," when she received a call from her mother thirteen months after admission, she became "quite cheerful, talkative, and communicative for the rest of the day." Left even more helpless by the death or removal of caretakers were feeble-minded, severely demented patients. [17]

Also a drain on familial resources were patients (mostly males) whose disorders (including syphilis, epilepsy, and drug addiction) ravaged both their bodies and their minds. Their numbers slowly increased at Utica and Willard over the course of the nineteenth century. Disproportionately middle- and upper-class in origin, their presence in state asylums revealed that even well-to-do families were limited in their ability to cope with behavioral extremes, especially when manifested by individuals who could not or would not take care of their basic physical needs. [18] Although New York's asylum superintendents willingly accepted syphilitics and epileptics, Superintendent John Gray of Utica bitterly resented the use of the asylum as a shelter for alcoholics and drug addicts, no matter how mentally and physically enfeebled. Yet, despite his disdain for such "moral weaklings," he was unable to prevent the admission of those whom families or local poorhouses could not control. [19] Of course, all demented and filthy patients did not end up in state asylums. The most notable exception before 1890 were the senile, largely cared for in county institutions or at home. Their absence reflected once again the extent to which many communities regarded commitment to a state asylum as a privilege reserved primarily, because of its expense, for two groups: the insane who showed some promise of recovery and future economic productivity (most of whom were between twenty-five and forty years of age) and those so disruptive that they made life at home or in the county poorhouse unbearable for their keepers. [20]

Somewhat surprisingly, although asylum doctors recognized (and often complained about) the extent to which economic factors affected communities' commitment decisions, not until late in the nineteenth century did they attempt to minimize such considerations by supporting the notion that the state, rather than counties, should assume the total costs of institutional care. As a result, before 1890, in New York State, only individuals whose families or counties were willing to pay for their institutional care ended up in state asylums. This situation was not unusual; according to Barbara Rosenkrantz and Maris Vinovskis, in nineteenth-century Massachusetts, the same factors affected the decision to institutionalize.[21] As early as 1844, Dorothea Dix found that some local poorhouse officials who had planned to send their insane charges to the new Utica Asylum changed their minds when they learned that counties would have to assume a portion of the costs of state care.[22] The expense of transporting patients further deterred some counties and families from relying on state asylums, just as it kept them from using general hospitals. As Paul Starr has pointed out, during the first half of the nineteenth century, the indirect costs of medical care (including transportation and time away from work) outweighed its benefits for many Americans. Even a ten-mile drive into town might mean the loss of a day's work for a farmer. As the means of communication and transportation improved over the course of the century, the balance of costs and benefits slowly shifted, and families became increasingly willing to use doctors and hospitals to care for both their physically and mentally ill members.[23]

Although the aged often were denied the Utica Asylum's therapeutic care, the institution received a number of young and middle-aged patients so physically weakened that they died soon after admission. Clearly their families had turned to the asylum only at the last possible moment for the medical resources they themselves lacked (or had become too exhausted to offer any longer). For example, a twenty-eight-year-old man who had "formerly been calm and affectionate" was sent to Utica by his father only after six months of violent activity, maniacal rages, and active delusions, all of which turned out to be symptoms of the syphilis from which he died six months later. Often physical problems, when added to long-standing emotional disturbances, provided the final blow to an individual's feeble grasp on sanity. For example, although the grief-stricken widow of a Civil War soldier wandered around the country looking for her husband's grave for a year after his death, not until she returned home, hit her head, and suffered a number of "epileptic attacks" was she sent to Utica. There, her epileptic seizures so increased in intensity that she had to be confined in one of the notorious "Utica cribs," where she died slightly more than a month after admission.[24]

93

It is not surprising that families turned to the asylum for assistance when members turned violent or became so disturbed that they could not care for themselves. Less attention has been paid to the fact that asylums occasionally were used to shield individuals from their families. Utica's casebook records contained many histories of abused women, often married to alcoholic husbands, who found a measure of relief at the asylum (although such a view of the asylum might be seen as a measure of their desperation). The following cases were typical:

> Aged 37. Married and has three children. Has had two husbands . . .—the present husband is a bad man and his conduct—spending her property, abusing and leaving her, are the causes of her insanity. Is violent and will strike.

> Aged about 31. Married and two children. Been deranged four months . . .—cause abuse of husband, after travail: she was proud-spirited and her husband shiftless—He provided very poorly—and one day she traded his coat for beans and an iron wedge for pork—eats irregularly—ranges about—sings, tears, strikes, breaks.

> About 32 years of age—married—no children. Native of Ireland. Been deranged three or four months. Supposed cause Bad conduct of her husband—he expended her money and abused her—She was arrested for stealing and found to be insane—Is not violent it is said except when she sees her relatives. [25]

The asylum provided a refuge of a somewhat different sort for the nineteen-year-old son of a wealthy upstate New York family who had been arrested for stealing money from the local post office. Although he showed no evidence of insanity (and a great deal of careful premeditation), the boy was institutionalized on the grounds of hereditary insanity. (His mother had had chorea for years, as well as repeated attacks of depression.) While at the institution, the boy wrote cheerful, flippant letters to his parents and friends about asylum dances and games. After nine months, he was released as "not insane," and his father took him home, criminal charges apparently having been dropped. [26] Even Willard was occasionally so used by middle-class families. When an eighteen-year-old local girl murdered her illegitimate infant, her father prevented her arrest for homicide by arranging for a quick medical examination by two physicians, who promptly ordered her committed to Willard. A contemporary journal remarked that it had cost the father five hundred dollars thus to settle the case out of court, but his daughter was subsequently released from Willard as "cured."[27] For the most part, asylum doctors resented the mixing in of those who had broken the law, even if declared incompetent to stand trial, with their other patients. The presence of such criminals interfered with the medical staff's efforts to portray the asylum as a hospital; by adding to the number of antisocial patients, it also frequently increased chaos on the wards.

In sharp contrast to the case histories of violent, threatening, or beleaguered patients are those which detail complex and confusing family conflicts. Some suggest the ease with which asylums could be used to get rid of eccentric or irritating family members; others present a tangle of intrafamilial conflicts impossible to unravel from the distance of one hundred years. The case of a thirty-nine-year-old housewife sent to Utica in the spring of 1869 exemplifies the latter. Her troubles dated from the death of a much beloved daughter seven years earlier. At that time, according to her husband, she had become markedly strange. Her eccentricities included a desire to have all of her teeth removed under chloroform and a tendency to make such rude remarks that he could not ask guests to dinner. In addition, she had a ten- to twelve-year addiction to laudanum; a constant desire to exaggerate; a tendency to circulate lies about her husband, daughter, and son-in-law; and an irritating secretiveness. He reported that she had struck him with a large stick, hit her son, and driven her own mother from the house by her abusive language. In self-defense, the patient claimed that her son had struck her hard enough to make blood flow, that he had turned her mother out of the house so that she and her mother had to creep back in through the cellar window, and that her husband would not let her have tea, forcing her to get it from neighbors. In a parting shot, the husband admitted that, while his wife had been more violent in conversation than in action, he himself had used physical violence against her (but only that which was justified, he argued). At admission, the patient claimed that she had come only because her son otherwise had threatened to put her in irons. Three months after this bitter turmoil had climaxed in her commitment, the wife was visited at the asylum by her husband and removed "cured." The reasons for her removal were as unclear as for her admission.[28]

A substantial minority of both Utica's and Willard's patients arrived at the asylum with no previous histories of behavioral extremes. These ambiguous cases included individuals with occasional hallucinations, depressed melancholics, and disorderly (but not violent) alcoholics. They ranged from those who suspected relatives of poisoning them or business associates of misusing their funds to unconventional women who took spiritualism too seriously and men and women worn out by religious excitement. Some had acted in a fashion considered by neighbors to be strange, albeit not dangerous; for example, the young laborer who covered himself with varicolored pockets stuffed with checks, which he made out for imaginary purchases. Others had offended community sensibilities in a number of ways, one of the most blatant being the public masturbating of a thirty-year-old man, reportedly begun after friends had prevented him from going out with the neighbors' hired girl. More difficult to understand on the basis of casebook histories alone were the institutionalizations of a forty-nine-year-old widow who felt surrounded by enemies and without a safe place in which to deposit her valuables, and of a thirty-year-old spinster whose main symptom, according to her sister, was the continual reading of old almanacs and quack medical books, on the basis of which she imagined herself afflicted with all the ailments described in them and took a great deal of medicine for relief.[29]

Why were such men and women committed? At least some seemed to be victims of nineteenth-century doctors' expanded definition of insanity (and its acceptance by at least part of the general public). According to the dictates of science and humanitarianism, such doctors declared, "almost every form of neurotic disorder that affects the moral powers in any way" merited hospital treatment. From their perspective, the insane included all those who had so lost self-control that they could no longer live in harmony with society, not just raving maniacs. Proof that many outside the medical profession agreed can be found in the increasing number of patient case histories between 1843 and 1890 which emphasized eccentric behavior as a shift from previous patterns. The quiet had become noisy and the loquacious quiet; the industrious had given up their work, and agnostics had become religious fanatics; the virtuous suddenly showed signs of promiscuity.[30]

From the "enlightened" perspective of nineteenth-century psychiatry, such shifts were clear evidence of a loss of reason meriting institutionaliza-

96

tion. In Victorian England, Elaine Showalter has observed, "Madness was no longer a gross and unmistakable inversion of appropriate conduct, but a collection of cumulatively disquieting gestures and postures.[31] In nineteenth-century New York it continued to be both, but at least some families and communities increasingly turned to state asylums like Utica and Willard to care for individuals who once had been allowed to wander the countryside or sit by the family hearth. These included women like the Willard patient who for some twenty years had gone from one poorhouse to another during the winter and camped out during the summer. When finally admitted to Willard, her commitment certificate noted only: "She is often uncontrolled in conduct, incoherent in conversation, noisy and insomnolent at night; at times extremely talkative, at other times silent and morose." Even Willard's walls could not constrain her, however, and she eloped shortly after admission. Eventually she was killed by a passing freight train. While newspaper articles after her death tended to romanticize her mysterious life, she herself had admitted fearing bodily harm. She still clearly preferred noninstitutional life, but not all in her position did. An Indianapolis paper from 1850 told of a similar middle-aged woman, ineligible for poorhouse care, who slept in open lots where she had been raped several times by groups of adolescents. Since Indiana in 1850 lacked an institution comparable to Willard, the paper could ask only "What can be done?"[32] More typical of Utica's patients was the young married woman with three children sent to Utica in 1870 because "at present she is different from what she formerly was; one week ago she acted very queer."[33] At the same time, medical rhetoric was not the only factor changing familial attitudes toward institutionalization. According to a Willard doctor, many families of the "middling sort" found the superior comfort and protection available in state asylums much more attractive than that offered in county poorhouses.[34]

The narrowing of the standards of acceptable public behavior for alleged insane persons had a parallel in the criminal justice system during the same period. According to Eric Monkkonen, while levels of violent crime (as measured by arrests) in urban areas decreased over the course of the nineteenth century, arrests rose steadily in that broad discretionary category called "disorderly conduct." He reviews a number of possible explanations for this statistical shift, finding most satisfactory the claim that cities, as they grew older, became more orderly.[35] An additional factor contributing to the comparable (although less dramatic) shift in the kinds of people sent to asylums may have been the growing acceptance of the asylum's therapeutic mission. Certainly, Utica's casebook records suggest that, an increasing (albeit small) number of individuals themselves sought psychiatric help at the institution. One such patient, a middle-aged man who had been devastated by the unexpected death of his young daughter, subsequently became paranoid and delusional. Eventually he asked his family to chain him up so that he would not kill anyone. When they refused, he tried to cut his throat. For him, admission to Utica meant a great easing of his own mind, as well as of his family's fears.[36]

The Medical Perspective

Even though they belittled families' tendency to attribute mental illness to relatively trivial events and attacked their reluctance to recognize the onset of mental disease, doctors realized that they vitally needed even the most imperfect casebook histories if they were to unravel the mystery of mental illness.[37] In their annual reports, Utica's superintendents used two kinds of charts to summarize their patients' preinstitutional histories: one called "causes of insanity" and the other "duration of insanity before admission." In the first, information was presented on nine causes of institutionalization: emotional stress (Fig. 4.1), economic stress (Fig. 4.2), sexual abuse (which mainly consisted of masturbation), heredity (Fig. 4.3), epilepsy (Fig. 4.4), paresis (Fig. 4.5), senility (Fig. 4.6), drug addiction (which included alcoholism), and an aggregated category of all physical causes (Fig. 4.7). Although such aggregate data mixed doctors' diagnoses with familial explanations in a fashion impossible to untangle, they revealed interesting patterns of change over time.

Not surprisingly, these figures show that, during Utica's early years, more men than women were admitted because of financial or job-related problems. More striking than such differences between the sexes was the overall drop, almost as soon as John Gray became superintendent of the Utica Asylum in 1854, in the number of patients with mental problems attributable to economic causes. Their percentage of the asylum population did not rise again (with the exception of the depression of the mid-1870s) until after Gray's death in 1886, a fact clearly more reflective of his opinions than of any real change in patients' preinstitutional prob-

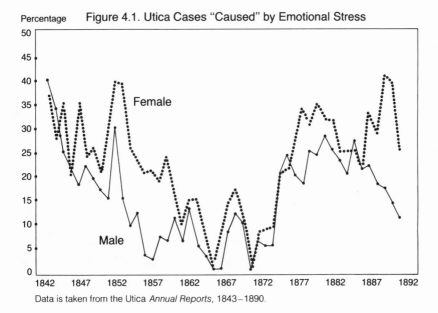

Percentage Figure 4.1. Utica Cases "Caused" by Emotional Stress

Data is taken from the Utica *Annual Reports*, 1843–1890.

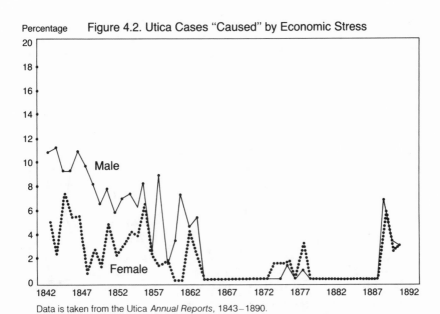

Percentage Figure 4.2. Utica Cases "Caused" by Economic Stress

Data is taken from the Utica *Annual Reports*, 1843–1890.

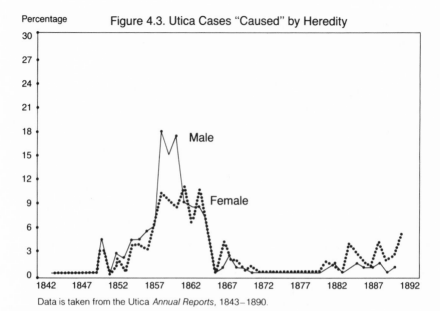

Figure 4.3. Utica Cases "Caused" by Heredity

Data is taken from the Utica *Annual Reports*, 1843–1890.

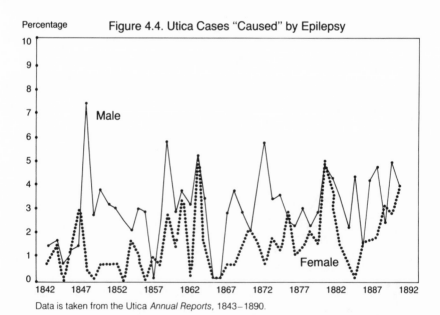

Figure 4.4. Utica Cases "Caused" by Epilepsy

Data is taken from the Utica *Annual Reports*, 1843–1890.

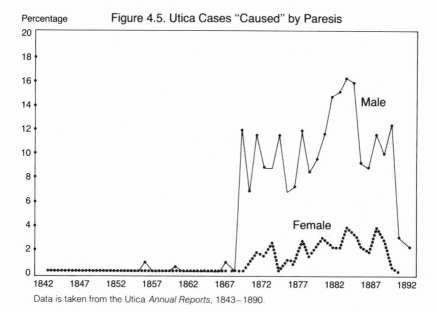

Figure 4.5. Utica Cases "Caused" by Paresis

Data is taken from the Utica *Annual Reports*, 1843–1890.

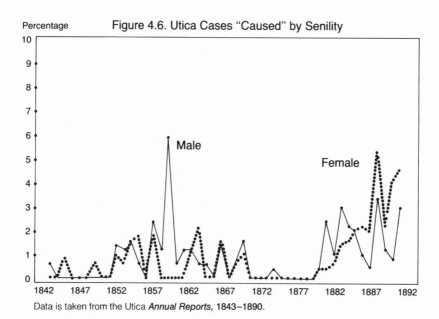

Figure 4.6. Utica Cases "Caused" by Senility

Data is taken from the Utica *Annual Reports*, 1843–1890.

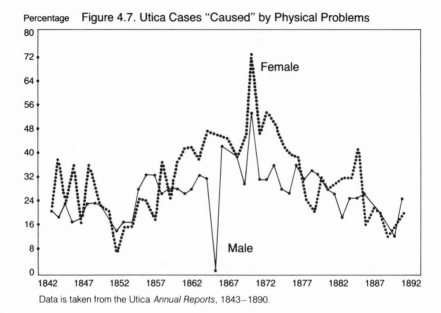

Percentage   Figure 4.7. Utica Cases "Caused" by Physical Problems

Data is taken from the Utica *Annual Reports,* 1843–1890.

lems. Gray strongly opposed attributing insanity to so-called "moral" forces, on the grounds that all mental illness had a physiological base. Yet he could not prevent the institutionalization of those whose derangement seemed to have emotional or economic roots, perhaps because the general public continued to believe in the accuracy of such diagnoses. Although more women were reported to suffer the ravages of emotional stress, the long-term variations in male and female susceptibility were quite similar.

Sexual abuse was presented as an almost exclusively male problem in Utica's annual reports, even though casebook records made were filled with stories of masturbating female patients. Somewhat surprisingly, given the large popular literature on masturbation's connection with insanity, masturbation generally accounted for only 9–15 percent of Utica's male admissions. Perhaps the young middle-class men most threatened by masturbational insanity did not often end up in a state asylum (although Utica did accept private patients).[38] Sexual excess was identified as a problem in many Utica and Willard casebook histories, but usually in

102

combination with other sorts of disruptive behavior. For example, one Willard patient who admitted to "unreasonable and unseemly sexual desires," manifested in habits of constant masturbation and a tendency to call on his wife "at all hours and in any presence to gratify his inclinations," was institutionalized only when he threatened his wife with violence. After several months in the institution, he showed "no unusual sexual desires," although he had become nervous and somewhat weak minded. Less than a year after his institutionalization, he was discharged "greatly improved" to live with friends.[39] When P. M. Wise admitted to Willard a woman dressed in male clothing, calling herself "Joseph Lobdell" and claiming to be the husband of a younger woman she had met during a county poorhouse stay, her case history suggested that it was her increasingly violent and erratic behavior, not community disapproval of her sexual mores, that had precipitated the commitment. (Of course, restrictive definitions of acceptable female behavior may well have contributed to the patient's psychic distress.)[40] Another Willard patient was readmitted after the birth of an illegitimate child because of "sexual weaknesses which would render her unsafe to be at large." If historian Peter Tyor is right, however, such women were more often described as feeble-minded than insane and were kept in county asylums or sent to the Newark State School.[41]

Heredity played a surprisingly small role in the Utica insanity statistics, largely because the Utica superintendents felt that, while a defective heredity might predispose individuals to madness, it did not by itself cause insanity.[42] More males than females were afflicted with epilepsy or paresis. Although such patients were a relatively small part of Utica's institutional population, they demanded a great deal of care and were seldom discharged, except to institutions for chronic cases, like Willard. There were very few senile patients of either sex at Utica during the nineteenth century; most patients were relatively young at admission and, if several years of treatment did not produce improvements, they were sent back to families or county facilities or transferred to Willard. Despite Gray's opposition to admitting drug addicts (whom he regarded as sinners, not lunatics), annual report statistics show that the Utica Asylum accepted a number of them, mostly male, over the course of the nineteenth century.

The ever-increasing numbers of patients of both sexes whose mental illness was attributed by John Gray and his assistant physicians to physical problems indicated not the declining health of the citizens of New York as the century progressed but the impact of Gray's somaticism on record keeping at Utica. Like his contemporaries, Gray regarded women as somewhat more vulnerable than men to physical disease. Although he attacked those who argued that most female mental problems had their origins in reproductive disorders, his staff tended to question newly admitted female patients closely about menstrual irregularities and problems relating to childbirth, whereas male patients were more often queried about the relationship between their physical ailments and overindulgence in alcohol, drugs, work, or sex.[43]

Sociodemographic Characteristics
of Patients at First Admission

Despite their complexity and variation, nineteenth-century patient casebook records offer a wealth of information about the timing of decisions to institutionalize the mentally ill and the factors which affected the decisions. Because of their complementary therapeutic missions, the Utica and Willard asylums attracted different sorts of patients, arriving at the institutions by a variety of routes. Like the details of individual cases, aggregate sociodemographic trends suggest which nineteenth-century New Yorkers were most at risk to be sent to a state asylum. A one-fifth systematic sample of patient casebook records reveals several interesting shifts over time. Utica's charges tended to be younger, more often native born, and less isolated from family and kin networks than did Willard's chronically insane paupers, many of whom had been transferred there from other institutions. These men and women often had lost their individual identities long before commitment to Willard. At Utica, both the mean and median age of patients at admission in the sample rose slightly over the course of the nineteenth century: from a mean of 36.4 years and a median of 34.5 for the period 1841–1868, to a mean of 38.8 years and a median of 36.9 for the years 1869–1890. For the second period, Willard's patients at admission were even older, with a mean of 41.2 years and a median of 39.1 At Utica, however, the proportion of patients over 60 during this same period remained about 7.5 percent, whereas at Willard, they constituted 12 percent of those admitted. (Since Utica continued to release patients more rapidly, its overall patient population also continued to be younger than Willard's.) Willard's age at admission was particularly high in 1869, the asylum's first year, when almost all of its patients were transfers from other state and local institutions.[44]

Willard had more foreign-born and Catholic patients (largely Irish), although Utica's foreign-born patient population grew slightly over the course of the century. (It constituted 26.2 percent of post–Civil War admissions.) Like poorhouse inmates, most asylum patients, whether native or foreign born, had at least a common school education. Although for the entire nineteenth century, unskilled workers (laborers and domestics) were the largest group in the Utica Asylum, by the end of the century, the institution admitted proportionately fewer professionals and white-collar workers and more from the ranks of skilled and unskilled laborers. While it is tempting to see this shift as evidence of the declining prestige of state insane asylums, it more likely reflected increasing pressure on Utica's superintendent during the 1880s not to admit private patients.[45] In general, Utica attracted patients of higher status (as measured by occupation) than did Willard, although the two institutions grew more alike toward the end of the century. For example, a substantial minority of Utica's patients had held professional or skilled trades positions before admission, whereas most of Willard's had been domestics or unskilled laborers. Although more of Willard's inmates also were first generation immigrants, the foreign born, institutionalized insane were not all alike. For example, Utica's foreign-born patients were more likely to have been skilled workers before admission than Willard's. At Willard, the Irish had fewer social resources than did other foreigners; they were more likely to be female, unskilled, Catholic, and poorly educated.[46]

That more cannot be said about the social and class background of New York's nineteenth-century asylum patients is disappointing but not surprising. At best, historians need to treat occupational trends based on institutional admission data with caution, whatever the institution. For example, the most common terms—"farmer," "housekeeper," and "laborer"—are highly ambiguous indicators of social class. Furthermore, according to nineteenth-century asylum doctors, those struggling with insanity frequently slid down the occupational ladder before ending up in an institution.[47] As a result, when families reported new patients' occupations at admission, they sometimes gave the most recent and other times the most prestigious or characteristic. (This can be seen, for example, in casebooks which describe individuals as farmers at the top of their records but then, in the case histories, make clear that they had not farmed for some time.)

Because of the shorter time span of Willard's records, sociodemographic changes in patient populations over time are less obvious than at Utica. More interesting than a look at Willard alone is a comparison of the Utica and Willard populations between 1869 and 1890. Both institutions held large numbers of the unmarried, although Willard had a greater percentage. The relationship between marital status and mental illness was a subject of considerable interest to nineteenth-century asylum superintendents. Amariah Brigham suggested that the Utica Asylum initially received large numbers of single patients for two reasons: some had gone insane before the usual age of marriage, and others were so strongly predisposed to insanity that marriage was not considered advisable.[48] Whatever the causal relationship between the single state and insanity, nineteenth-century records make it clear that those alone, whether single, divorced, or widowed, were particularly vulnerable to institutionalization. For example, according to Michael Katz, New York's poorhouses at this time held disproportionate numbers of widowed men.[49] Presumably, the large number of single women at Willard also reflected their more precarious social situation as much, if not more, than their weakened mental health. Since the Utica Asylum (like its counterparts around the state) was unwilling to release patients unless it was confident that they would not become an economic burden upon their home county, it more often sent home single men with job prospects and transferred to Willard those single women, particularly the foreign born, whose chances for finding domestic employment again were small and who had no kin willing to support them.

Neither of New York's first two state asylums received many nonwhite patients, although Willard had slightly more (2.2 percent in contrast to Utica's 0.8 percent). Like the old, blacks and American Indians were largely excluded from costly state-level asylum care. A look at the case records of some of the few black women whose families or communities paid for their care at Utica and Willard during the nineteenth century reveals that they closely resembled their white sisters. Typically between twenty and forty years old, they had worked in their own or others' homes.

They lived with or near relatives and friends. Their case histories are interesting primarily for what they reveal about the lives of nineteenth-century black women in upstate New York.[50] Several of the domestics had collapsed out of sheer exhaustion. For example, one twenty-four-year-old black woman became suicidal while simultaneously working as a domestic and preparing to become a schoolteacher. Described as initially "a healthy girl, industrious and quick at learning," she substituted study for sleep and eventually became both physically and emotionally debilitated. After several attacks of depression, she attempted suicide in 1861 and was taken to Utica by her brother.[51] Difficult family situations also contributed to emotional outbreaks among black women, as among white. One thirty-seven-year-old woman with three children lost much sleep after her second husband had spent all her money, abused her, and then deserted. Desperate and frustrated, she eventually became violent and ended up at Utica in 1872.[52] Despite their often violent and destructive behavior, such wife-abuse victims were described with sympathy by asylum doctors as moral, hard-working women betrayed by intemperate husbands.[53]

Black and white women at the Utica and Willard asylums all shared similar sociodemographic characteristics. In contrast, male and female patients, no matter what their race, differed considerably from each other. For the most part, it is easier to describe those differences than to assess their impact on institutionalization rates. For example, the greater propensity of females to claim church membership is hardly surprising. Somewhat more difficult to explain is the age differential at admission of men and women. At Utica, women tended to be younger than men at admission. According to Utica's annual report data on the duration of insanity by sex, in 1870, 1880, and 1885, women also generally were institutionalized more quickly than men. For example, between 1877 and 1878, the mean duration of insanity before admission (excluding outliers) for a sample of seriously disturbed females was reported to be 5.77 months and for males with similar kinds of preinstitutional behavior, 13.38 months. There are several plausible explanations for this differential. Possibly families, neighbors, and employers found violent behavior more inexplicable and socially unacceptable in women than in men. It also is quite likely that certain sorts of threatening men were sent to jail under the same circumstances as their female counterparts went to insane asylums. Finally, women were more vulnerable to institutionalization in an asylum as a result of their concentration in domestic positions. Because of their close proximity to employers, eccentric servants were more likely to be labeled insane than were unskilled male laborers.[54]

Here too, as in the case of occupational data, information on duration of insanity gleaned from patient case histories needs to be treated with care. While the overall patterns are suggestive, historians need to avoid making much of the exact numbers. According to asylum doctors, such information about patients' "duration of insanity before admission," when given by family members or friends, was often unreliable (a judgment supported by the accumulation of cases at the "one-year" and "two-year" points). Furthermore, because counties were supposed to send to Utica only recently ill indigent patients, Utica's doctors suspected that local superintendents of the poor sometimes misrepresented the length of time particularly troublesome paupers had been ill. Despite their unreliability, the asylums' medical staff felt that duration of insanity tables were of some worth. They clearly showed that the longer patients had been insane before admission, the less their chance of cure.[55] This was especially obvious in the Willard statistics. At least during the institution's first fifteen years, 46 percent of its patients at admission were described either as having been insane for ten years or more or as "chronic." In 1885 the proportion of recently afflicted to long-term patients shifted somewhat, as Willard began to attract more men and women from nearby counties (even though it was not supposed to accept such cases). Not until 1890 when it was designated a "mixed" institution by the provisions of the State Care Act did Willard become free to accept acute as well as chronic cases. The initial impact of the State Care Act at Willard was to increase the relative numbers of more promising patients. Indicative of this shift was the appearance for the first time in Willard's 1890 report of duration of illness categories as short as six months and even a few of five weeks, categories Utica had always used.[56]

In his much earlier annual reports, Amariah Brigham of Utica also had pointed out that a number of factors which had little to do with duration of insanity and behavior influenced the timing of asylum admissions, including the melting of canals in the spring and the opening of new buildings. Since most buildings or wings were sex segregated, the construction of new facilities often shifted dramatically (but temporarily) the relative proportions of men and women at the Utica and Willard asylums. For these reasons, Brigham warned fellow doctors against using month of admission data to conjecture about seasonal trends in mental illness; at best it indicated only the month when patients were brought to the asylum.[57]

Commitment Laws

While casebook histories taken alone seem to suggest that there were few constraints on families' and communities' decisions to send their members to state asylums, such was not the case. Even before the New York State Lunatic Asylum at Utica opened its doors, the legislature carefully spelled out the conditions under which involuntary civil commitments could take place. First, unless they could be cared for by families or friends, all insane persons "so furiously mad as to endanger their own persons or the persons or property of others" were to be sent within ten days of their first attack either to the State Lunatic Asylum or to a public or private asylum approved by county superintendents of the poor. Second, no one could be admitted to a state asylum without an order signed by a court, justice, judge, or supreme court commissioner. Third, before an alleged insane person could be confined, he or she had to be examined by two reputable physicians. Finally, if the insane, or friends of the insane, objected to a commitment order, they could, within five days of that order, appeal to a county judge for a jury trial of the facts of insanity.[58]

This statute was passed in April of 1842. In November of the next year, Charles Mann, head of the Utica board of managers, reported its provisos to the man about to become the first superintendent, Amariah Brigham. According to Mann, previous legislation pertaining to the "furiously mad" had been intended to secure rather than to cure. An important part of legislators' new recognition of insanity as a treatable physical disease was their insistence on a precommitment medical examination, a significant procedural innovation.[59] Yet, despite Mann's applause for this new requirement, it was almost immediately ignored in the commitment of two groups: paupers and private patients. According to Utica's doctors and to a later commentator on this law, paupers could be sent to the asylum simply by order of local superintendents of the poor; private patients, at the request of family members or friends. Only in the commitment of indigents (men and women but recently impoverished by their insanity) was the law enforced, primarily to keep the chronically ill out of the expensive state institutions.[60] Later in the century, reformers were to see this failure to have all alleged insane persons examined by medical doctors before commitment as a serious threat to civil liberties. But whatever their intent in passing the 1842 statute, New York's pre–Civil War politicians were not bothered by the way it was put into action. They viewed asylum treatment as an expensive privilege, not an imposition.

New York's 1842 lunacy statute was modified a number of times in the 1840s and 1850s, primarily so as to save local communities money. For example, in 1850, county judges were ordered to be more careful in their determination of the duration of illness and the financial status of alleged insane indigents before approving their commitment to the Utica Asylum. Thus legislators hoped to curb what they saw as a "too liberal or improvident" committing of the indigent at public charge.[61] While they did not object to the exclusion of chronic cases, the Utica Asylum managers strongly objected to the fiscal thrust of such policies. In only a few instances, they argued, had families persuaded judges to admit wealthy men and women at public charge. Furthermore, to consign to a county poorhouse "a very deserving but unfortunate class" before giving them the benefits of a therapeutic institution was "unwise as well as unjust." About one-third of the patients admitted to Utica between 1843 and 1848 had been such indigents, they claimed, and their cure rate had been the highest of any class of patients.[62]

In 1850 the legislature formally opened the Utica Asylum to another group already there: private, paying patients. Space permitting, the asylum managers were authorized to admit private cases in special need or which promised speedy recovery. For such patients, no formal commitment process was required. Here too the main concern of legislators was that the counties not be burdened with the costs of patient care. They waived the requirement of medical certificates for commitment but insisted that bank officers or other prominent individuals guarantee the financial reliability of those who promised to cover patient fees.[63] Families unwilling to pay such costs could care for insane members at home. While critics charged that such home care often was inadequate and abusive, by common law the state could not interfere in internal domestic affairs. As late as the 1870s, John Ordronaux, one of the leaders of the movement to reform New York's lunacy laws, argued that the family's right to privacy was more important than the occasional undetected abuse of dependent family members.[64]

During the 1850s and into the 1860s, civil commitment laws changed only in minor ways. Reformers continued to fight for expansion of state-funded asylum care, especially for the chronically insane accumulating in county poorhouses. Eventually, in 1863, legislators approved construction of Willard and it opened in 1869. In 1867 they also authorized the establishment of the Hudson River Asylum at Poughkeepsie, another acute care facility, and in 1870 a homeopathic asylum at Middletown and a mixed-care hospital at Buffalo. While most social reformers applauded this rapid expansion of state care, for the first time they also began to look carefully at its costs: this time defined in terms of personal liberties as well as tax dollars. Their concerns were not unique to New Yorkers. In 1882 the governor of Massachusetts commented sadly about postwar asylums: "Their doors open altogether too easily inward and with too great difficulty outward."[65] Even more alarming was the possibility that sane men and women were trapped behind those firmly closed doors. Newspapers and ex-asylum patients were quick to exploit such anxieties. And asylum doctors were equally quick to deny their legitimacy.

While newspapers across the country were running pro- and anti-asylum editorials in the 1870s, such talk of captivity and liberation, enchained reason and deprivation of liberty found a particularly receptive audience in post–Civil War New York. The state had one of the largest public insane asylum systems in the country and perhaps the most controversial superintendent: John Gray of Utica. It also was home to a vocal group of nineteenth-century asylum critics, the New York City neurologists who started the National Association for the Protection of the Rights of the Insane.[66] Finally, in response to reform pressures to tighten commitment procedures, John Ordronaux, the state commissioner in lunacy, re-codified the state lunacy laws so that for the first time formal commitment papers were required for all new patients, regardless of their status.[67]

After the New York legislature approved his new statute in 1874, Ordronaux published an analysis of his work in the form of a lengthy treatise. Under English common law, Ordronaux reminded his readers, anyone could detain, without legal process, lunatics dangerous to themselves or others, so long as they were treated humanely. Further, if relatives confined such persons at home, the state or other interested parties had no legal way to test the necessity for their continued detention.[68] Before passage of the laws of 1874, families and county governments also could confine pauper and private insane persons in state institutions without legal process, so long as it was dangerous to let them be at liberty. Ordronaux strongly objected to this situation on the grounds that the "physical status of insanity" could not produce civil disability until legally established. Furthermore, since an insane asylum was not simply a remedial but also a custodial institution (a hybrid of the ordinary hospital and the reformatory), no one should be committed to it except by due process of law. In practice, this meant that neither relatives nor doctors, whatever their knowledge of a person's condition, had the legal authority to commit an alleged insane person to the custody of an asylum. For the same reason, neither an insane person nor a sane person somewhat disordered in his nervous system could commit himself voluntarily.[69]

In such passages, Ordronaux asserted the supremacy of law and lawyers in the admitting process. After tightening procedural safeguards, however, he let his basic approval of asylum treatment resurface. Although many claimed that only the dangerous should be institutionalized, he argued that such a position reflected outmoded attitudes which stigmatized the insane. Initially he asserted that any insane person who might benefit from institutionalization should be committed.[70] By the early 1880s, he had further expanded his definition of insanity so as to include those "who are not perhaps in the estimation of the average community insane, but in whom specialists recognize a condition of . . . premonitory insanity; they see the incipient stages by reason of their skill in reading the prefatory chapters of insanity."[71]

To Ordronaux's regret, the New York legislature refused to encode his enormously broadened substantive definition of insanity, and for the rest of the century, lawyers and doctors were to argue about what kinds of behavior merited institutionalization. Several writs of habeas corpus involving patients from the Utica Asylum evoked the loudest debate. Typical was the trial of one James B. Silkman, a New York lawyer. According to Silkman's supporters, the question before the court was not whether Silkman was technically insane but whether he was so insane as to forfeit his liberty.[72] They felt strongly that, whenever possible, the insane should be spared the "forcible removal, deprivation of liberty, and odium" so integral to institutional commitments.[73] Not surprisingly, asylum supporters rejected this emphasis on the coercive aspects of asylum treatment, arguing that those who filed writs of habeas corpus on behalf of the institutionalized insane further stigmatized them by suggesting that they more closely resembled prisoners than hospital patients.

For the rest of the nineteenth century, lawyers and doctors continued to wrangle with each other and among themselves over the substantive definition of insanity. Asylum critics constantly complained that, in practice, many harmless (if a bit strange) people were being sent to state asylums. In 1888, in the case of Ayers v. Russell, O'Leary, and Gould, Judge Learned of the New York Supreme Court tried to tighten the definition once again, ruling that no one could be sent to an asylum unless he had been shown to be dangerous to himself or others. Subsequently, the plaintiff, Alfred Ayers, successfully sued the doctors who had signed his commitment papers, on the grounds that "physicians are liable for lack of ordinary care and prudence, and for failure to make due inquiry into the question of sanity."[74] But, in general, despite Learned's efforts, state asylums continued to accept a broad cross-section of the insane population.

The Social Impact

It is hard to ascertain the practical impact on families of the increasingly formal aspect of the certification process. Even asylum doctors admitted that it was fairly easy to find two physicians to sign a commitment certificate, and judges rarely, if ever, contested their judgment. As one asylum superintendent told an audience of medical students, families seldom wanted examining doctors to do an original appraisal of an alleged insane person; they wanted only ratification of the family's own judgment. (He went on to warn them to be careful at such examinations so as to avoid subsequent wrongful commitment suits.)[75] On the other hand, it did make the process more complicated and expensive, which no doubt made some families and communities pause. Ex-patients, however, felt that, so long as procedural reforms were combined with substantive expansions of the definition of insanity, the reforms offered little protection. For example, one Lewis Prudden, who felt he had been railroaded into the Utica Asylum by his wife, with the connivance of an unscrupulous lawyer, complained that, so long as sanity was defined as "soundness or perfection of mind," relatives would always be able to find some evidence of imperfection to justify the transfer onto the taxpayers of the burden of caring for difficult or dependent family members.[76]

Other patients echoed Prudden's complaints about the ease with which commitment laws could be manipulated. Many of their stories of persecution by relatives and business associates contain enough internal inconsistencies and bizarre details to justify doctors' skepticism as to their validity.[77] Yet several patient casebook records make clear that, however seldom asylums were used to incarcerate the sane, they did have that potential. One of the most horrifying examples of such injustice can be found in the story of the badly abused wife of a farm laborer. When she finally had her husband arrested for beating her, threatening her life, and neglecting to provide for the family, he retaliated while out on bail by having her committed to the New York State Lunatic Asylum. Like many of Utica's patients, the accused wife attributed her behavioral aberrations to having been poisoned by her husband—but in this case, the accusation was justified. Three months after admission, at the request of a county superintendent of the poor, who confirmed her story, the young woman was finally released as "not insane" to return to her children.[78]

Such a case demonstrates that, even though New York's nineteenth-century commitment laws were superficially sex and class neutral, they inevitably had a greater impact on the more powerless members of the community, who lacked the social resources to combat the institutionalization process. More important, even the most vehement asylum critics failed to solve the difficult problem of how to make it easier for recovered patients to reverse the commitment process and escape the institution. A few of the wealthier patients at Utica successfully used writs of habeas corpus to win their freedom, and several others simply ran away from the institution and subsequently tried to get official recognition of their sanity.[79] Few of those sent to the Willard Asylum for the Chronic Insane even left, except at death. Although the Utica Asylum managers were empowered to discharge (on the recommendation of the superintendent) both recovered patients and those harmless insane who no longer could benefit from institutionalization, the impetus for dismissal often came from patients' families or communities, not asylum doctors. Those who kept in

114

closest touch with their families had the best chance of being released.[80]

Not all of those who failed to keep in touch with institutionalized family members were heartless. Many had delayed commitment until their physical and emotional resources were exhausted. Feeling both guilt and anger, such relatives frequently distanced themselves (emotionally as well as physically) from family members after committing them. Such distancing created problems when patients were released, for it increased the difficulty of reintegration into family circles. Not surprisingly, the longer patients were institutionalized, the less likely became contacts with the outside world, especially if they were transferred from Utica to Willard, for often their case histories were not transferred with them. Willard's geographical location exacerbated patients' isolation, and few notations about visitors or letters can be found in its patient records.

The Family Re-formed

Many aspects of the history of the insane and their families in nineteenth-century New York have a timeless quality. Like the clients of the magician-doctor Napier in early modern England, like those of family counselors in twentieth-century United States, insane New Yorkers' case histories often focused on problems related to the emotional dynamics of family life.[81] Yet, in trying to restore familial harmony, nineteenth-century asylums unquestionably altered familial relationships. At the same time as they offered new forms of assistance to families trying to cope with the mentally ill, the ability of many of those families to deal with sick members decreased. The socioeconomic changes which accompanied industrialization and urbanization did not affect all New Yorkers equally. For some, but not all, the separation of work and residence, the increasing isolation of nuclear families, and the ever larger numbers of single men and women living alone and unable to care for themselves when illness struck, greatly increased their likelihood of institutionalization. Most affected were single foreign-born unskilled laborers, especially women, who even when healthy often barely escaped public dependency.[82] Yet, as late as 1889, New York's asylum doctors continued to complain about families' reluctance to turn to insane asylums, except in desperation. Even those most critical of asylums agreed with asylum superintendents about the need to "fight for the recognition of the fact that it is no disgrace to be crazy." For, as one reformer eloquently noted, "While the insane are thus regarded by the world in general as wild and dangerous animals, or as perverted mortals for whom there is no obligation of keeping faith, is it surprising that even at the asylum all superstition and ignorance cannot be done away with?"[83]

To reject what has become a favorite academic straw man—a simplistic social-control interpretation of nineteenth-century insane asylum—is not to deny that social control is an important theme in the social and medical histories of nineteenth-century welfare institutions. Large public asylums in nineteenth-century New York were molded, however, by the diverse demands of their client families as well as by their superintendents' medical ideologies and the increasing need of the society at large for public social order. As several historians have noted, the targets of reformers' manipulation themselves have a considerable ability to mold the institutions and agencies set up to improve them.[84] Patient case histories, whether looked at in the aggregate or individually, make clear that families looked to state asylums for help with a range of physical and emotional problems. The asylum–family relationship in nineteenth-century New York cannot be captured in a single formulation; it shifted from case to case, varied over time, and occasionally took some surprising forms. For example, in the 1880s, a young woman who had spent eleven months at Utica wrote to the doctors asking them to send her a "certificate" as to her sanity, for she kept losing positions as a domestic once employers found out she had been institutionalized. Having left the asylum family, she found herself alone in the world, for her mother had died during her institutionalization. Given her obvious social isolation and economic precariousness, it is perhaps not surprising that, less than a year after her release, she had returned to the asylum. Despite its obvious limitations, to her it had become the only "haven in a heartless world."[85] Both the institution and the community shared responsibility for her inability to live outside it.

5

Destiny in a Name

Some arrived in chains, raving and striking out at their attendants; others, withdrawn and silent, were brought by weeping family members. But whatever the circumstances of arrival, all newcomers to New York's nineteenth-century state insane asylums went through the same admission rituals. After entering into a spacious main hall, they were taken to a small examination room. There, admitting doctors chatted briefly with prospective patients and observed their behavior. On the basis of testimony from accompanying public officials, relatives, or friends, asylum doctors also took detailed notes about patients' past physical and behavioral problems. Especially after the Civil War, as public concern about wrongful commitments increased, they next scrutinized closely the civil commitment papers which were supposed to accompany all new patients. Typically these had been filled out by two local physicians, often in a cursory fashion, and signed by a judge. Finally, using these multiple sources of information, asylum doctors assigned diagnostic labels and sent new patients to a ward.[1] If New York's nineteenth-century state asylums ever turned patients away, their records make no mention of it. Occasionally Utica's patients were released as "not insane," but only after several months' stay in the asylum.

From the perspective of their critics, this admission ritual epitomized the efforts of the nineteenth-century psychiatric establishment to monopolize the definition (and confinement) of madness. Yet, while certainly through their diagnostic schema asylum doctors did their best to medicalize popular notions of insanity, asylum doctors most often simply acquiesced in a diagnosis made outside the institution. Families, neighbors,

117

and employers usually were first to label as "insane" markedly eccentric or threatening behavior, and committing doctors' papers most often parroted their observations. In turn, the asylum medical staff reratified (albeit in a more sophisticated form) diagnostic judgments made days or even weeks earlier.[2] Such a continuum of classification could exist because the technical terms of nineteenth-century psychiatry were drawn from the common stock of the language. The four most commonly used psychiatric diagnoses—mania, dementia, melancholia, and imbecility—all had clear roots in everyday language, and this comparatively close link between popular and professional conceptualizations of insanity added to the impact of extra-institutional forces on admission and discharge.

Modes of Treatment at
the Utica Asylum

Once asylum doctors accepted a new patient's commitment papers and collected case history notes, legal control passed from family or community to the asylum. A matron or supervisory attendant then took charge, removing all valuable jewelry, watches, and potentially dangerous personal possessions (although in one case Utica attendants missed, hidden in a patient's shoe, the razor blades with which he subsequently killed himself), and led often apprehensive patients off to their new "home" on one of the institution's many wards. With assignment to the appropriate ward, treatment of the alleged insane was considered to have begun, for appropriate "classification" (that is, the grouping together of patients with similar behavioral problems) not only made subsequent care easier but was considered a form of therapy itself.[3] The simplest classification systems separated the recently ill, considered most likely to benefit from treatment, from the chronic, who needed primarily custodial care. Furthermore, doctors felt, the sight of incurably ill patients might well discourage those with better prognoses for recovery. Its logical extension was the development of the Willard Asylum as a complement to that at Utica. While many European asylum doctors argued that mixing different sorts of patients uplifted all, New York's asylum doctors noted (and agreed with) the distaste felt by convalescent or quiet patients at the thought of mingling with their more disturbed brethren.[4] Under such a system, critics have suggested, diagnoses were essentially irrelevant because nineteenth-century doctors used their ward classification schemes more to ensure institutional order than to promote cures.[5] While classification was so used, the doctors themselves denied the existence of a conflict between their dual goals of effective patient management and therapeutic care. In addition, both their diagnoses and ward assignments were based on the same phenomenon, external behavior, and that fact reduced somewhat the potential for arbitrary mishandling of patients.

Of course, classification was not the only kind of treatment offered asylum patients in New York State. Although they disagreed about the relative importance of moral and physical explanations for insanity, all or Utica's nineteenth-century superintendents encouraged the use of both moral and physical therapies, albeit in varying proportions and for different reasons. Before 1860 Utica's doctors relied most heavily on labor and entertainment programs to calm and divert patients; during the second half of the century, they increasingly turned to a variety of drug therapies. Evaluating the relative worth of these various therapeutic strategies was, and continues to be, almost impossible. Not all of the doctors had the same therapeutic goals and, even when they agreed with each other on the relative merits of a specific course of treatment, they seldom could agree on the best measures of success or failure.

Moral Therapy under Amariah Brigham

Without giving up his conviction that insanity was a physical disease, at Utica Brigham modified his faith in depletion therapies, which calmed the mind by emptying the body, and in the value of phrenological head measurements. Instead, like most asylum doctors of his generation, he stressed the importance of diet, sleep, and environment. Even while issuing general prescriptions, however, he insisted that, because the causes of insanity are various and complex, so too must be the remedial measures.[6]

Highly conscious of his role as an innovator, Amariah Brigham described his therapeutic programs at Utica in great detail, in both his annual reports and the early issues of the *AJI*. He felt strongly that treatment should be tied to etiology but was unable to achieve this goal. For

119

example, he complained that the common nosological scheme of the day, which divided the insane into four categories: manics, melancholics, dements, and idiots, was defective because based on symptoms rather than on the faculties of the mind which were disordered. Although he tried, he never was able to develop a useable alternative system.[7] Similarly, he argued that "mad-doctors" should link their therapeutic prescriptions to the supposed cause of insanity, but once again he found it difficult to implement such a notion in practice. Insofar as he used medicines, he relied heavily on tonics for the physically debilitated (developing his own mixture of conium, iron, molasses, wine, and water), hyoscyamus for those with sleeping problems, digitalis and similar drugs for violent manics, and opiates for the noisy. He also continued several much older therapies, occasionally calming those with "cerebral excitement" by pouring cold water on their heads and putting others in warm tubs for the same purpose.[8]

More important than the use of medicines to Brigham, however, was the so-called moral treatment of insanity.[9] Although his annual reports stressed the importance of recognizing the physiological roots of insanity, Brigham developed an imaginative variety of "moral treatments" for his patients, intended to teach them new habits of self-control and positive thinking as well as to divert them from unhealthy preoccupations. These included manual and skilled labor workshops, formal schooling (especially important, he claimed, for the demented, whose "torpid" brains needed continual exercise), and even science lectures at an asylum museum. He kept a variety of animals at the asylum to amuse patients, including deer, rabbits, tame raccoons, canaries, and peacocks. Finally, Brigham let convalescent patients attend his monthly staff meetings, at which "the nature of insanity and its peculiarities" were discussed, in the hope that better educating them about their mental illness would help prevent relapses.[10] Clearly, during Brigham's administration, the New York State Lunatic Asylum was a much more entertaining and colorful place than under his successors.

Classification, Drugs, and Restraint under John Gray

During his short tenure as superintendent, Nathan Benedict devoted most of his energy to improving the buildings and grounds of the Utica Asylum, especially the ventilation system. When Benedict was replaced by John Gray, the kinds of therapies offered at Utica were changed to reflect Gray's heavily somatic interpretation of insanity. Gray wrote innumerable essays on the vital importance of good nutrition, exercise, and sleep for the retention of sanity. He also urged his fellow doctors to avoid weakening their sick patients, especially by purgatives and bleeding. Too often, he complained, patients arrived at the Utica Asylum so physically exhausted that their bodies were beyond recuperation and their minds doomed to a lifetime of insanity. To help such patients regain strength, Gray and his staff frequently prescribed tonics and dietary supplements and force-fed all patients who missed more than one or two meals, using a wedge and spoon or stomach pump (with the additional assistance of chloroform or ether if necessary).[11] Although Gray's views on the somatic origins of insanity were controversial, most of his early treatment programs at Utica relied upon the same measures used by general physicians of the time: good food, sanitary living conditions, stimulants like alcohol, and relaxants like opium.[12]

Because of the erratic nature of patient casebook notes, it is impossible to reconstruct the relative frequency with which specific drugs were used at the Utica Asylum at different points in its history, the kinds of patients most likely to be prescribed drugs, or the frequency of use of mechanical restraints (which Gray also was accused of letting his staff use too readily).[13] Yet, even if casebook histories cannot produce quantitative measures of treatment, they do suggest the kinds of behavioral and medical problems most bothersome to the Utica medical staff and usual staff responses to them. For example, after the Civil War, patients' casebook histories began to include more detail about digestive and reproductive problems in addition to the usual indicators of mental disorder. Utica's doctors were especially concerned about constipation, diarrhea, dysmenorrhea, amenorrhea, and menopause. (Although Gray felt that many of his peers put too much emphasis on the link between female reproductive disorders and mental illness, he and his medical staff never failed to inquire into the regularity of new female patients' menstrual cycles.) Having identified patients with such problems, doctors then devoted much effort to the curing of these physical ills. In addition to prescribing well-balanced diets and rest, doctors used a number of drugs, including cathartics, emetics, and emmenogogues (particularly ergot and ferricarbons) to restore normal physical functioning.

Amariah Brigham had experimented with drug therapies, most notably with *Cannabis indica* (marijuana), and Gray and his fellow midcentury superintendents extended the use of drugs at their institutions, keeping careful clinical records. Articles by assistant physicians describing the physiological impact of specific drugs used at Utica filled the *AJI*.[14] In contrast to Brigham and Benedict, who had relied heavily upon opium, morphine, and conium to quiet disturbed patients, Gray turned first to hyoscyamia and then to sedatives, including chloral and potassium bromide, as replacements for the addictive opiates. By calming patients without the undesirable side effects of opiates, such drugs not only suppressed the most violent symptoms of mental illness but made easier the maintenance of institutional order. Characteristic of Gray's approach to the use of drugs was his 1880 tribute to hyoscyamia, in which he carefully described its dampening physiological impact on nervous and muscular excitement. He felt it worked well with a wide range of Utica's patients, from a twenty-eight-year-old male with major physical problems ("emaciated and anaemic; circulation feeble; muscles soft and flabby; skin dry and harsh; bowels constipated; and breath offensive; as well as "gloomy, reticent, seclusive," and paranoid) to an overanxious, jealous, and suicidal middle-aged woman. After receiving the drug, the patients quieted sufficiently so as to benefit from the other treatments offered them, particularly good food and rest. They also became easier to control. Following ten days of twice-daily administrations of hyoscyamia, the female patient was "quiet, ladylike, neat in person and dress," thus evidencing her convalescence. Chronic delusional patients given to destroying their clothing and "fussing and mussing" similarly improved on small doses of this drug.[15] Their case histories also make clear Gray's propensity to consider improved manners and improved bodily functions appropriate indicators of physical recovery.

While Utica's patient records, especially during the second half of the nineteenth century, included many cases of patients institutionalized for drug addiction,[16] the institution itself perpetrated startlingly similar abuses. The same doctors attempting to cure patients addicted to opiates had few qualms about prescribing large dosages of experimental drugs to other patients. Although other AMSAII members expressed reservations about heavy usage of drugs such as chloral, Gray seldom let their misgivings moderate his practice at the Utica Asylum. While not indifferent to issues of appropriate dosage, he published in the *AJI* many more essays in praise of drugs than cautionary ones. When criticized, he responded aggressively as usual. Typical was his *AJI* reprinting of a report which claimed that, even when an acutely manic patient was mistakenly given a quadruple dosage of chloral (amounting to 120 grams) in a single night, she suffered no ill effects, even managing to sleep twelve hours. Her husband, an alcoholic, was supposedly cured of delirium tremens after taking 180 grams of chloral and sleeping continuously for twenty-four hours.[17] The earliest clinical experiments with chloral in the United States had been carried on at Utica in the late 1860s, and Gray was reluctant to modify his positive impression of this hypnotic, warning only that it should be prescribed with caution for patients with weak hearts.[18] At the same time, he and his staff opposed the substitution of drugs for mechanical restraints, arguing that opiates in particular were more likely to damage patients than were straitjackets and muffs.[19]

Utica's medical staff also treated a number of more serious medical problems, including tuberculosis, a contagious disease from which many patients died. Although their numbers were small, patients with epilepsy and general paresis especially challenged the nursing skills of the asylum staff. In his annual reports, John Gray devoted more attention to the causes of death among his patients than to the causes of chronic mental illness—an index of his concern with the threat of physical disease. He shared the general nineteenth-century fear of epidemics, and in 1865 he presented the protection of his institutional family from typhus, erysipelas, small pox, and diarrhea as a major achievement. He attributed its singular good health (in contrast to that of the citizens of Utica in the same year) to the asylum's efficient ventilation system and abundant water supply.[20]

Gray's emphasis on the medical functions of the asylum was so strong that in the early 1870s he began a campaign to call his institution a hospital. If legislative funding would so increase as to raise the Utica Asylum to the level of a general hospital, he contended, more of its patients would recover, and the incurable would become more comfortable. At the same time, improved facilities for clinical and pathological research would improve doctors' understanding of mental illness.[21]

Despite his heavy emphasis on medical therapeutics, Gray did not totally eliminate all moral treatment programs at Utica, although the vehemence of his rhetoric often led critics to exaggerate the difference between him and Brigham. Probably the most frequent form of "therapy" offered at Gray's Utica between 1854 and 1884 was classification and re-classification. Particularly troublesome patients might be moved from one ward to another as often as ten times in a year. Gray did discontinue Brig-ham's schools on the grounds that they were not worth the effort they en-tailed and even injured some recovering patients, whose brains needed rest; he also eliminated many specialized workshops from the patient la-bor program.[22] But entertainments continued to be offered to staff and certain patients, and Gray long campaigned for a larger, and more acces-sible amusement hall, finally completed after his death in 1886. Gray's lack of concern (rather than a formal policy decision) also led to the grad-ual deterioration of the patient library and the dwindling of newspaper subscriptions. His position was best stated in 1869, when he argued that true relief could come only from medicine and that the "moral appliances of isolation, amusement, and so forth should receive only secondary attention."[23]

Treatment Reform under George Blumer

George Blumer, Gray's successor, was typical of those late nineteenth-century superintendents who had moved up through the ranks of asylum psychiatry. Less inclined to theoretical speculations than their predeces-sors, for the most part they continued to offer the same sorts of therapeu-tics. Blumer looked like an innovator largely because he replaced Gray, who in his last years had refused to implement even the mildest sugges-tions for reform. Immediately upon assuming office, Blumer abolished the use of mechanical restraints in the wards and sent thirty-two of the notorious "Utica cribs" to the storerooms. He also eliminated censorship of patient letters and restored many of Brigham's early programs, includ-ing craft workshops and a patient school. In so doing, he carefully pre-sented himself not as an innovator but as a preserver of the oldest (and best) of the Utica Asylum tradition. He constantly quoted Brigham and his compatriots to justify his actions.[24] (The incongruity of relying on the wisdom of men born in the age of Jefferson to deal with the social prob-lems of the Gilded Age seemed not to concern him.) In the best American tradition of moving forward while looking backward, he simultaneously asked that the New York State Lunatic Asylum become the "State Hospital for the Insane." Such a name change would help general public realize that insanity was a physical disease like all others, or so he hoped.[25] Seemingly, he failed to appreciate the extent to which general hospitals and insane asylums were moving farther apart at the end of the nineteenth century. This could be seen most clearly in a comparison of their therapeutics: even as Blumer attempted to revive moral therapy, general hospitals were moving away from such strategies toward a heavy reliance on drugs and surgery.

Family Metaphor and Asylum Treatment

Even though they paid little attention to family circumstances in their analyses of mental illness, the Utica Asylum doctors all felt that the institution had an obligation to provide its patients with a surrogate family. They thus attempted to model asylum social relations on those of the family, but one lacking the disruptive elements that had driven patients to them. Within this ideal world, the superintendent was to serve as father; patients as children; and attendants as both sometime-parents and servants. Thus, Nathan Benedict often wrote to Dorothea Dix about the concerns of "our great family." Gray too enjoyed playing the role of head of household. He ruled the institution like a true Victorian patriarch, brooking no interference with his dictates, whether from patients or staff within the institution or reformers without. Like Benedict, Gray and his assistant physicians also involved their personal families in the care of their institutional children. For example, an 1881 literary and musical entertainment at Utica featured "Mrs. Dr. Gray," Gray's daughter, his son, and assistant physician George Blumer's daughter. When one of the assistant physicians took a leave in 1885, Gray replaced him with his son, Dr. John Gray, Jr.[26]

Occasionally, New York's asylums incorporated familial experiences which asylum superintendents would have preferred to exclude. For example, in 1863 a "demented woman" at Utica gave birth to a healthy child some six months after admission. The child was kept on the ward with its mother and cared for by an attendant until the mother was well enough to help. The presence of the child, the doctors argued, helped cure the mother, who previously had been homicidal and suicidal. (This was but one of several instances of patients giving birth while institutionalized at

125

Utica, although all had been pregnant at arrival. Thus, Utica escaped the scandalous illegitimate births among patients which occasionally plagued other nineteenth-century insane asylums.) In addition, relationships formed between staff and patients occasionally developed into marriages, and several husbands took jobs as attendants in order to stay with their wives at the asylum.[27]

Somewhat surprisingly, the Utica asylum doctors showed very little interest in the preasylum family lives of their patients or in the impact of institutionalization on patients' familial ties. (Perhaps the asylum "family" was considered an adequate substitute.) And yet that impact was often devastating. Most patients institutionalized any length of time gradually lost contact with the outside world, especially if they left one institution for another. Many Utica patients felt abandoned by family and friends. As one lamented in the patient magazine, the *Opal:*

A year is gone, and five months more,
My parent, since thy face I saw,
And full twelve months have past me o'er.
Since news from thee I heard or saw.

If you had loved me as you ought
A being you had given life,
Some note or message would you not
Have sent to cheer my prison life?[28]

The Utica doctors certainly did not improve patient–family relationships by their habit of censoring or confiscating patient mail. As a result, or so charged the New York neurologist William Hammond in 1881, its inmates were as cut off from their friends as if "buried in the tomb." Even a cursory glance through Utica patient records reveals innumerable letters both from and to patients which were never delivered but bound into the casebooks as further evidence of patients' problems. Many contained bewildered inquiries to relatives asking why letters were not being answered. A number also expressed maternal anxiety about children left at home. One agitated woman was told by a friend (in a letter apparently never delivered to her) not to worry but to "leave your children in God's care and he will take care of them"—no doubt scant comfort to the disabled victim of wife abuse, whose family had been too poor to get her the medical care she needed after a hip accident.[29]

Yet another illustration of the ease with which families abandoned institutionalized members is the letter written by a bereaved daughter who bemoaned her failure to visit her mother during the latter's three years at Utica. Indicative of her loss of contact was the question directed at doctors: "Do you think she was ever very homesick there?"[30] Such distancing was not always a reflection of heartlessness, however, for many families who had waited to institutionalize members until their physical and.emotional resources were exhausted subsequently found themselves reluctant to renew close contact with those who had caused such pain. Such distancing also created problems when such patients were released, for it made reintegration into family circles difficult. For example, the family of a twenty-four-year-old patient, on being informed of their daughter's improved condition, asked the asylum doctors to keep her "until she is perfectly well," for when she was home it had been difficult to keep track of her.[31] Few of those who lost touch with their families and friends, especially if they were women, subsequently returned to the noninstitutionalized world. And those bonds were easily broken, even by those who did not wish to do so. For example, in 1888 the commissioner in lunacy noted that he often received letters from friends of institutionalized patients asking about their whereabouts and condition, especially when such patients had been removed without notice to them.[32]

Patient Perspectives on Treatment

Although doctors left long descriptions of their therapeutic goals in annual reports and journal articles, patient perspectives on treatment practices are rare. Articles in the *Opal*, a patient magazine published in the 1850s, described amusements organized by patients for each other and the general public but only obliquely indicated patients' views of such events. Typical of the *Opal's* indirection was its description of the December 1855 "Ladies' Fair," at which "the fair daughters of Asylumia" sold crafts to staff and local citizens while the asylum band played. After thanking visitors for their patronage, the *Opal* editor suggested that, if they had not known in advance, they never would have guessed that the men and women serving them were asylum patients. He also noted that the "chilly gentlemen" of the asylum appreciated the opportunity to enjoy, however, briefly, the greater warmth of the ladies' side.[33] Similar in tone to *Opal* articles were the extracts from a patient diary published in the 1840 *AJI*.

Its author had spent eighteen months at Utica in a convalescent ward where patients were offered lectures on Monday (including a life of Franklin by a professor from nearby Hamilton College), cardplaying on Tuesday and Friday evenings, debates on Wednesdays (on topics such as "Are Early Marriages Beneficial to Mankind?"), and visits led by Brigham to the Asylum Museum. Although the author painted a colorful picture of his eccentric fellow inmates, in general his relations with them were pleasant. He clearly had experienced the asylum which Amariah Brigham and his contemporaries wrote about but seldom achieved: quiet and orderly so as to calm the manic, yet with a diversity of activities to stimulate the torpid mind and divert the melancholic.[34]

An extremely different view of life at Utica that same year was presented by another ex-patient, one William Hotchkiss. The frontispiece illustration of his published account was entitled "Scenes in Third Hall— Attendant Hunt pounding a patient" and made clear the horrors of backward life, even in the asylum's early decades. Locked into an eight-foot basement cell and frightened by the screams of his fellow inmates, Hotchkiss had his leg ulcers scrubbed with a broom by a sadistic attendant, who also "playfully" threatened him with a knife. When moved upstairs to the third hall, he was attacked by a fellow patient, who in turn was hit by an attendant. Whenever his delusions returned, he was strapped into a muff: when he attempted to resist, he was chased around the room and jumped upon. Although asylum trustees occasionally inspected the hall, they refused to listen to complaints made by obviously crazy men. Eventually, Hotchkiss was removed to the first hall, where the chief attendant, himself a former patient, ran a calm and kind operation. He noted that visitors were always shown this model hall, although they were not told it was kept clean by compulsory patient labor. Hotchkiss was finally released when he followed advice given him several times during his stay: he admitted to his insanity and spoke favorably of the institution and its treatment.[35]

Hotchkiss's casebook history confirms many of the details of his book, such as his continuous restraint for the first fifteen days of his stay because he was "excited and noisy." According to his medical records, even after he began to improve and was moved to the third hall, he sometimes mistook physicians and attendants for people from Buffalo who supposedly had injured him and became very angry with them. Offered little moral

128

therapy (besides reclassification), he took endless cathartics and endured a seton in his neck for bloodletting (at which, he claimed, attendants would tug until he bled profusely). His record suggests that some of the harsher eighteenth-century methods of treating insanity persisted well into the nineteenth century, despite prominent physicians' disavowal of them.[36]

Hotchkiss ended with several perceptive criticisms of the assumptions behind moral treatment. He challenged the notion that the insane needed to be isolated from family and friends, claiming that their very hypersensitivity was likely to be better tolerated by those who loved them. Most of the asylum doctors (except Brigham), he complained, had received no special training in asylum care, and Brigham was often away. Although many families sent sick members to be treated by Brigham, they failed to realize that he himself was unable to treat (or even to take interest in) most of the patients under his charge. Finally, Hotchkiss concluded, while many of the doctors and attendants were kind, they could not eliminate abuse and violence, for the asylum "is an unwholesome and unpleasant place for all: doctors, patients, and attendants."[37]

Another relatively early account of life at Utica was published in 1855 by an ex-patient named Phoebe Davis. She too complained bitterly of patients being forced to work on threat of punishment and also of the tyranny of the asylum routine, the stench of the water closets, and the attendants' rough treatment of difficult patients. Superintendent Benedict, she felt, would have preferred a better class of patients and disliked "the grubs and the low order of bipeds" with whom he had to deal at this public institution. Whenever she disagreed with Benedict or his assistant Cook, she deliberately acted in a vulgar and coarse manner just to annoy them. Like Hotchkiss, Davis was told by an attendant that she would never be released until she treated the doctors more politely, but she claimed to have responded that, if she treated such "fashionable brutes and murderers with respect," she would feel guilty for the rest of her life. Her eventual cure, she felt, was due only to the unusual kindness shown her by several other female patients on her ward.[38]

Patients also complained of overmedication; their descriptions of doctors' indiscriminate use of drugs contrast sharply with the picture presented in *AJI* of carefully controlled experiments. One patient, Hiram Chase, claimed that a Utica doctor had ordered him to take medication for a specific problem and then continued that prescription for three years without once inquiring about its effects. He also resented having been forced to imbibe alcoholic drinks for several years, noting that he was lucky not to have become a drunkard.[39] At an 1884 legislative investigation into the management of the Utica Asylum, other ex-patients confirmed Chase's complaints about the institution's careless use of powerful drugs. Too often, untrained attendants at their own discretion ladled out doses of sedatives from quart bottles despite strict rules to the contrary. At the same hearing, a female patient also complained of having been attacked sexually by a doctor while heavily sedated. While the investigating legislators had trouble corroborating her story, they did use her testimony to rebuke asylum doctors for their excessive reliance on calming drugs.[40]

Obviously, these patient memoirs offer a skewed picture of treatment at nineteenth-century Utica, for most of their authors were patients with grievances, several of whom subsequently took to the lecture circuit with tales of the horrors of asylum life. Only the better educated patients at Utica wrote about their experiences. (None of Willard's inmates, poorer and often sicker than their Utica counterparts, left published accounts of their asylum lives.) Patients who testified at legislative investigations also stressed the darker side of asylum life. Never printed were the positive letters sent to asylum doctors by ex-patients, such as that they received by Gray in 1872 from a forty-one-year-old cabinetmaker, who thanked him for the "kind and attentive treatment" for melancholia he had received during his two and a half years at Utica. Although at admission his health had been so poor he had despaired of recovery, the ceaseless efforts of the assistant physicians had restored him to work again. Another ex-patient wrote: "I shall carry with me many happy memories of you and other friends at the Asylum."[41] Of course, such testimonials from the recovered also were unrepresentative. Utica's chronically insane, assigned to back wards until transferred to county poorhouses or Willard, left no accounts of their experiences; yet, these extremely difficult or severely incapacitated patients were most vulnerable to neglect and abuse.

Modes of Treatment at the Willard Asylum

Work Programs

The content of Willard's therapeutic programs differed substantially from Utica's for a number of reasons, including differences in patient populations, budgets, and administrators' therapeutic philosophies.[42] The roots of the differences lay in Willard's early history. In his 1860s campaign for legislative approval of Willard, John Chapin had argued repeatedly that New York taxpayers did not want to replicate for the chronically insane Utica's expensive therapeutic care but would support their cheap, humane maintenance at a large, primarily custodial asylum. Chapin and his colleague George Cook also had stressed the fiscal advantages of employing the quiet chronically insane so that they could contribute to their own maintenance costs. Since everyone agreed that moderate, regular labor was therapeutic for able-bodied patients, what was the harm, they had asked, of so arranging and systematizing that labor as to make it profitable? While they never expected the Willard Asylum to become totally self-supporting, they hoped that low per capita costs would prove that the state could offer asylum care to large numbers without violating principles of "sound political economy."[43]

Once his building campaign succeeded and he became head of the new Willard Asylum in 1869, Chapin remembered these early promises. In his annual reports, Chapin showed less concern to explicate his views on insanity and its most appropriate treatment than to reiterate, year after year, the cheapness of the care he offered at Willard. His concern to control expenses was fruitful; he spent about one-third less per patient on drugs than did John Gray, and he involved large numbers of patients in regular employment: primarily housework for the females and farm work for the males.[44] Such work opportunities were intended to contribute to patients' general well-being while in the institution but not to ease their transition back into the noninstitutional work world, for few expected the chronic afflictions of Willard's patients to be reversed. Instead, while Willard's superintendents noted the therapeutic (as well as the economic) advantages of patient labor, they expressed its therapeutic benefits in very different terms than did Utica's leaders. Rather than speeding patients' recoveries, Willard's employment programs were intended to relieve the intolerable boredom of asylum life, channel patients' physical energies into constructive pursuits (thus reducing the need to rely on restraints), and at least partially lead the chronically insane back into more rational modes of thought and health.[45]

Willard's medical staff also attempted to increase the benefits of their work programs by integrating them into institutional classification schemes. Even before Willard opened, George Cook proposed dividing its chronically insane into two groups: "the excited, paroxysmal, and grossly demented" (who would require expensive, intensive care) and the much larger "quiet, cleanly and industrial" class. Members of the latter were to be housed in economical detached buildings, according to their occupations. For example, all the farmers would live together in one cottage and the gardeners in another.[46] While Willard's work force never became sufficiently specialized to permit the full implementation of this scheme, whenever possible Chapin grouped together attendants and patients with similar work assignments. Such classification, he hoped, would improve the quality of daily life by increasing efficiency. When criticized for exploiting rather than curing his charges, Chapin counterattacked by deriding those who preferred "gilding public reports with extravagant expectations" of cures to providing for the ever-increasing numbers of chronically insane. New York's politicians, he asserted, wanted practical schemes for dealing with the chronically insane, not medical daydreams. Only cost-effective programs had any chance of winning legislative approval.[47] Bluntly he accused his critics of indifference to the chronically insane, "the most suffering, friendless, and helpless" of the dependent populations of New York.

To demonstrate the economic viability of his therapeutic programs, Chapin annually published detailed statistical summaries of the quantity of manufactured and hand-sewn goods produced in Willard's workshops, the value of its farm produce, the profits made from slaughtering pigs and cattle, and the total number of days of patient labor. This practice was continued by his successor, P. M. Wise, who proudly reported the following accomplishments for 1885.[48]

Activity	Total Number of Days of Patient Work
Farm, garden, and grounds	45,385
Barns and piggeries	7,277
Laundry and kitchen	37,288
Needlework	42,479
Tailors and tailoresses	1,277
Hall work	77,090
Carpenters, painters, shoe-makers, etc.	4,017

These statistics are somewhat difficult to evaluate, for neither Chapin nor Gray attempted to assign a dollar value to patient work nor explained how they calculated patient workdays. Casebook records suggest that many patients worked only erratically or for short periods each day. For example, one middle-aged epileptic, who became confused and somewhat violent during convulsions, worked hard "between fits." Another extremely demented female patient, though in poor physical and mental health, occasionally managed to polish ward floors. Most of those Willard patients able to work did unskilled labor, as they had before institutionalization.[49] As the 1885 statistics show, women were assigned different tasks from men and worked longer hours, largely because they labored indoors, unaffected by bad weather and darkness. Occasionally, Willard's doctors lamented the lack of outdoor work for restless female patients, but they felt that even light gardening was not suitable for women.[50]

While annual reports stressed the voluntary nature of patient labor, asylum doctors strongly encouraged unwilling but able-bodied patients to join their more industrious fellows. For example, Chapin admitted during a legislative investigation that his staff sometimes used incentives ranging from verbal suasion to the promise of tobacco rations to persuade the reluctant to work.[51] He also criticized those patients and their friends who felt that the involuntarily committed owed the state nothing. No principle of social ethics, he proclaimed, exempts certain individuals from the duty of contributing according to their capacities to their own support; furthermore, work was the activity "most conducive to health, happiness, and contentment."[52] The first New York State commissioner in lunacy similarly defended Willard's work programs: "Man was intended to labor at all periods of his life." Employment programs, he went on, not only saved money but shortened the duration of insanity, improved digestion, and lightened the spirit.[53]

Obviously, Willard's superintendents, like most nineteenth-century officials, strongly supported traditional work values and attempted to persuade all able-bodied patients to follow suit. Yet, even the most heavy-handed "moral suasion and influence" could not convince all patients to labor, and those who absolutely refused were permitted to stay on the wards. For example, one forty-eight-year-old farmer, who had been institutionalized twice before, initially worked but then stopped, claiming he had done all the work he intended to do at Willard.[54] (Here, asylums differed from nineteenth-century prisons, whose inmates did not have the luxury of preferring "listless idleness" to work.) And, of course, many patients were too ill to work. Willard's 1883 report categorized 801 patients as "able and willing to work"; 261 as "able but not willing" because of delusions or laziness; and 714 as "incompetent for mental or physical reasons."[55] These statistics substantiate the frequent complaints of Willard's superintendents that county poorhouses often sent only their most difficult patients to Willard, keeping the quiet chronically insane who made the best workers. Although even the most demented sometimes worked part-time, they could not be expected to become self-supporting.[56] Yet, even a number of actively delusional and violent patients managed to clean halls and work in the kitchen. One middle-aged woman was transferred to the main building, where she could be supervised closely, after threatening to kill fellow patients, but she continued to work in the laundry. She worked there for another twelve years until a painful cancer sent her to the infirmary and then to her death. Similarly the paranoid ravings of a young Irish farmer who claimed enemies had "pumped out his brains" did not keep him from working daily with an attendant on the asylum farm. He too left his labors only when weakened by illness.[57]

Despite their physical and mental limitations, Willard's patients made an important contribution to the institution's internal economy. The men helped in the construction of new buildings and worked on the farm; the women sewed everything from dresses and sunbonnets to bed sacks and shrouds and, at least during the institution's early years, did all the washing and ironing for more than one thousand people. In addition, fresh-air

134

employment got male patients off the wards and offered an outlet for pent-up physical energies. Skilled workers took pride in the high quality of their products, and Willard's administrators boasted of their workers' responsibility. For example, they pointed out that, although axes, picks, shovels, crowbars, and blasting powder all had been used to grade a new railroad bed, not a single patient had been injured.[58] Because patients and attendants together did almost all the construction work required for a new infirmary, it was one of the most cheaply built brick buildings in the county, or so Willard's superintendent claimed.[59] Such was the success of the Willard program that even politicians and reformers generally critical of asylums praised it. In 1880 the neurologist William Hammond suggested that New York City's insane asylums, where too many patients just sat and brooded all day, should emulate Willard; E. C. Spitzka, another neurologist well known for his attacks on state insane asylums, likewise praised Willard's management.[60]

Perhaps the major flaw in Willard's employment program was the preponderance of monotonous, physically demanding jobs. Although working patients' daily lives were more pleasant than those of patients who spent their days hunched unmoving in chairs or slumped at the side of large, barely furnished day rooms, the unrelenting tedium and hard physical labor required of those who washed clothes or sewed sheets all day did little to divert demented minds. Willard's leaders were not unaware of this problem and noted with favor the great diversity of employment available in English and Scottish asylums.[61] In 1882 the state commissioner in lunacy, Stephen Smith, recommended that New York's state asylums diversify their employment programs, in particular by expanding opportunities in mechanical trades. He offered no concrete suggestions, however, as to how superintendents constrained by limited budgets and inefficient workers might offer imaginative training programs without incurring large deficits. In general, economic considerations tended to override therapeutic ones. For example, when staff members suggested that female patients begin making clothing for male patients, Chapin agreed to support such a diversification of employment opportunities only if it saved the institution money.[62]

Clearly, employing the largest possible number of patients for maximum profits was Willard's primary objective. This goal enjoyed wide popular support. While a few critics worried about exhausting already physically and mentally weakened patients, more complained that the asylum was too lenient with those unwilling to work. For example, in 1883 the commissioner in lunacy criticized Willard's employment practices, noting that during the preceding year the asylum had employed only 38.2 percent of its male inmates and 37.6 percent of its females. In contrast, some county institutions had managed to put as many as 75 percent of their chronically insane patients to work.[63] While he agreed that patient labor should be voluntary, he suggested that financial compensation of a limited sort might motivate the reluctant to work. Once again, his recommendations ignored several important realities of the Willard situation. For example, when he urged Willard's doctors to adjust labor assignments daily, he did not explain how they were to add this new task to their already heavy daily responsibilities.[64] His critique highlighted without resolving the contradictory aims of Willard's labor program: to make money at the same time as it met the individual therapeutic needs of large numbers of patients. Unskilled nineteenth-century labor seldom satisfied both these goals, either inside the asylum or outside.

Like Chapin, his successor, P. M. Wise, also spent most of his time trying to keep his charges clean, active, and in good health. He, too, stressed the advantages of decent custodial care for those who had been abused and neglected in county poorhouses. As Willard moved closer to becoming a "mixed" institution, however, Wise revived the rhetoric of moral treatment to justify his continued heavy reliance on work programs. The "proper application of moral and industrial conditions to the specific requirements of individual patients," he claimed, was what distinguished Willard from county asylums. Willard could offer such care because it has a one-to-ten attendant–patient ratio, in contrast to most counties' ratio of one to twenty-five.[65] Principally a caretaker, not an innovator, Wise managed to preserve the positive public image of Willard built up by Chapin. Of course, in many respects Willard was not held to very high standards. As one newspaper noted, so long as the institution was clean and its patients reasonably healthy, few were willing to criticize Willard. Cure or release rates were considered irrelevant to its mission.[66] Not until after 1890, when the institution began to accept acute as well as chronic cases, did it find itself subject to the critical public scrutiny under which Utica had operated for most of the century.

Moral Treatment

Classification Schemes. Like all nineteenth-century asylum doctors, the Willard staff saw classification as an important part of their moral treatment program. Most consistently, Willard's medical staff divided patients into two groups: the "orderly, harmless, and industrious" and the "turbulent, noisy, and violent."[67] Such simplistic schemes were not unique to Willard; outside the institution, reformers and the general public alike tended to think of the insane as consisting of two equally broad and heterogeneous groups: the acute and the chronic mentally ill.[68] While this brace of dichotomies was not congruent, it did reflect a general tendency within and without the asylum to see the insane in either the cheering light of hope or the gloom of resignation. Furthermore, as Superintendent Chapin predicted even before Willard opened, the larger an institution's population, the more rigid must be its discipline. Inevitably, at an institution like Willard, "the individual is submerged in the mass."[69] Yet, so powerful was the ideal of individualized treatment in nineteenth-century psychiatry that he continued to dream of providing each of his almost two thousand patients with a personally tailored moral treatment program. Here his comments suggest an important reason for the popularity of classification schemes in nineteenth-century asylums: they promised that standardization and individualization were not incompatible.

Perhaps Willard's most famous classificatory achievement was its development of an elaborate "cottage system." Rather than keeping all patients in a single, massive building, its doctors sent the quiet chronically insane to detached buildings scattered across the grounds, while keeping the violent and physically ill in a central administrative unit. In theory, once assigned to a detached building, patients had more independent, less routinized lives. Yet this ideal was seldom achieved. Typically manics, melancholics, the demented, the epileptics, whose only shared quality was their offensiveness, were all jumbled together into detached cottages. And Willard's overworked physicians showed relatively little interest in training such chronically insane people to handle freedoms they were unlikely ever to enjoy. From the beginning, the primary rationale for Willard's congregate system was fiscal, not therapeutic. As a result, with the exception of a parole program which involved only small numbers of patients, the rhetoric of individualized treatment which occasionally surfaced in annual reports bore little resemblance to practice. While the daily lives of those patients who helped with the farming certainly differed from those of bedridden syphilitic and tubercular patients, for both groups the days were organized around an unchanging routine, for both work and leisure hours.

The regimented quality of daily life at Willard validated those who had argued that large institutions were bound to substitute regimented control for individualized treatment. Yet, while Willard's overworked doctors may readily have relied upon rigid daily schedules, they certainly never achieved total control over those in their charge. Attendants drank or slept on duty; patients ran away, struck each other, and mutilated themselves. Violent patients posed a particularly troublesome challenge. Their casebook records overflow with stories of patients attacking one another. Such conflicts could produce serious bodily injuries as well as fear and humiliation. For example, one woman suffered a severed artery when a fellow patient struck her over the forehead with an earthen vessel.[70] A male patient was bitten on the forefinger by "a vicious epileptic" with whom he was having "some difficulty." His entire hand became inflamed before doctors noticed the injury and treated it.[71] A third patient, himself a violent epileptic, in the course of "some trouble with a patient named Brown" was struck on the head with a chair so that two-thirds of his ear was severed from his head.[72] Not surprisingly, such ward violence exacerbated many patients' tendency to withdraw. As doctors characterized one middle-aged man in 1881, "He keeps aloof from everyone and refuses to talk with others for fear that they will undermine or injure him."[73] Other patient records note with relief: "makes no assaults unless provoked." Despite the description of Willard's quiet daily routine offered in annual reports, medical and casebook records make clear that the crowding together of large groups of disturbed people frequently produced a frightening and disheartening living situation.

According to Willard's superintendents, their high attendant–patient ratios supposedly were sufficient to ensure "constant watching" and thus to prevent untoward incidents. Casebook records make clear that, even when present on the ward, attendants often could not intervene quickly enough to protect their charges from each other. While many outbursts were unpredictable, some assaultive patients had a long history of violence. A few were restrained physically, particularly if destructive at night, or moved to single rooms. Most often, if on a quiet ward, noisy, violent patients were transferred to one filled with like men or women. Such moves protected those left behind but created a new sort of hell for the transfers. Surrounded by shouting demented people, those with tendencies toward destructive behavior frequently worsened. And the old and others who needed extra care because of physical weaknesses found themselves particularly vulnerable to attacks. Here, the therapeutic limitations of classification once again became obvious. One demented woman was "quarrelsome and abusive" to her weaker associates for some six years in the 1880s; not until she started to attack doctors and attendants as well was she transferred to the main building for close observation.[74]

Ironically, only therapeutic inefficiency kept the situation in such wards from becoming intolerable. No matter how hard they tried to create a perfect classificatory system, Willard's physicians failed to do so. Wards intended for one type of patient quickly became mixed owing to overcrowding and shifts in patients' behavior. Thus, on the one hand, neither the daily lives of the insane nor the details of their environment were fixed and stable, despite doctors' best efforts to make them so.[75] On the other, no one ward contained only screaming or filthy demented patients. Most (to varying degrees) had a mixture of patients in quiet and agitated stages. In cases of intrapatient violence, inadequate supervision worked to patients' disadvantage, but in other cases it permitted a welcome break from daily routines. Male attendants and patients who worked in the fields found it particularly easy to circumvent institutional surveillance. A number of patients housed in detached buildings managed to "elope." One such patient escaped twice, the first time while going from the Assembly Hall to his cottage in the late evening and the second on his way to the vegetable cellar.[76] Patients most often tried to elope early in their stay at Willard, and many returned voluntarily, content to have seen once again family members and friends. That attendants failed to notice until the early morning the absence of a patient who had run away the evening before suggests again that regulation of daily life was less than total.[77]

Because the aggregation of chronic patients was a new experiment, traditional classification schemes also did not take into account the special medical needs of many of Willard's patients. Almost as soon as the institution opened, the medical staff realized that the effective care of physically debilitated or extremely demented patients required a separate infirmary, with extra bathing and washing facilities and better ventilation.[78] They began to lobby for funds to build an infirmary in the 1870s, but it took more than a decade to get the necessary appropriation from the legislature. Without infirmary care, offering helpless patients even that minimal requisite of moral therapy—a healthful, well-organized environment—became a draining responsibility. Staff members were required not only to contain the noise and chaos created by such patients but also to keep the incontinent clean, restrain the violent without excessive physical force, and watch over convulsive epileptics around the clock.[79] Although only about one-quarter of Willard's patients could not care for themselves, the custodial burden of that group absorbed institutional energies disproportionate to their numbers. For example, in 1880, despite close surveillance by attendants, a ward of 42 demented men reportedly required 532 baths and destroyed 2,996 separate pieces of clothing and bedding in a single week. Large numbers of Willard's patients were wet or dirty at night, had to be dressed and undressed, and fought off efforts to care for them.[80] Without an organized night service for the "filthy insane" until late in the century, attendants found such men and women each morning "literally wallowing in their own excrement." Patients also frequently injured themselves during the unsupervised evening hours. For example, when a paretic fell from his bed one night and fractured his clavicle, he lay in pain until attendants unlocked the door in the morning. The patient never recovered from the resulting paralysis.[81] When New York State's commissioner in lunacy confronted such early morning sights and smells during an inspection visit in 1880, he expressed amazement that staff members were willing to tackle such cleaning tasks at any price.[82]

Given such daunting therapeutic challenges, in many respects Willard's patient care was remarkably good. In addition to keeping death rates relatively low,[83] Chapin's most impressive accomplishment as its superintendent was his successful campaign to limit use of mechanical restraints. While John Gray of Utica bitterly attacked English experiments in the abolition of restraints, Chapin eagerly investigated them and in 1881 introduced similar reforms at Willard. By requiring daily reports from wards on the number of patients in restraint, eliminating the system of charging damages to patients' home counties, and improving the quality of attendant care, he managed to reduce the average number of patients in restraint from 5 percent of the daily population in 1874 to .5 percent in 1881.

Years later, he attributed much of his success to the support he had received from a young "God fearing but not man fearing" Irish attendant. When challenged by Chapin to take care of four particularly noisy and destructive patients without the use of restraints, she did so with ease. Her success proved to fellow attendants that even the most refractory of patients could be tamed.[84] Once Chapin left Willard, his successor continued a modified version of his policy. In 1885, for example, 6 patients (out of a daily average of 1,835) were restrained, and only 4 in 1886 (2 of whom had attempted to tear off surgical dressings).[85] Instead of bundling difficult patients into straitjackets or cribs, Willard's doctors transferred them: from dormitories to single rooms, from detached buildings to "Main."

Entertainments. In addition to work and classification programs, Willard offered a modest recreational program based on "the proper application of moral and industrial conditions to the specific requirements of individual patients," or so its doctors claimed. Yet, despite such boasting, the range of diversions offered to patients was quite narrow, and with the exception of work programs, the number of patients involved was small. For example, although Superintendent Wise boasted of his school for patients (established many years after Gray had eliminated such classes at Utica), no more than forty of his almost two thousand charges ever attended classes at one time.[86] Although his initial instructional goals were modest—not education but the stimulation of "thought in connected ideas" so as to slow or reverse patients' deterioration into dementia—he subsequently limited them even further. With 33 of Willard's 2,255 patients attending school, Wise commented, at least it got a few patients off their wards each day.[87] Similarly, during all of 1882, fewer than half of the patients even were taken "in squads of forty or more" on group walks, despite the beauty of Willard's rolling acres. A handful with "parole" privileges were allowed to take brief walks by themselves or with approved companions.[88] Religion played an equally minor role in the asylum's daily routine, although three local clergymen, including an Irish Catholic priest, were available to minister to patients' spiritual needs, especially at the point of death.[89]

Willard's requests to the legislature for a library for their many patients who enjoyed reading was turned down, perhaps because legislators found it hard to imagine that the chronically insane might enjoy reading. Also turned down were requests for funds to improve the grounds, although

141

doctors argued that even poor, intellectually disordered patients could appreciate the beautiful and had a right to minimal ornamentation of their "life abode." [90] Only superficial efforts were made to give a homelike aura to the massive halls. One visitor pointed with delight to a few rocking chairs, two canaries, and the lack of patients sleeping on the floor as evidence of Willard's success in recreating the appearance of home on one of the better wards. [91] Chapin greeted the hanging of pictures on the asylum walls with similar elation: "We cannot measure the imperceptibly good influence such objects exert, and the relief from asylum monotony they insensibly produce. [92] Of course, life on the wards for violent or ill patients lacked even these amenities.

With the help of private donations, plays and concerts were put on for the benefit of quiet patients and the staff. At various times, local philanthropists also financed a patient library, decorations for ward walls, landscaping, and Christmas presents for patients. [93] But such privately funded amenities tended to reach only a small number of the almost two thousand patients. And the extraordinary attention given to the Christmas celebration of 1888 suggests the rarity of such festivities at the asylum. According to one local newspaper reporter, most of the patients had long ago been forgotten by their friends and had not celebrated Christmas in many years. When Superintendent Wise's appeal for gifts and money evoked a generous response, he was able to provide presents for everyone. The resulting celebration seemed "to awake the dullest intellect and bring smiles to faces to which smiles are strangers." Patients long forgotten by families were overjoyed to receive even the smallest token. One elderly woman broke into tears when she received gifts from her son, saying, "Oh Look! My boy has thought of me—see, each has written on it 'From _____ to Mother'; that is better than all the rest." In a telling analogy, another reporter infantilized the inmates, describing them as "happy as any children among the cozy homes of our state." [94]

When criticized for inadequate recreational programs, Willard's doctors always responded that, however tedious their lives, patients were better off in a state asylum than in a county poorhouse, and in a number of respects they were right. At Willard, many of the physically weak regained their health; drugs eased the pain of dying; a few acute manics and melancholics even recovered. Nonetheless, as the attention given the 1888 Christmas party suggest, life in a nineteenth-century asylum for the chronically insane was still painfully circumscribed. For the most part, patients were left to their own highly limited resources. They lacked even access to the alcohol which solaced so many attendants. Casebook notes record in fatalistic detail the various ways in which patients gradually lost interest in the unchanging life around them. Content to attribute such worsening mental states to the progress of disease, doctors did little to reawaken those who withdrew. So long as they bothered no one, patients were allowed to sit for hours at a time, often with faces averted or covered. One such woman, an Irish domestic, had been admitted in 1869, with periodic mania. Although initially sociable, by 1874 she refused to move from her favorite spot in the hall. There she sat, day in and day out, with her head bent and eyes closed. Yet, doctors insisted, she was "usually happy" and in good bodily health. Her condition changed little over the next twelve years, and she finally died of tuberculosis. Similarly, when another patient spent almost two years with her face covered with a handkerchief, the staff did not interfere.[95]

Such cases suggest that mass custodial care, no matter how well intentioned, often had negative results. Yet weighing its relative advantages and disadvantages was as difficult in the nineteenth century as in the twentieth. Two newspaper reporters who visited Willard in the 1880s came away with dramatically different impressions. One saw patients sitting tranquilly on the lawn in "blissful inactivity," protected from the "toil and weariness" which had driven them to the institution. For them, he speculated, Willard must seem "a haven of rest, a land of pleasant dreams."[96] The other exclaimed, "It is appalling. It is pitiful. Gray-haired old men playing at innocent games like children of four years. Venerable ladies happy with a piece of string and a bright bit of tin. There is mental ruin everywhere." He, too, found patients sitting on the lawn, staring out over the lake, but noticed not "the low murmur of the waves" but the massive officer who stood watch over them.[97]

Medical Care

Because of their patients' many medical problems, Willard's doctors and attendants paid as much, if not more, attention to their physical as their psychic needs. In theory, they felt strongly that the two were closely related; in practice, keeping patients alive was a more immediate challenge than controlling their delusions.[98] As a result, doctors took almost as many notes about patients' physical vitality as mental health, noting improvements with joy and deterioration with dismay. In some cases, the maintenance of physical well-being was the institution's only accomplishment. For example, a patient admitted in 1870 was described in both 1875 and in 1877 as in good bodily health although he had not spoken since admission.[99] In addition to casebook records, notes about patients' health also were made in the clinical recordbooks Willard's doctors began to maintain in 1886, only two of which are extant. That for male patients in the main building shows the medical staff responding to a wide range of problems, from life-threatening diseases like cancer and angina to acute conjunctivitis, scurvy, fractured bones, and bruised ribs. Together with annual report statistics, it makes clear that tuberculosis, pneumonia, and diarrhea were the doctors' most persistent medical challenges.[100] Tuberculosis, in particular, killed large numbers of men and women, a number of whom apparently contracted the disease after coming to Willard. Their casebook records suggest that Willard's doctors often failed to notice the symptoms of tuberculosis until afflicted patients were at the point of death. Yet they knew it was a major institutional problem, for when they performed postmortems, doctors almost always looked first for tubercular deposits in the lungs. Like their peers outside the institution, Willard's doctors could do little for their tubercular patients except ease physical discomfort. Pneumonia, diarrhea, and dysentery were less often fatal, unless patients were already enfeebled. Typically doctors treated such illnesses with opiates and nourishing diets.[101]

Perhaps the most demanding of Willard's patients were those with epilepsy or tertiary syphilis. They often arrived at Willard in acute physical distress, like the epileptic patient brought in unconscious on a stretcher, his right side twitching convulsively. He was but one of the increasing number of terminally ill patients transferred to Willard from New York's acute care asylums toward the end of the century.[102] While at the institution, epileptic patients often injured themselves during convulsions. Those with frequent convulsions were prescribed sodium bromide or chloral to control seizures. After taking a forty-gram dose, one such epileptic stopped convulsing but sank into a stupor and suffered partial paralysis of the glutineal muscle. Paretics seized with convulsions were treated similarly. When one begged for medicine to stop his fits, the doctors first prescribed thirty grams of potassium bromide every hour and, when that dosage failed, another twenty grams of chloral hydrate. Not surprisingly, the patient then "passed into quiet sleep." Epileptics, in particular, both discouraged and irritated the Willard medical staff, who felt they should be segregated from all other patients.[103]

Like their Utica counterparts, Willard's doctors also lived in constant fear that contagious diseases might infect their closely knit community. As Chapin pointed out, even the aggregation of several hundred healthy people posed sanitary problems. When a large proportion of a population was bedridden, helpless (from physical debility, old age, or paralysis), low in vitality, and filthy in habits, the potential for medical disaster was enormous. While he refused to admit patients from areas known to be infected with smallpox or measles and, beginning in 1874, vaccinated old and new patients, occasionally these preventive measures failed.[104] Imperfect sanitary arrangements also created health problems. In 1872 large numbers of Willard's staff and patients succumbed to a typhoidlike fever which they attributed to a polluted water supply. The problem was solved temporarily when sewage pipes were renovated directly into Seneca Lake, but typhoid fever itself appeared in the mid-1880s. While John Gray measured success in terms of the numbers of patients who recovered each year, at the end of 1881 John Chapin was content to sigh, "It is a relief to have passed through it without any serious calamity to persons or property under our charge."[105]

For a long time, the legislature refused to fund an infirmary for Willard on the grounds that its patients needed only the most minimal care: fresh air, adequate food, clean clothing, and suitable employment.[106] Meeting even these basic needs of heavily demented patients was not, however, always easy. Several refused to eat because they feared being poisoned and fought off stomach tubes so strongly that doctors could not force sufficient nourishment upon them. Furthermore, asylum doctors, like their counterparts in private practice, were stymied when tonics and nutritious foods failed. The emaciated frames of such patients frustrated physicians who often measured good health in terms of ample flesh. Typical was the fifty-five-year-old woman who, despite daily doses of morphine, iron extract, and stimulants, had "scarcely more than a skeleton left" when she died in January of 1871. Baffled doctors attributed the deaths of such patients to "exhaustion resulting from chronic mental disease."[107]

For the most part, Willard's doctors practiced reactive, not proactive,

145

medicine. Constrained to offer the cheapest possible care, their annual per capita expenditure on drugs was substantially lower than Utica's. Chapin also was less enamored of chemical solutions to psychiatric problems than his Utica counterpart, Gray. He preferred to allow noisy patients to rant and rave and the demented to tear their clothing. Perhaps because drugs were considered a last resort, however, once they decided to prescribe, the Willard medical staff used a wide range, often in combination. They seemed little concerned about possible overdoses or negative interactions, despite the many published discussions of such complications. For example, one manic male was given forty grams of sodium bromide at admission. Still boisterous the next morning, he was given a hot bath, *Cannabis indica*, and thirty more grams of sodium bromide three times in ten hours until he finally fell asleep. Another acute manic was given milk, whiskey, and thirty grams of sodium bromide four times a day. The first patient, a middle-aged man not otherwise ill, recovered; the second, an aging paretic, died.[108] Willard's doctors in the 1870s and 1880s prescribed what Eric Carlson and Maribeth Simpson call (in reference to opiates) the "short heroic treatment": large doses of sedative drugs given for a brief time.[109] Such a practice was cheaper than long-term drug programs and lessened the risk of addiction.

Treatment of Sexual Disorders.   Perhaps the most controversial medical treatments offered at late nineteenth-century asylums were those devised for patients with sexual problems or abnormal sexual appetites. The New York asylum doctors devoted little special attention to such patients, however, and neither the Utica nor Willard asylums performed clitoridectomies. When a thirty-one-year-old male imbecile was castrated at Willard, the rare operation was performed at his mother's request.[110] Although many nineteenth-century doctors physically restrained masturbating patients, Willard's doctors for the most part treated excessive masturbation as a sign, not a cause, of mental disturbance and simply moved the most demented of such patients to intensive care wards, where attendants relied upon surveillance to break them of their "filthy" habits. Occasionally the abuse they prevented was genuinely harmful. At the daily bath of one female self-abuser, an attendant removed from her vagina a ball of cotton yarn, two thimbles, one large spool, a hair pin, the stem of a leaf, and quantities of paper and rags.[111] Occasional masturbators, if they showed no other signs of disturbed behavior, were left alone. For example, in

1875 an assistant physician noted the masturbatory habits of a delusional young Irish man but also described him as "always quiet and orderly" and permitted him to go to and from his work at the branch alone. A man institutionalized because of his unnatural sexual appetites, too often inflicted upon his unwilling wife, quieted quickly at the institution and was released.[112]

Some of the Willard doctors' relative indifference to masturbation may have reflected social attitudes toward their mainly lower-class patients. Vieda Skultans suggests that, for nineteenth-century psychiatrists, young middle-class men were most vulnerable to masturbational insanity because they needed self-control in order to succeed.[113] More likely, however, they could see no point in disciplining extremely demented masturbators, such as the man who sat all day looking at the floor, unable to give his name and making hissing sounds with his mouth.[114] At the same time, they always noted instances of masturbation in individual patient records. One single female patient admitted for the second time in 1878 was described as "foolish in manner" with a "sexual weakness which would render her unsafe to be abroad." She masturbated frequently and exposed herself to male patients. Although Willard's doctors clearly did not approve of this behavior, they did nothing more than note its continuation for the next twelve years.[115]

Generally, Willard's doctors wrote of sexual and gynecologic problems in a straightforward fashion. Consistent with the notion that female insanity often was limited to problems with reproductive organs, Willard's female physician (hired in 1885) spent much of her time giving patients vaginal and uterine examinations. She filled an entire clinical record book with detailed descriptions of her findings. Of the 389 patients examined between September of 1885 and November of 1886, only 4 were described as having "normal" reproductive organs. The rest suffered from lacerated perineum or cervix, prolapsed or retroflexed uterus, vaginal discharge, or fibroid tumors. Having noted these problems, the doctor did little for them beyond painting cervixes with iodine and soothing irritated areas with glycerin pads. Embarrassed patients often resisted such gynecologic examinations. One protested that she felt disgraced; another responded by first fainting and then becoming hysterical.[116] Even questions embarrassed patients, especially when they came from male doctors. When asked about her dysmenorrhea, one middle-aged woman protested that other patients could hear the question.[117] Occasionally, patients resisted so violently as to make examinations impossible, but usually doctors overcame their resistance by force if necessary. At the other extreme, even female doctors found that patients occasionally became "erotic" during examinations; they also found evidence of masturbation in swollen and tender vaginal areas. For the most part, however, Willard's doctors drew no link between sexual habits or delusions and uterine conditions. Despite the large numbers of female patients who died of tuberculosis, only two instances of tubercular problems occur in the eighth volume of the women's clinical record book. Several tumors were noted, and occasional heart problems. But, whatever the presenting symptoms, Willard's female doctor performed pelvic examinations on her patients.

Patient Views on Treatment

Despite their limitations, memoirs by ex-asylum patients offer glimpses of daily life within the asylum not available in annual reports. Unfortunately, because so few of Willard's patients were ever released, they left no published accounts of their stay. In addition, because their correspondence with family members and friends was not restricted, no unmailed letters home remain in casebook records. Thus it becomes necessary to look for indirect evidence of patients' feelings about their lives in documents such as the reports produced by local superintendents of the poor after their visits to Willard. In 1887 county supervisors checking on the care of Westchester patients found themselves besieged with patients asking, "Are you going to take me home?"[118] Patient casebook records make clear that a number of patients tried to run away, but most lacked the social skills and physical strength required to live outside the institution. Within it, at best they were treated like unpromising children. One assistant physician described his patients as "ignorant, uneducated, and naturally of simple tastes." Manual labor, preferably out of doors, he declared, was the most appropriate form of moral treatment for such men and women, who neither required nor appreciated "extravagant surroundings and grand and palatial structures."[119] Whether or not patients agreed, no one knows.

Discharges and Cures

Most nineteenth-century critics measured insane asylums' success or failure in terms of cure rates, although asylum doctors constantly complained about the inappropriateness of such imperfect measures. As one noted, asylum doctors variously labeled patients "recovered," "restored," "cured," "in usual health," "improved," "very much improved," "unimproved," and so forth without specifying what they meant by such terms.[120] Although New York State's discharge laws specified that only asylum trustees could release the institutionalized insane, they did not define what was meant by "completely recovered" or "incurable." One judge tried to clear up the confusion by ruling that the insane could not be released from asylums just because relatives agreed to keep them at home. He trumpeted that they first must be judged harmless "beyond the possibility of a doubt,"[121] but he failed to indicate how such an unmistakable determination might be made.

At both the Utica and Willard asylums, doctors and managers struggled to established uniform definitions of recovery, and they participated in the national discussion about discharge policies carried on at AMSAII meetings. But neither the New Yorkers nor their counterparts elsewhere succeeded in producing a valid, reliable definition of mental health, any more than they could agree on one of mental illness. Initially, Brigham offered some fairly simple guidelines. Upon "complete restoration of mental powers," patients were declared to have recovered. Discharged as "improved" were the "nearly well" and those who, though still insane, had become amenable to control by friends.[122] Brigham's successor, Benedict, was more cautious, preferring to label many cases "improved" rather then "recovered," especially those whose insanity had been caused by intemperance, epilepsy, senility, and fits because of the frequency with which such patients relapsed.[123] Early in his career, Gray also began to discharge as "improved" those who had received all possible benefits from institutionalization. Though not fully sane, they were now able to make themselves useful at home.[124] Well aware that public outrage swelled as readily when released patients relapsed as when recovered patients were not released, Gray increasingly preferred to release patients as "improved" rather than "recovered." Evidence of his caution can be seen in

149

the stories of two patients released in 1857 as "improved but not recovered" and who promptly got demanding white collar jobs.[125] With the help of such deft turns of terminology, the Utica Asylum was able to move patients in and out more quickly, without risking community wrath for certifying as cured those who subsequently relapsed.

All across nineteenth-century America, the so-called cult of curability encouraged asylum superintendents to inflate their patient recovery rates. Like most of his fellows, Gray argued that the best measure of his treatment programs was the annual ratio of those released "cured" to new patients that year (Fig. 5.1), for such a ratio eliminated those long-time inhabitants of the institution whose insanity had become entrenched even before admission. Each year, however, he also calculated recovery statistics based on the average and total number of patients treated that year (Fig. 5.1). But no matter how such statistics were calculated, the number of patients released as recovered declined over time at Utica. After 1856 it never went above 16 percent, and by 1890 it had fallen below 11 percent. By themselves, however, recovery figures understate patient turnover. While each successive year saw fewer of the "recovered" discharged, the percentage of residents who left the institution remained comparatively stable. Predictably it peaked at almost 44 percent in the early decades of Utica's history, but it remained between 35 and 40 percent for most of the nineteenth century. These rates suggest that there was a substantial annual turnover of patients each year at the New York State Lunatic Asylum for most of the nineteenth century.

Not surprisingly, the situation at Willard was dramatically different. Most patients, once admitted, never left. Two British historians found that, at the Colney-Hatch Asylum, the patients most likely to recover were those suffering mild forms of mania and melancholia not complicated by dementia, paralysis, or fits.[126] The same was true at Utica, but there, exit-level statistics clearly reveal less about the curability of certain forms of mental illness than about diagnostic patterns. Patients initially diagnosed as acute manics or melancholics, who then did not recover within a year or two, were often rediagnosed as chronically afflicted or as demented. (Even if their degree of mental illness did not intensify, long-term institutional life seemed to have a negative effect on many patients.) Those arriving in poor condition bore such diagnostic labels from the beginning. The one notable exception was the category of violent, even

150

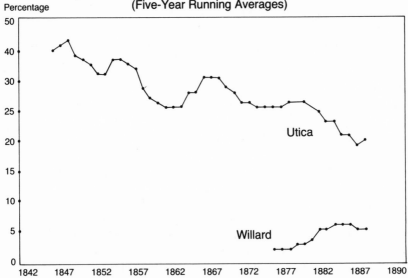

Figure 5.1. "Recovered" as a Percentage of Admissions (Five-Year Running Averages)

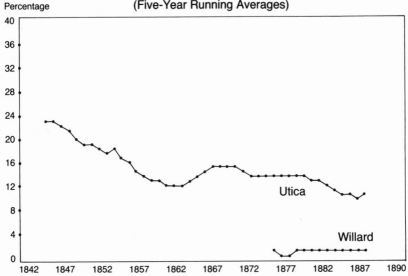

Figure 5.2. "Recovered" as a Percentage of Those Treated (Five-Year Running Averages)

Data is taken from the Utica *Annual Reports*, 1843–1890.

"delirious" manics whose agitation was relatively recent. Under the influence of tranquilizing drugs, such patients (even at Willard) frequently recovered.

However much the patient movement in and out of Utica, its therapeutic success still was much less spectacular than that anticipated by its early supporters. In anticipation of criticism from disappointed legislators, Gray argued for a broader conception of his institution's function. Many long-term inmates slowly improved their personal habits, if not their minds, as a result of exposure to the Utica Asylum's discipline, he claimed. Others, before they improved, passed through stages of such acute mania that their friends could never have controlled them;[127] thus the asylum served a protective as well as a therapeutic function. Many of Gray's points were important ones. Although nineteenth-century asylum critics considered recidivism rates evidence of medical failure, twentieth-century historians need not repeat their mistake. As Gray noted, all diseases are liable to recur, especially if their original causes persist. Given the frequency with which released patients plunged themselves back into routines of overwork, poor diet, and lack of sleep, he marveled that recurrences were not more frequent. Asylum superintendents also recognized the contribution of poverty to relapses. The poor, they argued, "harassed by the wants of poverty," isolated from friends, frequently rejected by former employers, easily became first anxious and sleepless and then relapsed.[128]

Despite Gray's recognition of the need for them, few nineteenth-century asylum doctors attempted to set up aftercare programs for released patients to help prevent such relapses. But they did attempt to make sure before release that patients had the resources necessary to sustain financial and emotional independence. Utica's patient casebook records suggest that most patients were released only if and when their families promised to take subsequent care of them. In marginal cases, families had to post bond as surety. The Utica superintendents knew well that those same newspapers which excoriated them for supposedly detaining "sane" patients like James Silkman and Clarissa Lathrop against their will became equally savage when "prematurely released" patients turned violent in their home communities.[129]

While nineteenth-century doctors may have had some influence over their admission policies (albeit a very limited one at state asylums), they certainly did not control discharge decisions. Both the state and patients' families demanded a voice in the release process. Initially, by legislative fiat, the New York State Lunatic Asylum was supposed to hold indigent patients at least six months but no more than two years.[130] Those who did not recover within two years were considered unlikely to do so. Because state care was expensive, legislators reasoned, it should be reserved for those most likely to benefit from it. Asylum doctors did not like to release patients unimproved, for they knew that many would spend the rest of their lives in a county poorhouse. In addition, they pointed out that patients who had remained at the Utica Asylum for years sometimes recovered unexpectedly. If such patients had been relegated to a poorhouse, they might never have recovered. Private patients could stay as long as families continued to pay for their care and the asylum had sufficient space for them; paupers stayed longer than two years, if their home counties did not complain. When, however, local superintendents of the poor arrived at the asylum to take long-term patients back to county poorhouses, where the costs of care were lower than at Utica, the asylum doctors had to release them. Other times, they initiated such transfers themselves (albeit reluctantly) to make room for the ever increasing numbers of newly stricken insane persons.[131] Once Willard opened in 1869, Utica's doctors immediately transferred many chronic cases there. Late in the century, in response to local political pressures, they also let return home a few men and women whom they considered to be "harmless and probably to continue so and not likely to be improved by further treatment in the asylum." They hoped that such individuals, even if not "cured," would contribute to their own support and eventually become independent.[132] John Gray also regularly released a small number of patients, mostly hysterics, alcoholics, and drug addicts, as "not insane," for he attributed their afflictions to moral weakness, not mental illness. He also used the rubric "not insane" in some more puzzling ways, as when he discharged the female chlorotic whose diet of spices, cloves, chalk, slate-pencils, and limes had several times induced a state of hysterical catalepsy so profound she was considered dead. Feeble and pale, hemorrhaging from the lungs, she also had attempted to commit suicide by taking overdoses of opium. Her release as "not insane" suggests the arbitrariness with which diagnoses were occasionally made.[133]

Whatever their feelings about release policies, doctors' discussions showed no concern for the patients' perspective on the issue. Yet many patients were extremely homesick, and others deeply hated institutional life. One male epileptic at Utica in the 1880s wrote to his sister: "I feel very lonesome here. I feel very lonesome for Lizzie and the baby, but they wont let a person go home without the consent of the person that sent them here. I want Lizzie to write to them and tell them to let me go home. I would be better to home." [134] The letter was never sent; we know of its existence only because one of the assistant physicians quoted it in an article as an example of the echo sign in epilepsy. Others complained that patients were kept long past recovery, a charge whose truth Brigham admitted in his fourth annual report. Such patients, he claimed, often served as a useful class of assistants to the staff and thus contributed to the good order and comfort of their fellows. [135] Patients, however, sometimes regarded such use of their talents as exploitative. One who spent two long years on the so-called convalescent ward tried several times to convince visiting friends of his sanity, but his entreaties had only embarrassed them. All patients and attendants knew, he noted bitterly, that if a man claimed not to be insane, he thereby proved he was. Another managed to gain interviews with both John Ordronaux and Stephen Smith, commissioners in lunacy. Although the two were friendly and listened attentively to his story of having been railroaded into the asylum by unscrupulous business associates, they took no action. More successful in gaining the initiative for their release were the very few patients who, after the Civil War, won habeas corpus suits against the asylum. While their trials attracted much newspaper publicity, few other asylum patients had the financial or social resources to use the legal system to gain their freedom. [136] Whether sane or insane, patients correctly perceived that asylum doctors wished to keep discharge judgments in their own hands. When occasionally families removed private patients against medical advice, doctors not only expressed concern for the patients' subsequent welfare but also threatened to lobby for the statutory power to monopolize removal decisions. [137]

Willard's doctors less frequently struggled with the difficult task of defining recovery because they expected most of the chronically insane paupers to remain at the asylum until death. To deal with those who showed potential for release, they proposed several times that state legislators legalize the conditional discharge of "harmless patients who have homes, or friends willing to take them."[138] Politicians' reluctance to grant their request again reflected the general public's fear of asylum patients, whatever their mental condition. While waiting for political action, Willard initiated a parole system designed to give convalescent patients slowly increasing amounts of personal freedom. Since such efforts reached very few patients, Willard's recovery rates seldom rose above 1 percent for the entire period 1869–1890.

To add to the confusion about discharge policies, at both Utica and Willard, casebook notes about the behavior of the released differed little from those about patients retained. Since doctors tended to make only brief comments about nontroublesome patients, the superficial similarities between the two groups may be real or artifacts of inadequate record keeping. Whatever their behavior, patients whose relatives or friends expressed an interest in them were more likely to be discharged than those with no extra-institutional ties. For example, an epileptic whose parents waited twelve years to institutionalize him was returned to them once a sudden outburst of violent behavior subsided, less than a year after admission. Another patient, a fifty-three-year-old delusional woman, was discharged unimproved to her county poorhouse at the request of a sister, reported also to be "nearly insane," who wanted to be able to visit her.[139] Unfortunately for most of Willard's patients, their residence there was the last in a long series of institutional commitments; in many cases their families long ago had either forgotten about them or given up hope of their recovery.

Despite ever increasing numbers of chronic cases, asylum doctors continued to insist that such men and women were not necessarily incurable. Occasionally, seemingly miraculous cures at Willard substantiated their claims. For example, in 1890 a thirty-seven-year-old woman who had been insane for "some years" unexpectedly improved. Long filthy, incoherent, and kept in "strong dresses" because of her destructiveness, she suddenly became quiet, industrious, and well mannered. Allowed to leave, "recovered," with her sister, she never returned.[140] Such cures were relatively rare, however; the majority of the Willard patients allowed to return home were discharged as "unimproved, but harmless" or "improved." Perhaps because of the sheer numbers under their supervision and their isolated location, Willard's medical staff expressed much less concern about "eloped" patients than did Utica's. For example, in 1889 a thirty-eight-year-old German peddler who had become paranoid and delusional after losing twenty dollars worth of the matches he sold for a living, was sent by county officials to Willard. Several days after his arrival, he slipped away from an entertainment; after locating him a month later in a distant town, both the Willard doctors and his local superintendent of the poor decided not to fetch him back.[141] Occasionally, "eloped" patients were subsequently discharged as "recovered" or "improved" from both the Utica and Willard asylums.[142]

As nineteenth-century asylum doctors asserted, a full understanding of their asylums' discharge and retention rates could not be read from charts of discharges and cures. Annual reports alone also were inadequate. It needed to be pieced together from a multitude of sources and speakers. Consider, for example, the Utica patient who had struck himself seventeen times with an axe before admission, under the delusion he was possessed by the devil. His wounds healed, and this violently deranged man returned "recovered" to his wife and son only nine months later. More tragic were the life experiences of a thirty-four-year-old "physically healthy and industrious" man driven by financial worries to acute depression. Once at Utica, he became so agitated by his commitment that attendants shut him up in the notorious Utica crib. There he slept little, grew exhausted and emaciated, masturbated constantly (for which he was "blistered"), and less than six months after admission, died of acute mental exhaustion.[143]

Such case histories suggest why nineteenth-century asylums aroused such a range of emotions in those they served and in the general public as well. They also remind twentieth-century scholars of the intricate interconnection of events in patients' life histories, inside and outside the asylum. Patient recoveries, often considered an asylum's highest achievement, did not guarantee future happiness for the newly restored. "The world avoideth the insane as the pestilence that walketh in darkness" warned one *Opal* editor. Many, in a phenomenon with which twentieth-century mental patients are only too familiar, found it difficult to readjust to extra-institutional life. One three-time patient stayed on for a while as an attendant after her last admission. When doctors first suggested she go home, her symptoms worsened, but she ultimately did go. And other ex-patients found the stigma of insanity difficult to lose. A school teacher who unsuccessfully had tried to hide his asylum experience found parents reluctant to send small children to him (especially as he also had been known to lecture on the abolition of slavery). When a recently released young woman returned to her hometown church one Sunday, she found her every action watched, her every word stored up for future scrutiny. Written on all the faces surrounding her was the question: "I wonder, if she is *quite right?*" And though many were willing, there was no one— not in her family, in her community, or even back in the Utica Asylum— fully able to answer it.[144]

Therapeutic Anomalies

In 1883 the commissioner in lunacy attempted to summarize the differences between acute care and chronic care state asylums. He made the following points:

1. Acute care facilities which accepted many new patients each year had to offer more medical care (particularly in the form of preliminary physical examinations) than did institutions for chronic cases. For example, in 1882 Utica had received 412 new cases, whereas Willard had accepted only 217, 92 of whom were transfers from other state hospitals.

2. Acute care facilities needed a higher patient–attendant ratio than did institutions for the chronically insane, in part because they received patients of all classes, not just paupers.

3. Acute cases required a more varied and often richer diet than did chronic ones.

4. General hospitals like Utica dealt with many more visits from, as well as correspondence with, patients' relatives and friends than did custodial asylums.

5. Acute cases demanded more constant classification and reclassification than stationary chronic cases.

6. As a result of such differences, both capital expenditures and daily maintenance costs were higher at hospital facilities such as Utica than at custodial institutions like Willard. [By 1883 New York State had four acute care hospitals and two institutions for chronic care.][145]

His observations certainly made clear why Utica's legislative funding was so much higher than Willard's, but he missed a number of important points of similarity and difference between the two institutions. For example, while the Willard Asylum produced much of its own food, clothing, and other necessities, its doctors still lacked sufficient funds to set up adequate moral treatment programs. Willard's patients certainly were more isolated from families and friends and much less likely to return to them than were Utica's. On the other hand, their therapeutic needs often were even greater than those of Utica's patients. An overwhelming majority at Willard had been labeled demented. Short of general paresis or epilepsy, this was the most pessimistic diagnosis which could be made in nineteenth-century America. Utica's and Willard's comparative discharge rates suggest again that the diagnosis most critical to the nineteenth-century insane was not of a specific syndrome but of curability or chronicity.

Strong philosophical and personality differences between Utica's and Willard's most influential superintendents, John Gray and John Chapin, intensified preexisting institutional difference due to different patient populations and funding levels. Yet, although Gray and Chapin certainly never consulted with one another, both asylums shared a number of similar problems. The commissioner in lunacy was wrong in his assumption that Willard's chronically insane patients needed substantially less attention from attendants and doctors. Although there were more doctors per patient at Utica than at Willard, the attendant–patient ratio was about the same at both institutions. It averaged one attendant to ten inmates, although the ratio varied from ward to ward. While Willard could not afford to offer the same level of medical care as did Utica, doctors at both institutions paid careful attention to the seriously ill or disturbed and relied on the nonprofessional staff to look after the rest. As at Utica, many of Willard's patients needed (and were given) substantial diets, supplemented by tonics, to rebuild their weakened bodies.

While both nineteenth- and twentieth-century observers have interpreted this post–Civil War emphasis on dietary programs and medical care as evidence of the increasingly custodial nature of insane asylums, physicians at Utica and Willard would have disagreed. As early as 1843, Brigham testified to the importance of diet and rest for the restoration of reason. Under Gray, Utica admittedly abandoned many of Brigham's early experiments in moral therapy but replaced them with what he considered to be a more promising stress on medical treatment. If insanity was a physical disease like other physical diseases, Gray felt, it was best treated by medical means, including drugs, iron tonics, and dietary supplements. He also used chemical and mechanical restraints to rest the minds and bodies of overexcited patients (as well as those of their neighbors and attendants) and hoped that pathological research, including postmortems, would provide the key to the physical mysteries of the brain.

Willard was even less able than post–Civil War Utica to offer its patients individualized treatment (whether medical or psychological), but members of its medical staff still considered their work to be therapeutic. They sharply criticized county poorhouses for their largely custodial programs, under which former Willard patients, even those released "unimproved," deteriorated further. In contrast, Willard aimed to elevate even its most demented patients "to higher planes of mental and intellectual life." By offering employment and recreational programs, medical care, and an adequate diet, Willard hoped "to eliminate much of what is intractable in many cases, and render dangerous and homicidal and destructive patients quiet and orderly and industrious."[146] While their goals were less appealing to taxpayers and politicians than Utica's curative aspirations, Willard's doctors resented being delegated to the role of mere custodians.

The complexity of nineteenth-century definitions of "therapeutic" adds to the difficulty of comparing the quality of care offered at these two asylums. On the one hand, Gray's medical/pathological emphasis, however immediately unproductive, would in the hands of his successors lead to substantial improvements for certain categories of the mentally ill. His insistence on good food, medical care, and an orderly environment for patients saved many lives and enabled postpartum mothers and overworked laborers to recover their physical as well as emotional balance. On the other hand, Gray's unvarying hostility to noninstitutional forms of treatment, his refusal to listen to criticism of any sort (which led him to ignore serious incidents of patient abuse), and his reluctance to increase patient liberties, even by minimizing the use of mechanical restraints or eliminating censorship of patient correspondence, made the inevitable burdens of institutional life intolerable for a number of his charges.

Although Willard's doctors released few of their patients back to the community, they took great pride in their low death rates and the fre-

159

quency with which they nursed almost moribund patients back to health.[147] The needs of the filthy and demented, even when these constituted only one-third of the patient population, were enormous and absorbed much staff energy. Yet such unfortunate men and women often received better care at Willard, an asylum set up for their special care, than they did at Utica, where they dramatized doctors' therapeutic inadequacies and undermined the institution's formal mission. Willard's administrators also expended much effort in devising a patient employment program, which involved even the extremely demented and attracted national attention. On the negative side, Willard's patient casebooks record multiple incidents of patients injuring themselves or others, many of which might have been prevented. The frequency with which doctors did not notice patients' serious illnesses until several days before their deaths suggests that, on daily medical rounds, they ignored all but the most flagrant physical symptoms. They often expressed surprise when patients died "quickly" of enteritis, painful cancers, or tuberculosis. To an even greater extent than at Utica, patients received little individual attention unless they became acutely ill. Seemingly little effort was made to distract or engage very withdrawn patients, many of whom sat immobile, day in and day out, on ward floors for years. The condition of most long-term patients slowly worsened over time, although it is hard to separate the extent to which such deterioration reflected an inevitable progression of their illnesses from patients' response to the monotony and lack of hope characteristic of their institutional lives.[148]

Patient memoirs and casebook records make clear that there was no uniform standard of care at these two asylums. The extent to which patients were offered specific therapeutic programs varied greatly from ward to ward, particularly at Utica. Imaginative treatment programs characterized wards for quiet and convalescent patients; restraints, drugs, and brutality prevailed on many back wards. (Although the relative numbers involved in each are unknown, there seem to have been proportionately few of the better sort of wards.) Even at the end of the nineteenth century, the Utica Asylum continued to offer a mix of therapeutic and custodial care; the extent to which patients received one or the other depended on both medical and social factors. Whatever their disorders, at both Willard and Utica all patients were expected to conform to highly structured routines. Particularly in the twentieth century, such institutional efforts to cure through the heavy-handed imposition of order and routine have been sharply criticized. Yet, whenever their coercive routines faltered, a swift, negative public and political response reinforced nineteenth-century superintendents' commitment to them. Asylums were much more likely to be criticized for not watching patients carefully enough than for excessive supervision. When one patient (who eventually won a suit against the Utica Asylum for unjust incarceration) escaped, his alarmed relatives wrote hasty letters of protest to the institution. When another evaded attendants long enough to break off a table leg and kill a fellow patient, newspapers criticized Utica administrators' reluctance to keep all potentially dangerous patients in heavy restraints.[149] Fear of destructive patients haunted asylum administrators, whose worst fears were realized in 1857 when a patient burned down the asylum barn and much of its main building. Although originally committed for criminal arson, the patient had seemed to be recovered and been given positions of responsibility in the institution.[150] Such events did not have to occur very often to persuade asylum doctors of the righteousness of their demands for regimen and discipline.

By the end of the nineteenth century, both Utica's and Willard's diagnostic and treatment practices were undergoing close scrutiny from many groups: from the institution's own medical staffs; from reformers of all sorts (including New York's neurologists, the State Charities Aid Association, and the National Association for the Prosecution of the Insane and the Prevention of Insanity); from a number of state regulatory agencies; from state legislators; from the medical profession at large; and from the parents and friends of patients. These groups agreed neither on what the institutions were or should be doing. In their public arguments with each other, they often seemed to lose sight of the private realities of New York State insane asylums. And Gerald Grob's study of twentieth-century American mental health care suggests that this turning away from the real needs and concerns of the institutionalized insane only increased in subsequent years.[151] Despite the substantial inadequacies of diagnosis and treatment at the nineteenth-century Utica and Willard asylums, their medical staffs remained committed to helping the institutionalized insane. Then as now, balance in attitudes toward and treatment of the mentally ill was difficult to achieve. Asylum superintendents seldom sought help for their charges beyond the asylum walls; their critics were equally unwilling to explore the therapeutic potential, however limited, available within those same walls. Finally, while they seldom spoke to each other, both supporters and critics alike never listened to patients' suggestions or comments. Their debates, however well intentioned, had little effect on the daily lives of patients like the Willard woman who sighed softly to her attendant: "I am an angel with a broken wing, and I can no longer fly." [152]

6

Attendants and Their World of Work

Attendants occupied an ambiguous position within the asylum work world. Nineteenth-century asylum superintendents liked to think of their institutions as homes, places of refuge which offered a healthy, happy domestic life to patients. Within this world, the superintendent was clearly the patriarch, a father with almost unlimited authority. His children were the patients; although adult in age, they lacked not only responsibility for their actions but also the right to self-direction. Attendants had a vital role within this family structure. Since doctors spent at most a few minutes a day with patients, attendants had the greatest opportunity to shape their behavior. They cared for them night and day, as for a sick spouse or child. They prevented them from injuring themselves or others and re-taught the habits of adult self-control. Each ward or cottage was considered a distinct (if single-sex) family whose health as a unit depended upon attendants' unceasing vigilance.[1]

Despite their awesome therapeutic responsibilities, attendants most resembled not members of the family but domestic servants, for whom the duty of child raising had been added to their usual chores. Like nineteenth-century mothers, attendants were asked to provide a loving and moral environment for their patient-children, but they were deprived not only of the housewife's domestic autonomy but also of the many rewards of child rearing. Many of the attendants' "children" never grew up; of those who left the asylum cured, few felt much gratitude toward the men and women who had overseen their darkest days. Finally, despite the limited legal position of nineteenth-century housewives, they had more social status, both inside and outside the family, than did asylum attendants. Close to the bottom of the asylum work hierarchy, even the most devoted felt the burden of their public image as brutish abusers of helpless patients.

Conditions of Daily Work

Arduous and poorly paid, attendants' work seldom attracted the kind of skilled caretakers considered essential to the success of moral therapy programs. Asylum superintendents complained about incompetent attendants just as middle-class housewives complained about servants. They failed to perceive the contradictory nature of their expectations. While they required attendants to make beds, scrub floors, and bathe filthy patients, they also expected them to offer moral guidance and psychological counseling. The ideal attendant, one New York State official proclaimed, had "all the higher attributes of a refined nature, such as patience, benevolence and sympathy . . . conjoined to a firmness that will not waver—a decision of character that will command respect in the midst of the wildest excitement—and a forbearance that cannot be thrown off its guard, even by personal assault."[2] Equally demanding was the Utica board of managers. Attendants, they proclaimed, must always be "tender and affectionate" to patients, calming the irritated and cheering the depressed. If abused or struck, they should never retaliate. To prevent suicides and escapes, attendants were commanded never to leave their charges, even briefly, unless relieved by other attendants. Such individuals were not easy to find.

The board attempted to regulate attendants' lives as strictly as those of patients. Attendants had few personal freedoms and could not leave the institution without permission of the medical officers, to whom they owed total obedience. Forbidden to criticize the asylum or its officers, no matter what the occasion, they were enjoined never to forget that "the whole time of the attendant and assistants belongs to the asylum." In addition to such restrictions on behavior, Utica's managers tried to control attendants' thoughts. "Let a smile habitually light up your countenance," they admonished; "cultivate a humble self-denying spirit," they urged (a practical necessity given the conditions of work). The board's list of attendants' duties and responsibilities was endless. It was five times longer than the comparable list of duties prescribed for medical officers.[3]

Similar injunctions applied to Willard's attendants. Their official "Rules and Regulations" specified such details as the frequency with which water closets were to be cleaned and bed clothing changed, the importance of making sure that no patient entered a bathtub until both hot and cold water were turned off, and the procedures to be followed in case of fire.[4] According to Willard's Employment Recordbook, at least some asylum work supervisors attempted to enforce these lengthy lists of rules. Their own duties were too demanding to permit frequent inspections, but egregious violations were promptly punished. For example, they dismissed several attendants for leaving their halls without permission and fired a middle-aged married woman, whose two daughters also worked at Willard, for not reporting the entry into her room of an intoxicated male attendant. Most such regulation of attendants' morals and behavior was left to assistant physicians and supervisors, but occasionally, the superintendent himself took on the task of monitoring his employees' work habits. One night in 1888, P. M. Wise watched for hours a night attendant whom he suspected of neglecting his duties. When he found that the man visited patients only twice during the night, Wise declared this "a distinct breach of faith in a confidential position," suspended the offender for a week, and demoted him.[5]

As a result of these rules, attendants had the heaviest work responsibilities in the asylum but little formal power. Typical of the medical staff's attitude was the comment "An attendant is good in proportion as he obeys the superintendent. The superintendent should be the brain, the attendants the hands." Gray objected to hiring attendants older than forty because, with maturity, men and women often lost the will to "spontaneous obedience and to the execution of fixed rules." Gray was so obsessed with his own authority as to insist (to the horror of a legislative investigative committee) that attendants who visited wards other than their own without permission, even to investigate allegations of patient abuse, should be fired. Such unofficial activities, he contended, bred "insubordination and disturbance," for they usurped the prerogatives of the medical officer.[6] In practice, since Gray and his fellow superintendents rarely appeared on the halls after 1860, attendants exercised many initiatives expressly forbidden them, such as ordering restraints and forced feeding for patients. Overworked assistant physicians acquiesced in, and even tacitly encouraged, these practices. Yet, attendants knew that such informal powers were theirs only by default and might be rescinded at any time.

While all attendants worked long hours for low pay, their experiences varied with their ward assignments. Work with convalescent patients could be pleasant and rewarding; that with severely disturbed patients in back wards often involved the threat of physical danger in a chaotic and noisy setting. At Willard, Chapin preferred to assign only experienced and skilled attendants to patients requiring intensive care, but at Utica, supervisors reserved for the newly hired attendants the least desirable wards. Although state officials had hoped that the Willard Asylum would need fewer attendants for its chronically insane, in 1885 the overall ratio at Willard was one attendant for every eleven patients. Here, too, administrators found that patients had varying needs. Although halls with quiet patients averaged one attendant for sixteen patients, those for physically ill demented patients assigned each attendant to only six patients. When funding permitted, both institutions maintained a high attendant-to-patient ratio on difficult units and limited their overall size. For most of the nineteenth century, the Utica Asylum averaged one attendant for every ten patients, but specific ratios varied greatly from ward to ward.[7]

Over the course of the nineteenth century, the number and kind of staff positions at both Utica and Willard grew along with patient populations. The resulting occupational specialization changed attendants' work and increased opportunities for job mobility. For example, the hiring of dining room girls for some Willard wards in 1872 decreased attendants' domestic responsibilities. In 1888, when additional attendants were hired to care for patients at night (and in particular to help keep them clean), daytime workers for the first time could enjoy evenings of uninterrupted rest. This innovation had been introduced first on an experimental basis in 1883, when Chapin assigned two night attendants to a department of one hundred males, many of whom were incontinent. The two men made a continuous round of the wards, helping patients to the water closets when necessary. If patients were wet or soiled, they cleaned them and replaced their bedding. With such assistance, the number of dirty patients on the ward dropped by 50 percent, and sanitary conditions were improved greatly. Yet, despite the experiment's success, night service was not extended to the other Willard wards until 1886, largely because of its expense.[8] At Willard, in particular, the care of incontinent patients was a never-ending task for many attendants, as well as for their patient-assistants.

Despite the continuous cleaning, the smell of urine pervaded certain halls. When Stephen Smith visited one such ward in 1883, he was horrified to encounter large numbers of demented patients smeared with filth, despite the night watch's efforts to keep them clean. Work in such wards, according to Chapin, was "trying and repulsive." In 1889 George Blumer of Utica argued that the clean and self-aware among the chronically insane should not be forced to associate in the same ward with "helpless, filthy patients in the last stages of terminal dementia." To protect the sensibilities of the well-behaved patients, he requested legislative funding for a separate building for their more disturbed brothers and sisters. Willard, too, tried to segregate helpless patients in special infirmaries, with high staff–patient ratios. Here suicidal patients could be cared for without restraints, and convulsive epileptics could be watched at night.[9] Such changes, and the attitudes behind them, had a mixed impact on patients. Willard's doctors hoped that, by isolating their most disturbed patients, they could offer them better care. They also thereby improved somewhat the living conditions on the remaining wards. Yet, by the 1880s, both asylums doctors and state officials retained little of their antebellum predecessors' sensitivity to the basic humanity of their most demented charges. Given asylum leaders' distaste for such patients, it is perhaps not surprising that some attendants translated this repugnance into contempt, and even abuse.

While annual reports offered a wealth of detail about attendants' duties and work schedules, neither asylum doctors nor official visitors tried to capture the less formal aspects of attendants' lives: their friendships, amusements, and feelings about their work. Chapin's request to the legislature for funding of a new amusement hall at Willard was a rare exception. In it, he commented on the problems created by his many young unmarried attendants' social isolation and suggested that an amusement hall might lessen the attraction of local taverns. Once built, the hall did indeed become the site of numerous events, organized and attended by staff members and the "better quality" of patients. In addition to frequent musical evenings, doctors, staff, and the townspeople of Willard also organized dramatic recitations, short plays, and presentations by the "Willard Minstrels." Occasionally, visiting troupes appeared, but they more easily

167

found their way to Utica than to the isolated asylum on Seneca Lake. For the most part, Willard's doctors and staff had to create their own entertainments. One young assistant physician, particularly beloved by patients and attendants, became as celebrated for his vocal solos at asylum concerts as for his conscientious therapy. Doctors, attendants, and townspeople worked together on such productions as "The Shakespeare Water Cure." That particular play, a resounding success, had characters to appeal to all: a financially devastated Macbeth, staying at the Cure to escape creditors; a depressed Hamlet; the doomed romantic lovers Romeo and Juliet; even Shylock and Othello.[10] Such activities were vital to staff morale at Willard. To help promote them, the steward between 1886 and 1890 began to ask job applicants about their musical abilities. To records of age, nativity, and place of former employment, he added such comments as "sings well and plays cornet" or "has no musical talents." Although both musical and unmusical attendants were hired, in competitive situations the steward clearly preferred those who had not only good references but also skills with such instruments as the drums or organ.[11]

In 1887 the Willard Asylum began to publish a monthly guide to its entertainments. Typical was the schedule for May of 1887:[12]

May 1	Concert and readings	Hall
May 4	Dancing party	Hall
May 8	Stereopticon exhibition	Chapel
May 11	Dancing party	Hall
May 15	Concert and readings	Hall
May 18	Dancing party	Hall
May 22	Stereopticon exhibition	Chapel
May 25	Dancing party	Hall
May 29	Concert and readings	Hall

Although such activities engaged many members of the staff, they did not eliminate the excessive drinking which created serious problems at both Utica and Willard. While Utica's administrators could not keep off-duty attendants away from city bars, Willard's fought a bitter political battle in the state legislature and with the governor to prohibit the sale of alcoholic beverages within several miles of the asylum. They also bought the only nearby hotel, primarily so that they could prevent its sale of alcoholic beverages to their employees.[13] Such actions were taken primarily out of a concern for patients' welfare, although several board members also supported the temperance movement. The detailed "discharge list" for 1889 appended to the official Willard Employee Recordbook reveals that attendants drank not just during their free time but also while on ward duty. For example, three ward employees became so intoxicated and disorderly early one October morning that their antics drew the attention of a night watchman and one of the doctors. Initially all were dismissed for intemperance, and the ward supervisor also was charged with patient neglect. Although one of the three was rehired on the grounds that he had been least to blame for the incident, he first had to pledge never to touch alcoholic beverages again. His reprieve was only temporary, for this "willing and gentlemanly" young man subsequently lost his job when a female attendant accused him of having fathered her illegitimate child. As his dismissal indicates, the Willard authorities also tried to control the sexual activities of their staff. Here, too, their reasons were both moral and pragmatic. When one young woman was discharged for "disregarding the advice about receiving personal visitors," her employers simultaneously condemned her moral laxness and the neglect of patients which resulted when she left her hall "to visit with young men." [14]

Insubordination, moral laxity, and patient neglect were considered by asylum superintendents equally serious threats to their institutions' authority structures. As a result, at Willard, employees were fired for attempting to organize a strike, conflicts with doctors, and insubordination as well as for neglect of duties. Unfortunately, the steward in charge of employee records did not bother to note the issues which led to the threatened strike. When he dismissed a laundry attendant for "incompetency, insubordination, and improper language to the Superintendent," he also failed to record the circumstances under which this lowly drudge happened to encounter Wise. [15]

Qualifications, Retention Rates, and Salaries

Asylum doctors frequently referred to such incidents as proof of their inability to find well-qualified attendants. Yet, beyond formulaic statements about attendants' importance, the superintendents at Utica and Willard paid little attention to the qualifications of those actually hired at their institutions. They delegated that responsibility to the asylum steward, whose hiring procedures were highly informal. According to Horatio Dryer, Utica's steward for over thirty years, during times of depression he was swamped with job applicants, but when the economy flourished he had none. Most often he judged candidates simply on the basis of their appearance. Those hired confirmed Dryer's remarks. One young farmer applied for a job on a whim in 1881, while visiting an attendant friend at the asylum. Never asked to submit letters of reference, he simply talked briefly to one of the doctors and then to the steward, who promptly offered him a position. The matron used a similar process to hire female attendants. She looked first for evidence of "good health and a good nature." If applicants also could write their age and place of former employment and do simple sums, she employed them. While she preferred candidates with letters of recommendation, she often found herself forced to hire all those with a respectable and trustworthy appearance.[16]

Such informal hiring procedures, characteristic of most state institutions in nineteenth-century New York, led to newspaper charges that state jobs were handed out as a form of political patronage. Although the civil service regulations of 1883 were intended to improve the quality of state employees, they had little effect on asylum hiring procedures. The requirements for attendants' work continued to be minimal. Applicants had to be healthy; able to furnish satisfactory recommendations; schooled in reading, writing, and basic mathematics; and of an "equable and humane disposition." The only major civil service innovation was the introduction of strict age requirements, which limited applicants to those between twenty and forty-five.[17] Utica's administrators felt such general hiring guidelines were sufficient, but a state legislative committee disagreed, arguing that prior work experience needed to be considered. On these grounds, it criticized the employment of a former hostler as an attendant. Yet, in its final report, that same committee merely repeated the time-worn recommendation that attendants' work hours be diminished and pay increased, while the more knotty question of appropriate but realistic job qualifications was not addressed. And, subsequently, both the asylum management and their fellow legislators ignored even these two simple recommendations.[18]

Although Willard's steward left no formal description of his hiring procedures, the information collected in his Employees Recordbook suggests the job qualifications he valued. Most of those he hired were relatively young: the median age for men was twenty-four and for women twenty-one. Like Utica's attendants, Willard's had little if any professional work experience. Most males had been farm laborers, and females, house-workers. Only 9 percent of those hired between 1886 and 1890 reported previous asylum employment, thus suggesting that Willard was too isolated to attract the "asylum tramps" complained about by other super-intendents. Such lack of expertise bothered neither the steward nor his superintendent. Even those with relevant job experience began at the bottom of the occupational ladder, as did 89 percent of all new employees. Those few applicants who had held skilled or white-collar jobs before becoming attendants stayed only a short time, seemingly having turned to asylum work as a temporary expedient.[19]

Between 1869 and 1886, Willard's steward noted little in his records about new staff members except their age. Beginning in the late 1880s, he also began to make occasional comments about their health, perhaps in response to the new civil service requirements, although such concern about the physically demanding nature of attendants' work was not new. Many years earlier, Gray had written of a job candidate, "I hardly know how she would bear the fatigue of an attendant's life." Despite its casual quality, Willard's preliminary screening seemed to have had some effect, for few employees left because of poor health. Also frequently noted in the post-1886 records of successful female applicants was their size. The steward divided them into two groups: those of "small stature," most often assigned to kitchen and laundry jobs, and those of "good size," more often made attendants.[20]

In the mid-1880s, the steward also began to note for the first time the nativity of those he hired. Increasingly, attendants' work, like domestic service, attracted newly arrived immigrants who lacked the social skills required for better paying positions. Both the Utica and Willard asylums hired attendants who could not speak English, once again demonstrating their lack of concern (despite rhetoric to the contrary) for attendants' contributions to the therapeutic process. The resulting ethnic differences between patients and staff exacerbated ward tensions. Several Utica patients complained about being forced to associate with coarse, ill-bred Irish attendants. At Willard the situation was reversed; since most employees continued to be recruited from small towns near Willard, largely native-born Americans cared for the asylum's disproportionately foreign-born patient population.[21]

A comparison of Utica and Willard attendants is not easy, for comparable records do not exist for the two groups. Yet, in general, Willard's attendants seem to have stayed longer and engaged in less patient abuse than did Utica's. Since both groups were poorly trained and overworked, such differences were probably due to the relative availability of other kinds of employment and the somewhat different supervisor–employee relationships at the two asylums. For example, the Utica Asylum after the Civil War experienced great difficulties in attracting and keeping high-quality attendants from the growing Oneida County area. While Gray blamed the rapid turnover on the stigmatizing effects of legislative investigations into patient abuse, his own strong opposition to work-hour reductions of any kind no doubt exacerbated staff discontent. "Attendants should be *made* to understand that they are the companions and constant associates of the patients, and they must be with them day and night," he asserted [emphasis mine]. That so few attendants died while working for the asylum, he claimed, proved that their work was not too arduous. Yet, by his own count, 493 of the 583 attendants hired between 1869 and 1884 left the asylum.[22]

Early in Willard's history, its managers bragged of the ease with which they attracted "first class attendants," but by 1882 its superintendent also complained that attendants seldom stayed even four years. Their restlessness, he claimed, was a peculiarly American trait, for English and Scottish asylums managed to keep excellent attendants for many years at much lower wages. Although Chapin's complaints echoed those of his fellow superintendents, they were not substantiated by his institution's employee records. Of those nonprofessional workers hired at the Willard Asylum between 1869 and 1890, most worked at least four years; 20 percent of the men and 10 percent of the women made a career of asylum work, leaving only upon death or retirement. Although most of those employees who worked for more than twenty years were men, women as a group worked longer at the asylum than did men, perhaps because they had few alternative job possibilities. Whatever their persistence rates relative to workers at other asylums, Willard's attendants certainly stayed at their jobs much longer than did domestic servants, a group with whom they were often compared. Although nineteenth-century women complained about their servants' "restlessness" in almost the same terms as did asylum superintendents, household employers had more reason for dissatisfaction. Between 50 and 60 percent of domestic servants stayed less than a year, and very few lasted as long as eight years.[23]

Although asylum hours were even longer than those of domestic work, and the pay no better, perhaps working with chronically insane paupers was easier than with temperamental mistresses. Attendants had only limited formal power, but the overworked medical staffs were seldom able to supervise them as systematically as asylum rules mandated. In contrast, domestic servants had little privacy or independence. Domestic work also lacked the job security and occupational mobility characteristic of asylum employment. Almost all of Willard's employees started at the bottom of the asylum's occupational ladder, but more than half made at least modest moves up it. Although far from typical, one long-term employee advanced her career in a fashion impossible in the most pleasant of households. When twenty-year-old Mary Ryan first came to the asylum in 1881, she began as a lowly dining room girl. After six years, she advanced to the position of attendant; four years later she became a supervisor; then a charge attendant. By the time she retired on a state pension in 1932, she held a high-ranking administrative position.[24] Attendants at Willard also had ample chances for employment diversity. The frequency with which the steward offered exhausted ward attendants lateral moves when promotion was not possible may have helped the institution hold employees. Fewer than half of all nonprofessional employees held only one position, and most of that group left during their first two years of employment. At both Utica and Willard, promotions came from within the ranks, so that the longer individuals stayed, the greater their likelihood of job mobility. This is not to suggest that, at Willard at least, the ineffective were promoted simply as a reward for length of service. In contrast to Dryer at Utica, Willard's steward closely monitored his employee's work. Not only did he move them frequently from job to job, but in several instances, he demoted those who had been promoted beyond their competence.[25]

Perhaps another reason rural New Yorkers sought Willard employment was the asylum's willingness to hire husbands and wives and to rehire former employees with good work records (a boon for women who had left during their early childbearing years and for men who had experimented with but failed at farming). For example, one woman, who began working in the kitchen in 1879, left to be married in 1888. She was reemployed in 1889, left again in 1890, returned in 1893, and left again pregnant that same year, "at the advice of her physician." The asylum was equally willing to hire widows with small children. Most of these mothers took jobs that did not require residency, like ironing and laundry work, but a few left their children with relatives and moved onto the wards. By the late 1880s, some of their children had joined the asylum work force as well. Such family ties among workers became increasingly common at the end of the nineteenth century. As Willard's Irish community grew, young men and women began to migrate directly from Ireland to Willard, where relatives got them jobs at the asylum. The work force also included a small but cohesive group of Danes hired in the mid-1880s, most on the recommendation of a family patriarch, one Jens Jensen. In this manner, among certain families a tradition of asylum work emerged which persisted well into the twentieth century. At the same time the size of Willard's work force stabilized. Although Utica, too, occasionally hired employees' siblings and children, it failed to develop the stable local work pool on which Willard depended. Not only were its superintendents markedly less interested in issues of employee morale, but the city of Utica and its environs offered a wider variety of alternative employment opportunities than did rural Ovid.[26]

For the most part, attendants' wages were the same as those of day laborers and domestics, and in the best free-market tradition, Willard salaries clearly reflected fluctuations in the local demand for unskilled workers. When wages in Seneca county dropped in the early 1880s, Willard's cost-conscious board of trustees immediately reduced institutional wages as well. Although large numbers of attendants immediately left, the board attributed such defections to the "migratory disposition" of asylum employees. Nothing could have induced such unreliable employees to remain, they claimed, even higher wages.[27] Not surprisingly, Willard's salaries embodied the same sex-biases as did the general labor market. Male attendants averaged 42 percent higher salaries than females, and male supervisors almost 100 percent higher, while male cooks received double the stipend of their female counterparts. Those positions held only by women, such as dining room girl and chambermaid, were the lowest paying in the institution. Finally, men monopolized the highest paid, nonprofessional staff positions, such as clerk, accountant, butcher, carpenter, and locomotive engineer (whose incumbent made eighty dollars a month the same year kitchen girls made nine dollars).[28]

As striking as the gap between male and female salaries was that between poorly paid attendants (whatever their sex) and most other asylum employees, including such unskilled workers as teamsters and porters. Possibly attendants suffered financially from the frequent comparison of their work to domestic service. In any case, administrative rhetoric about the importance of their work was never translated into monetary rewards, even though state legislative committees several times recommended pay increases. At Utica, the board of managers regularly raised the salaries of its professional staff but refused to do the same for attendants. On one rare occasion when they considered attendants' wages, discussion stalled when one manager insisted that no general wage increases be considered until female attendants were paid the same as males. When a number of Utica's most highly qualified attendants threatened to quit if they did not get either higher wages or additional privileges, John Gray angrily fired them. Such selfish and unreliable employees did not deserve a place within his asylum family, he asserted, for they were too self-centered to be entrusted with the care of others.[29]

Late Nineteenth-Century Tension and "Reforms"

Although attendants' wages remained low for the remainder of the nineteenth century, a number of other reforms helped to improve working conditions. In 1887 the Utica board for the first time gave two weeks' vacation with pay to all attendants who had worked a full year, a much-needed reform. With the establishment of nighttime care at the end of the century, the state asylums also began to construct sleeping accommodations for attendants separate from patient wards. For the first time, attendants could retreat for short periods from the noise, confusion, and excitement.[30] A reform somewhat less appealing to attendants were the uniforms adopted at Utica in 1887. Even the managers divided over the issue of whether or not the wearing of uniforms was inherently un-

American. Superintendent Blumer's arguments, however, finally produced a four-to-three majority in favor of this innovation. Disagreeing that uniforms were a sign of servitude, he argued that they made easier the maintenance of the "semi-military" discipline so essential in a large state institution. He also hoped that wearing uniforms would somehow improve attendants' estimation of their status and thereby encourage them to consider their work a lifetime profession.[31]

After several legislative investigations of patient abuse at the Utica asylum in the 1870s and 1880s, a coalition group of social reformers, politicians, and neurologists campaigned for the improvement of asylum staffs. For years, managers and superintendents had responded to all criticism by arguing that no hiring test could separate those with the requisite qualities of human kindness from those lacking them. Yet, as one journal editor noted in 1880, the kind of educated, refined men and women skilled at nursing were seldom willing to endure asylum working conditions for domestic servants' wages. And the senators who cross-examined John Gray about patient abuse at Utica in 1884 suggested pointedly that Gray might have paid less for the expensive purebred bull and cow he had recently added to the asylum herd and more for a better class of attendants. Gray and his colleagues ignored such protests, perhaps because they realized that, however frequently legislators complained about attendants' low pay rates, they seldom suggested raising them.[32]

Yet reformers' proposals, even if implemented, would not have eliminated attendant–patient tensions. Although they assumed that if "better sorts" of people became attendants, abuse would disappear, patient abuse was rooted in social phenomena appreciated by few asylum outsiders. Elitist critics often attributed attendants' brutality to their class and ethnic origins, but asylum records tell a different story. No matter what the class or ethnicity of attendants, they found working with violent, abusive patients difficult. Not infrequently, delusional patients saw attendants as demons and attacked them. Less threatening but more exasperating were those patients so demented that they could not converse coherently nor control their bodily functions. Under such stresses, the metaphor of the asylum as a happy family broke down. Unlike parents, or even tutors and nannies, asylum attendants too seldom saw their "children" mature and grow up. Instead many found themselves trapped in situations similar to those which produced abusive mothers, seldom relieved from care of

their difficult "children." As a result, with a frequency impossible to estimate, overworked, harassed attendants responded impatiently, roughly,
sometimes even brutally to difficult patients, even when their only offense
was an unwillingness to eat or to sleep at night.[33]

In short, while cries of outrage filled leading newspapers, those most
agitated about the need for reform knew little about the social realities of
patient care. They also made no serious effort to challenge asylum superintendents' almost total authority over staff. At Utica, Gray's position on
attendants changed little during the thirty-two years that he ruled the asylum. While he felt that their kind, loving care was vital to patients' recoveries, he fought bitterly all attempts to cut hours or raise pay. When reformers suggested that attendants might take better care of patients if
freed from domestic duties, Gray again disagreed. Like many nineteenth-
century asylum superintendents, he wanted attendants to be both loving
companions to the insane and efficient domestic servants. Not infrequently, the second role (which best matched the attendants' social status
within the institution) overwhelmed the first. Once attendants finished
their housework, many considered their responsibilities met and chatted
with each other or read instead of working with patients.[34]

In contrast, Willard's superintendents personally attempted to strengthen
staff morale. They also showed more interest in and concern for attendants' daily performances. In 1875 Chapin mandated that attendants report daily to him as well as to their supervisors. He hoped thereby to
increase their sensitivity to patients as well as help them develop systematic habits of observation. Then in 1876 he appointed a well-respected
member of the local community to act as "inspector" of the men's wards, a
strategy, he claimed, which improved patient care. (John Gray, who
fiercely opposed any outside interference with the running of the Utica
Asylum, would never have contemplated such a step.) Furthermore,
Willard employee records suggest that, at least by the late 1880s, Willard's
doctors monitored even relatively minor instances of patient mistreatment. When, in 1892, a twelve-year veteran handled an idiot roughly, he
was warned that repetition of such behavior would lead to dismissal despite his record of long and faithful service and the patient's lack of physical injury. Most often, Willard doctors presumed that an accused attendant was guilty, whereas Utica's took the opposite stance. For example, in
1890 a Willard patient claimed that a young female attendant had struck

her on the forehead with a shoe. Although the attendant denied the charge, her explanation was considered "not satisfactory" and she was fined. Several other attendants who used "excessive force" to protect themselves against violent patients also were reprimanded. In 1879 Chapin recommended that patient assault become a legal misdemeanor. Such legislation, he argued, would anger only those who violated it and would protect the reputations of the kind, hard-working attendants who constituted the majority of the work force.[35]

That attendants often treated their work duties as comparable to those of domestics should not have surprised their supervisors. Even the New York State commissioner in lunacy agreed. "The service is peculiar, and far more domestic in its real character than public," he noted. As the 1884 legislative investigation of Utica revealed in painful detail, the Utica Asylum during that period did little to train its attendants beyond handing them a printed list of duties and responsibilities, although such had not always been the case. During Utica's first few years of operation, Amariah Brigham had brought together his medical officers, attendants, and assistants for monthly discussions about proper management of the insane. Through such sessions, he had hoped not only to instruct but also to deepen the interest of his staff in the welfare of those assigned to their care.[36] But such personalized instruction stopped with Brigham's death in 1849 and was never resumed.

While Gray also thought of himself as the institution's patriarchal head, he lacked Brigham's fatherly concern. The continued expansion and specialization of the institution's work force also diminished the usefulness of such general meetings. Gray continued to think of his staff as a family, but for him, it was an extended family, with each hall an individual unit. Gray and his fellow superintendents argued that training was a continuing, practical process. New attendants learned by watching their more experienced fellows, just as children emulated older brothers and sisters. Although asylum doctors frequently complained about parents' indifference to the socialization of their children, they failed to see their similar failures. Yet, within the ward family as within the biological family, knowledge gained from slightly more experienced members was often inadequate. The first (and sometimes last) instruction of most attendants was in self-defense. One Utica attendant best remembered lessons in how to kick recalcitrant patients in the stomach so as to leave no marks. Another candidly, if naively, described her limited "therapeutic" strategies: "If patients are refractory we try to hold them in a chair, and after awhile they will probably behave themselves, when we let them go again." She added that, while the doctors never officially informed attendants of their duties, they did so "whenever it is necessary." Not surprisingly, such haphazard education seldom produced attendants who could cope with mentally ill patients' diverse physical and psychological needs.[37]

Despite the obvious need for more formalized instruction, asylums in New York State (as elsewhere) hesitated to establish formal training schools. As late as 1890, Henry Hurd charged his fellow superintendents with criminal negligence for expecting competence from the uninstructed. Too often, he commented caustically, when attendants did poor work, superintendents comforted themselves with the cliché that "all the Christian virtues could not be obtained for sixteen dollars a month."[38] While the Utica and Willard doctors never openly discussed the reasons for their reluctance, Utica's superintendents in particular seemed to have feared the development of a professional identity among their attendants. In 1888 Superintendent Blumer commented that, while willing to sponsor "simple lectures in which no attempt is made to take the nurse beyond her depths," he was opposed to the unfortunate tendency in many asylum training schools to feed classes' self-esteem by using words like "student," "graduate," and "diploma." In an *AJI* editorial that same year, his staff blasted the Essex (New Jersey) Training School for Nurses for giving out both diplomas and prizes to their best students. "Love of display," they pontificated, "is not a desirable accomplishment of the higher education."[39]

At Willard, the medical staff expressed less opposition to the idea of a training school, although they still lagged behind the national movement. Part of their reluctance stemmed from the small size of their overworked medical staff. When in 1887 they finally opened a school, they recognized the need to offer inducements to prospective students and thus promised a diploma and more rapid job advancement to all those who took the two-year course and passed a final set of exams. Under the guidance of several assistant physicians, Willard's students acquired a smattering of knowledge in such areas as anatomy, physiology, hygiene, and diet. They also received clinical training in diagnosis and treatment. Although this attempt to upgrade attendants into nurses promised better future care for patients, only two women and fifteen men graduated in 1889. Utica, too,

179

offered classes to its attendants starting in 1883, but not until 1890 did it begin a formal school.[40] By that point, its doctors had become persuaded of the help trained nurses could offer them. But, while eager to exploit the new nurses' skills, the medical staff did not abandon their condescending attitudes. Typical was the Utica-trained head of Willard who criticized those lecturers who tried to teach asylum nurses such scientific facts "as only students of medicine can comprehend." "It is much better," he added, "to tell them a few simple facts than confuse them with scientific theorizing."[41]

While training by itself did not eliminate patient abuse, a Scottish doctor, A. Campbell Clark, offered in the *AJI* a perceptive analysis of its benefits. Informal contacts with attendants had persuaded him that even the most mechanical had perceptive diagnostic insights (about superiors, he notes wryly, as well as patients). Too often, social biases prevented officers from recognizing their attendants' mental and moral capabilities. Until medical training raised the social and industrial status of attendants' work, Clark warned, few would view it as a reputable lifetime occupation.[42]

According to Gray, journalists frequently aggravated the low status of attendants' work by their sensationalistic coverage of atypical patient abuse cases.[43] Certainly such articles reinforced public fear of asylums. When appalled state legislators leafed through Utica's ward "injury books," they found instances of both serious negligence and overt violence. Similar problems plagued Willard, despite its overseers' efforts to avoid them. For example, in 1882 a feeble-minded patient scalded himself to death, when he stepped "unseen" into a tub while the attendant was still running the water into it.[44] Yet, the legislators themselves shared responsibility for the therapeutic inadequacies of state asylums. Always stingy with funding, for many years they even refused to fund a second shift of attendants, so that sick patients had to be locked in their rooms at night. Left to fend for themselves unless they could awaken their exhausted attendants, many patients seriously injured themselves during the night.

In the nineteenth century, as in the twentieth, those patients with the fewest resources were most vulnerable to attendant abuse. While Utica's doctors claimed its few widely publicized abuse cases were atypical, legislative investigations uncovered an institutional conspiracy of silence about abuse. According to one new Utica employee, when he saw his head attendant kick a patient, he did not report the incident out of fear that he himself would be discharged on a trumped-up charge. Once a patient was injured, floor attendants rehearsed together a manufactured explanation of the injuries. Most attendants felt that informing was as despicable as abuse. When one horrified attendant saw a patient die from injuries inflicted by his fellow workers, he resigned rather than report the incident. As he told a Senate investigating committee, "It is the general rule that if a person . . . makes it a practice to tell the doctors any thing, he is [pause] well, he is called a sucker . . . and they all get down on him; so it is a general rule that one does not tell what happens."[45]

Occasionally the prohibition within the attendant subculture against informing broke down, but those most willing to violate it tended to be marginal employees motivated by discontent about their work. For example, when a Buffalo State attendant reported an abuse case to his superintendent, he did so because "those Utica boys [his superiors] are down on me, and are going to get me out, and I am going to defend myself."[46] Many attendants considered the rough treatment of patients fully justified. Not uncommon (except in his frankness) was the Utica attendant assigned to the most violent ward (known colloquially as the "dead house") who claimed that everyone knew "a madman would kill you if he got the chance." Pointing out that fights disturbed his ward almost daily (one battle between attendants and male patients had lasted three and one-half hours), he argued that attendants should be allowed to "do a little fighting" when necessary. Such open acknowledgment of the need for physical force, he claimed, would eliminate the bleaching out process (whereby a patient was soaked in cold water so as to prevent the formation of bruises), which often produced more harm than a "thumping." This same attendant also gave the legislators a practical demonstration of how to choke patients with towels without leaving a mark. Utica's administrators seemed to agree tacitly that three men could not care for twenty-five insane patients without some use of force, for they were reluctant to fire attendants accused of abuse or even to probe very deeply into patients' allegations of mistreatment. As even one ex-patient noted, if force were not sometimes used to control Utica's violent inmates, there would be no rest for the quiet men there. The excessive use of force was a particularly acute problem on the male wards, where general patient–staff tensions were exacerbated by male attendants' need to defend their masculinity. Most of Utica's male attendants seemed to share the attitude of a Phila-

181

delphia attendant who, when told by his superintendent that he should run and call for help when attacked rather than strike a patient, responded defiantly, "I'll never run."[47]

While patient deaths at the hands of attendants were relatively rare, incidents of petty harassment, aimed at bolstering attendants' authority, were common. One victim of such treatment remembered vividly the feeling of being "unmanned" when forced to eat an extra bowl of soup even though he was already full. Another, who had taught newly freed blacks in the South after the Civil War, complained that patients had no more rights than slaves and often were forced to submit to unreasonable tasks. Neither doctors nor attendants regarded them as individuals, she complained. Tired and overworked attendants, such as the one who pushed her hard for not going upstairs fast enough, frequently lost their tempers.[48] Ex-patients recalled feeling particularly vulnerable during baths, and several complained about the frequent forceful plunging of feeble patients into cold baths, where they were scrubbed with a corn-stalk broom and soap so harsh that it blistered the skin. Patients also felt degraded when forced into bath water already used by four or five other patients. Once bathed, patients reported, they often received additional bruises while being dressed.[49] Whereas nineteenth-century newspapers attributed such incidents to inhumanity, Erving Goffman has suggested that mental patients are particularly vulnerable to abuse while being made presentable against their will. Forcible bathing and dressing, Goffman argues, violate the basic cultural rule that adults freely choose to present an appropriate physical appearance. When attendants take over that task, patients give up both dignity and deference. While nineteenth-century asylum superintendents lacked Goffman's insight, they, too, recognized the frequency with which patients were mishandled during bathing and, in a few instances, assigned doctors to oversee that activity.[50]

Injuries also were frequent during the forced feeding of patients who refused to eat. While doctors supposedly supervised all forced feeding, they often failed to do so. At Utica, one young attendant broke a patient's teeth while using a pine stick to hold open her mouth. Another patient died from injuries received during the repeated rough insertion of stomach tubes. None of these Utica cases, however, attracted the newspaper attention given a New York City incident. When an inept attendant at Blackwell's Island mangled the roof of a female patient's mouth during

182

forced feeding, the victim's husband took the hapless attendant to court. Although he lost the case, at least momentarily he focused public attention on the ease with which less lethal forms of maltreatment than murder pervaded asylum life.[51]

Of course, not all patient–staff ward interactions were negative. Both Chapin and Blumer gave dedicated attendants credit for the successful implementation of a number of important reforms, including the abolition of mechanical restraints and the diversification of patient work opportunities. When a smallpox epidemic threatened the Utica Asylum, two Utica attendants voluntarily spent almost two months isolated with four smallpox victims in hospital tents pitched on a remote part of the asylum farm. Willard's attendants responded with similar bravery when an epidemic resembling typhoid fever swept the institution in 1871. Despite widespread apprehension, not a single attendant left the asylum service or refused to work around the clock.[52] Other Willard attendants, including those assigned to chronically demented patients, responded to their charges' helplessness and dependency with much pity and affection.

In addition to citing such individual achievements, both Willard and Utica doctors defended their attendants by noting the heavy physical and emotional demands of their work. The majority of attendants, doctors proclaimed, were hard-working, reliable, and compassionate. Their daily good deeds were too often overlooked when patient–staff tensions erupted into the popular press.[53] Still, "good" and "bad" attendants resembled each other more closely than doctors cared to admit. Dedicated, energetic teachers of convalescent patients easily deteriorated into irritable, harsh autocrats after several weeks on a ward for the noisy, incoherent, and incontinent. The frequency with which the same individuals assumed the dual roles of loving parent and harsh patriarch reflected the conflicting demands of attendants' work. Like parents, attendants sometimes loved, other times struck out at, their difficult children.

When asylums were small, superintendents managed to keep such erratic behavior within reasonable bounds. By the end of the century, the conceptualization of the asylum as a family in which attendants lovingly cared for the childlike patients was increasingly anachronistic. Brigham's cohesive Utica community, with its fifty employees, had mushroomed in size and complexity. To function efficiently, the institution required more than three hundred staff members. As they marched patients from ac-

183

tivity to activity to the blaring of bugles, attendants more closely resembled prison guards than kindly companions. The Willard Asylum was even more overwhelming, a small world unto itself with a population of more than two thousand patients, doctors, and staff. And while even the most preoccupied of Victorian patriarchs recognized his own children, by 1890 Willard's superintendent knew few of his charges.[54]

Such growth had been gradual, but asylum administrators never fully adjusted to it. In their annual reports of the 1880s, they experimented with a variety of new metaphors—medical, industrial, and military—to characterize their activities, but they had difficulty reconciling their therapeutic objectives, as well as their self-image, with notions of a military encampment or industrial plant. And so they continued to rely most heavily on familial rhetoric.[55] Both Utica and Willard administrators refused to abandon the vision of their institution as a home away from home, where patients and staff lived together in large and contented families. As a result, attendants remained trapped within the confines of what was at best an inadequate and partial vision of their work.

The medicalization of lunatic asylums at the end of the nineteenth century did little to improve attendants' status or to clarify the ambiguities of their position. When the 1890 legislature changed the names of New York's lunatic asylums to "state mental hospitals," asylum doctors hoped that the prestige of both their own work and their institutions would increase. Yet, they never seriously considered redistributing internal asylum authority to accommodate their shifting mission. Instead, they emulated their colleagues at general hospitals. Despite the recent professionalization of nursing, large social and power differentials continued to separate doctors, nurses, and patients in general hospitals.[56] Within mental hospitals, this hierarchical structure was even more rigid. Hence the continuing popularity of the family metaphor. It helped to blur power differentials exacerbated by the increasing emphasis given to a strictly medical approach to mental illness. It also made easier institutional psychiatrists' justification of the continuing therapeutic differences between caring for the mentally and physically ill. For attendants, however, its effects were less benign. Although the most promising patients confined within the asylum family were encouraged by doctors to mature and break away, attendants were given few opportunities for change. The medical staff continued to show little interest in extending the benefits of professionalization to these lowly members of the hospital hierarchy, despite their vital role in patient care and therapy. Asylum doctors either could not or would not see the contradictions inherent in asking employees simultaneously to counsel and to clean, to befriend and to discipline, to follow and to lead. Even as mental hospitals moved into the twentieth century, attendants remained frozen in their old, conflicting roles: as children themselves in need of continued supervision by the medical staff, as the surrogate parents of patients, and as the domestic servants of all.[57]

7

The Politics of Maintenance

After the Civil War, the New York State asylum system found itself in a somewhat peculiar position: simultaneously under attack for a number of internal management problems and lauded for its superiority to county-level institutions. As a target of criticism, it was not alone. Nationwide the prestige of insane asylums was decreasing as their early therapeutic promise dimmed and their facilities filled with seemingly incurable pauper insane. Reformers long concerned with the plight of those excluded from state care now began to worry about those confined within the rapidly expanding institution. "Who Shall Guard the Guardians?" asked the *New York Times* and others.[1] When asylum superintendents refused to listen to their complaints, they formed groups such as the National Association for the Protection of the Insane and the Prevention of Insanity (NAPIPI). In New York, they also helped to launch a series of legislative investigations into patient care and administrative practices at state asylums.[2]

In large part as a result of such critiques, between 1865 and 1890, New Yorkers experimented with a variety of strategies intended to improve supervision of state institutions. For example, in 1867 the governor named eight commissioners of public charities to oversee state-funded social welfare institutions. In 1872 the legislature authorized appointment of a special state commissioner in lunacy to oversee the internal affairs of both state and local asylums. Finally, in 1889 this commissioner was replaced with a three-person commission in lunacy, whose members imposed uniform standards of patient care, fiscal accountability, and attendants' employment and training on all of New York's state-level insane asylums (by that date called hospitals).[3]

The long-term impact of the reforms was limited. For the most part, state officials were more concerned about the inadequacies of care at the remaining county-level institutions than about problems at state facilities. While legislative investigations of the state asylums, especially those of Utica, attracted much attention, they had little impact on patient care. For, while stories of abused and neglected patients had a powerful initial impact, they produced few long-term changes. Between 1870 and 1890, investigations increasingly took on the flavor of morality plays in which stock characters (defensive doctors, angry ex-patients, and overworked attendants) always appeared playing predictable roles. The testimony offered from one investigation to the next varied so little as to suggest, over time, that the asylums' flaws were inevitable. Yet, although they seldom produced substantial reforms, such investigations permitted New Yorkers to exorcise their guilt about relegating family members to massive, overcrowded institutions without digging deeper into their pocketbooks to improve funding or accepting such disruptive individuals back into the community. They seemed to disturb the daily functioning of the state asylums only momentarily, if at all.[4]

Also during the second half of the nineteenth century, the long battle between advocates of local and state care of the insane came to a climax. In support of their campaigns to improve and to extend state-level care of the mentally ill, late nineteenth-century reformers used somewhat different language than had their antebellum counterparts. Continuing to repeat the attacks on county care developed decades earlier, they moved the chronically insane into center stage, the position previously monopolized by the acutely insane. Concerned about the ever-increasing numbers of incurably insane paupers, politicians and reformers began to develop a new "politics of maintenance" (a logical, if one-sided, development of certain themes implicit in the "economics of compassion") to justify to New York taxpayers state-level care for all chronically insane paupers. Although George Cook and John Chapin had developed the outlines of this argument in the 1860s during their lobbying to get funds for the Willard Asylum, not until after the Civil War did it come to the forefront in New York. Somewhat ironically, late nineteenth-century reformers found themselves engaged simultaneously in two challenging battles: an attack on state asylums' abuse of their powers and an attempt to extend those same powers to all insane paupers in New York. They partially resolved their dilemma by creating a new level of bureaucracy at the top of the system (a state commissioner of lunacy) even as they fought to eliminate the bottom level: county asylums.

The same asylum doctors who opposed the intrusion of centralized state authority into state institutions supported its extension to county facilities, in part because such a move bolstered their own authority. Although post–Civil War county politicians fought to keep the chronically insane in their own institutions, they eventually were defeated.[5] In 1890 the State Care Act ordered the transfer of all insane paupers, except those in three exempted counties, from local to state facilities.[6] The State Care Act was to revolutionize New York's treatment of its mentally ill men and women, albeit in a different way from that anticipated by its framers. Once county-level facilities closed, state hospitals were overwhelmed with the difficult-to-care-for chronically insane, many of them senile or syphilitic. In struggling to cope with the resulting overcrowding and understaffing, state institutions found almost impossible the fulfillment of their therapeutic mission. Refuges they sometimes continued to be; hospitals for sick minds they certainly were not.

Proposals for Regulation and Reform

Three decades of debate, experimentation, and reform preceded the successful passage of the State Care Act in 1890. The first state-level regulation of insane asylums, both local and state, began in the late 1860s, under the direction of the Board of State Commissioners of Public Charities (later renamed the State Board of Charities).[7] New York was not unique in setting up such a state-level coordinating agency to oversee its charitable activities. According to Gerald Grob, the establishment of such board was part of the growth of rationalized bureaucracies in late nineteenth-century America, developed in partnership with the expansion and specialization of the activities of the state.[8] Initially, the New York board floundered as its members attempted to translate its broad mandate into concrete policies. By the early 1870s, however, its executive secretary,

Charles Hoyt, had developed into a strong leader, and the board began to replace earlier coalitions of journalists, lawyers, and former asylum patients as the leader of New York's forces for institutional reform.[9] One of Hoyt's first actions was to conduct a statewide survey of the insane, whether at home, in county facilities, or in state asylums or hospitals. Like his antebellum brethren, he hoped that the resulting "statistics of insanity" would inform policy and allow him to establish a more rational and effective regulatory system. His survey, especially insofar as it dealt with the insane at home or in the custody of friends, was much more thorough than that made by state and national census leaders because it relied upon local doctors (rather than families) to report private patients.

The result was a detailed sociodemographic profile of the insane, inside and outside institutions, which helped to clarify the dimensions of New York's insanity burden.[10] By themselves, the statistics did not reveal the best way to deal with that problem. They made clear that county institutions still held large numbers of the chronically insane, but they said nothing about the quality of their care. Nonetheless, upon being reminded of the magnitude of county care, the state commissioners responded with horror (reflecting longstanding prejudices in reform circles about county care in general). All too frequently, when individual commissioners visited such institutions, they found that even the best lacked resident physicians—for the medical establishment, a benchmark for effective care in the 1870s.[11] In subsequent legislative reports, both members of the State Board of Charities and the commissioner in lunacy emphasized the neglect and abuse of the insane which could be found in the worst of the county facilities. While they also inspected state asylums, the inadequacies they found there were less glaring and could more easily be explained away by attending physicians who shared the class origins of board members (as county officials most often did not). After 1872 the State Charities Aid Association, a voluntary charitable groups whose local visitors inspected county social welfare institutions, took over much of the board's investigative work. For the next three decades, the two groups worked closely, if not always in harmony, to replace county care of the dependent insane with that of the state.[12]

Thus, the anti-county, pro-state rhetorical tradition started by Dorothea Dix and Sylvester Willard continued into the post–Civil War decades. Yet, even while few criticisms of state asylums surfaced in the State Boards' annual reports, by the 1870s and early 1880s such institutions were no longer completely shielded from critical appraisal. The State Charities Aid Association, in particular, felt that all public institutions, whether state or local, needed some external supervision, and its members joined with the New York Neurological Society and the State Board of Charities to lobby for a number of reforms, including creation of a lunacy commission on the English model.[13] In response, asylum sympathizers eulogized the shelter and care offered by "our noble, palatial state lunatic asylums" and argued that political interference with their internal management would hurt, not help, their inmates.[14] New York politicians, caught between critics and defenders of the status quo, left the asylum system and commitment laws untouched but created a new supercustodian (in emulation of the English), the commissioner in lunacy. This new official, along with members of the already existing State Board of Charities, was asked to investigate "any situation in which there was reason to believe that a person was being unjustly confined or improperly treated in a New York institution for the insane, whether public or private." He also was ordered to investigate the condition of the insane and idiotic in the state, especially in asylums, but only in such a way as "not to prejudice the[ir] established and reasonable regulations." If he found abuses, he was to recommend reforms through the State Board of Charities.[15]

What from a twentieth-century perspective seem to be the mixed values of this statute accurately reflected the ambivalent feelings of even the most rabid critics of New York's insane asylums. Whether lawyers, doctors, or ex-patients, none of them wanted to eliminate such institutions, particularly at the state level. They simply wanted assurance that asylums would be reserved for, and take good care of, those in most need of them (especially if poor and socially disruptive). Here, nineteenth-century Americans resembled twentieth-century ones. As a contemporary legal scholar observes, the general public fears wrongful noncommitments even more than wrongful commitments.[16] As a result, even those asylum reformers who realized the inherent limitations of the new commissioner applauded the legislature's move. Initially, New York asylum superintendents opposed the notion of external supervision, for they feared interference with their almost absolute institutional control. (In New York, at least, local boards of trustees seldom interfered with asylum management.) The superintendents quickly learned, however, that the commissioner in lunacy (no matter who he was) at worst only tinkered with their internal affairs and at best became one of their most fervent apologists.

Thus, the ambivalence built into the 1873 enabling legislation worked to their advantage.[17] In New York as in England, the establishment of an external supervisory agent helped to legitimate, not constrict, state insane asylums.[18]

In addition to the statutory restrictions on his power, the man who became New York's first commissioner in lunacy was further limited by his own personality and intellectual propensities. A graduate of both Harvard Law School and the National Medical College of Washington, D.C., John Ordronaux had excellent formal qualifications for the new position. After serving as an army surgeon in the Civil War, he had written two much-cited books on medical jurisprudence. According to his contemporaries, however, Ordronaux was a shy man, intimidated by the slightest hint of hostility, physical or verbal. In court, he could be reduced to tears by harsh cross-examiners. The emotional strain of his work sometimes made him ill, and when seriously depressed, he withdrew from even his closest friends.[19] Such a person, even if he had been given more power than that granted the commissioner in lunacy, was hardly the best choice to tackle New York's powerful and firmly entrenched state asylum superintendents.

Though trained in both medicine and law, Ordronaux preferred to deal with legal, not medical issues. Such an inclination was understandable. Commitment laws and the insanity plea, however controversial, were straightforward in comparison with sagging cure rates, debates over therapeutic strategies, and attendant–patient abuse. Therefore, Ordronaux's first move as commissioner was to plough through New York's chaotic insanity statutes. Enlisting the help of the state's attorney general, Daniel Pratt, he began to eliminate duplications and contradictions and to bring all of the relevant legislation together into one place. Within a month, Pratt and Ordronaux had ready for the legislature's scrutiny a lengthy proposal for a new chapter in New York law, plus a report presenting the rationale for the codification.[20] In both the report and the proposal, Ordronaux and Pratt put special emphasis on the need to reform New York's commitment procedures. They wanted to make sure that never again could a person be confined in a New York asylum without medical certification and court approval. The doctors who signed such certificates needed to be well qualified and therefore, Ordronaux and Pratt limited the power to examine the allegedly insane to graduates of reputable medical schools who lived in the state and had practiced there at least three years.

Thus the insanity laws of 1874, quickly approved by the New York State Legislature, far from restricting the power of the medical profession in the commitment process, strengthened it. Ordronaux, like his English counterparts, in many respects legitimated "the perpetuation of medical hegemony" in institutional response to madness.[21] Still, Ordronaux did not give the asylum doctors everything they wanted. In an 1883 essay on the rights of the insane, Superintendent Gray argued that as with any disease requiring hospital care, doctors alone should determine whether or not individuals were proper subjects for asylum treatment. The "real rights of the insane," he orated, should include "the right of being protected against the danger of the disease and of being cured as speedily as possible."[22] Despite his great admiration for Gray, Ordronaux the lawyer could not accept such a statement of nineteenth-century liberal paternalism.

Just as they removed medical certifying power from marginal doctors, Ordronaux and Pratt also took the power to sign commitment papers away from justices of the peace. Only judges from courts of record were now permitted to approve commitment orders. Although the justices' power to commit "upon their own view" had been designed for cases of sudden and violent insanity, they refused to so confine themselves, alleged Ordronaux, and too often committed even quiet and harmless people. Ordronaux did not object to such a process per se but rather to the infringement it represented on the jurisdiction of superintendents of the poor, to whose care such harmless paupers had been given. Others noted that local justices of the peace were much more likely than court judges to be aware of and swayed by neighborhood opinions of alleged lunatics.[23] Finally, Ordronaux and Pratt argued against the use of jury trials in commitment cases, on the grounds of expense and lack of professional expertise. Here, they were in agreement with asylum superintendents and in sharp conflict with a number of reformers.[24]

Ordronaux's revision of state commitment laws satisfied many who had worried about the possibility that "sane" men and women might unjustly be sent to state asylums. But the struggle to improve the lot of those within the institutions, however demented, continued. Active in this campaign was Hervey B. Wilbur, the head of the New York State Asylum for Idiots. In 1874 Wilbur, a long-time enemy of John Gray and his friends, had been sent by the State Board of Charities to England and

Europe to see if any aspects of their asylum management profitably might be emulated in New York State. Upon Wilbur's return to New York in 1875, he offered first to the State Board of Charities and then to the National Conference of Charities and Corrections what one historian has called "the first clearly-articulated program for reforming the system of insane asylum management in the United States." [25] Wilbur described admiringly the work programs of British asylums, their efforts to increase patients' personal liberties (through such innovations as uncensored correspondence, the abolition of mechanical restraints, and the removal of bars from asylum windows), and Scotland's family-care experiments. He blamed the reluctance of many American institutions to introduce such reforms on their superintendents' unwillingness to relinquish even the smallest portion of their autocratic powers or to restrain their fiscal extravagance. [26]

Wilbur's proposals for change engendered much controversy, within New York State and across the country. Nationally, the fight for asylum reform was led by NAPIPI and the National Conference of Charities and Corrections (NCCC) and countered by the AMSAII. So many of the NAPIPI and AMSAII leaders came from New York State that New York events and personalities dominated the debate between the two groups. In particular, Gray, president of the AMSAII in the middle of this critical period, became (for both his friends and enemies) a symbol of opposition to change. New York City neurologists, like William Hammond and E. C. Spitzka, as well as such public officials as Wilbur, launched vitriolic personal attacks on Gray in both the New York and national press. Gray responded in kind. [27]

Legislative Investigations

1880–1881

Although the pro- and anti-asylum factions most often fought out their battles in the pages of professional journals and on the floors of conference meetings, they also took their conflicts to the people of New York

State through two widely publicized legislative investigations: one beginning in 1880 and the other in 1884. These were not the first legislative inquiries into the internal affairs of New York asylums. For example, in 1869, three senators and five assemblymen had journeyed to Utica for a day-long investigation of complaints made by George Cook against his former superintendent, John Gray. Although the committee's report did not reveal Cook's specific charges, presumably he had alleged financial mismanagement, for the legislators paid particular attention to the asylum's accounts. They also briefly checked patients' appearance and "the general manner of conducting the affairs of the asylum." Finding no legal proof of irregularities, they praised Utica's humane and progressive policies toward the insane. Although conceding the inadequacy of a single day's probe into Cook's charges, the eight politicians then returned to Albany. Not surprisingly, asylum critics attacked the investigation as a whitewash.[28] They similarly characterized the next inquiry, carried out in 1873 by order of the governor. Although serious charges of improper commitment procedures and patient abuse had been levied against several New York asylums, the three appointed commissioners did little to investigate them. They felt that they had neither the authority nor the qualifications to comment upon asylums' treatment and disciplinary programs. After clearing the institutions of wrongdoing, however, they recommended appointment of the state commissioner in lunacy, to alleviate unjustified public mistrust, and their bill to do so was passed that same year.[29]

More critical was the 1879 state comptroller's analysis of the fiscal affairs of New York State's charitable institutions. In submitting to the legislature what became known as the Apgar Report (after its chief investigative agent), the state comptroller urged forceful state supervision of insane asylums. In visits to seventeen state-funded charitable institutions (including the Utica and Willard asylums), his agent had found inconsistent accounting systems, few property inventories, enormous cost differentials, and evidence of manipulation of financial records so as to cover up waste and extravagance. In comparison with state asylums elsewhere, per capita expenses at New York's three acute care insane asylums (Utica, Poughkeepsie, and Middletown) were extremely high. In conclusion, Apgar argued for fiscal retrenchment and increased state budgetary control. His supervisor, the comptroller, also proposed that all institutional receipts be paid directly into the State Treasury, from which he would advance appropriations when necessary, and that all requests for legislative assistance first be submitted to the State Board of Charities for certification. The recommendations of the Apgar Report were only partially implemented at this point. Most important, the comptroller and the State Board of Charities had to approve specific proposals for additional construction at state institutions before legislative appropriations could be spent. Although these institutions also were ordered to provide detailed annual expense reports to the State Board of Charities, the Utica managers refused to do so for many years.[30] Yet the Apgar Report was an important augury of the future; it reflected the growing conviction of bureaucrats and reformers that state-level control would be more cost effective and less vulnerable to corruption than local autonomy. Although Gray and several of his fellow superintendents protested that officials in Albany could not respond flexibly to local needs and opportunities, by the late 1880s they had lost the argument. Whatever the ultimate merits of tight state fiscal control, it was never seriously challenged, once given statutory embodiment. In subsequent years, whenever fiscal irregularities reappeared in institutional budgets, outraged reformers and newspaper reporters invariably responded by calling for more of the same, that is, further increases in the regulatory powers of the comptroller.

The Apgar Report had indirect results as well. In 1880, in response to the Apgar Report, complaints from the New York Neurological Society, and growing public distrust, the New York State Senate began its first thorough examination of public insane asylums. A three-person committee spent over a year interviewing superintendents, attendants, trustees, independent medical experts, and the state commissioner in lunacy.[31] Their hearings brought onto the same platform men who had been battling through the written word for almost a decade. Although they never confronted each other directly, the neurologists (especially Hammond, Spitzka, and George Beard) and their opponents (especially Gray and Ordronaux) used the hearings to focus public attention on their arguments with each other. Their testimony invariably mingled theoretical differences with personal animosities.

Judging from contemporary accounts, the neurologists and their allies dominated the hearings, their testimony eventually helping to fill a thousand-page report. Typical were Beard's comments, which summarized points also made by Spitzka, Hammond, and Seguin. As an officer of

NAPIPI, Beard called again for a number of the reforms Wilbur had advocated five years before. These included central governmental supervision of state insane asylums by a paid commission of three experts; more and varied labor for patients; reduction of the use of mechanical restraints; minimization of locked doors, barred windows, and censored correspondence; construction of asylums composed of small, separate buildings, rather than massive monoliths; and higher pay for asylum officers.[32] To highlight the need for reform, the neurologists described in horrified tones current asylum practices, especially at Utica. Attendants used the notorious Utica crib upon the slightest provocation. Utica's doctors as well as attendants worked little, and the institution lagged far behind in the scientific study of insanity. Although it employed a trained pathologist, his work was of little, if any, value. Worst of all was the dishonesty and manipulativeness of John Gray. Two of his upstate enemies, Louis Tourtellot, a one-time assistant physician at Utica, and Hervey Wilbur of the New York State Idiot Asylum at Syracuse, repeated once again those rumors about Gray's personal finances and asylum management which had prompted the 1869 investigation. Tourtellot, in particular, charged Gray with misuse of asylum resources for his own financial benefit and with refusing to call for coroner's inquests in suspicious cases of sudden death or suicide among patients. Wilbur, too, criticized Gray's budgetary maneuvers and attacked his asylum's heavy reliance on restraint to calm patients who might better have been controlled by labor programs comparable to those used so effectively in Europe. Wilbur's hostility toward Gray had a long history, and he claimed that, when he had attempted to visit the Utica Asylum the preceding year, an assistant physician had asked if he came as friend or enemy. When he rejected both designations, the doctor refused to let him enter.[33]

Gray was not the only target of criticism at these hearings. The other principal villain, somewhat ironically, was the first commissioner in lunacy, John Ordronaux. Although both the neurologists and the State Board of Charities strongly supported the notion of state-level supervision of insane asylums, they disliked equally strongly the first man appointed to hold such an office. Initially they had expected Ordronaux to work closely with the State Board of Charities to monitor abuse at state and county asylums. Yet Ordronaux, a former professor of medical jurisprudence at Columbia University, preferred to devote most of his first year in office to

196

recodifying the state insanity laws.[34] Once this task was completed, his critics charged, he became little more than a tool of the asylum interests, and a not very industrious one at that. Of course, as Edward Spitzka admitted, Ordronaux's powers were limited by the laws which created his position so that, for example, he could supervise only those asylums which kept insane paupers. He also had been enjoined to perform his duties in such a way as "not to prejudice the established and reasonable regulations of such asylums and institutions." Yet, the neurologists complained, Ordronaux's habit of warning superintendents of his impending visits and his reluctance to inspect wards at night represented an excessively pro-asylum interpretation of the word *reasonable*. According to John C. Shaw, a reformer in charge of the Flatbush Asylum who had attracted national notoriety by burning its camisoles and muffs. Ordronaux always asked Shaw to accompany him on his perfunctory inspection tour of the asylum. He never probed into the asylum's policies nor made any specific recommendations, although he did agree to support Shaw's request for additional room.[35]

Ordronaux's self-defense at the 1880 hearings further tarnished his reputation. He offered the investigating legislators a judicial history of his office, making clear his cautious operating style. Typical was his account of an 1873 incident. Asked for help by a local reformer in collecting information about abuse at the Kings County Insane Asylum by a Brooklyn reform committee, Ordronaux agreed to cooperate. He warned, however, that he had no clerical help and that his final report had to be submitted to the Board of Charities before being shown to the governor. Although the State Board probably would not forward the findings before its annual report was due, Ordronaux claimed his responsibilities would end with its submission to them. The reformer then left Ordronaux's office in a huff, claiming that Ordronaux's proposed plan of action (and inaction) was "too circuitous a way of reaching the remedy."[36]

As the questioning of Ordronaux proceeded, it became increasingly clear that the senators knew of the allegations of his incompetence and intended to probe into them on the witness stand. Their commitment to more substantive action was unclear. After all, state legislators themselves had been responsible for many of the limitations on Ordronaux's powers. Furthermore, these were not the first indications of his incompetence. For example, a member of the State Board of Charities had complained two years earlier that when Ordronaux came to his district to investigate, he had stayed no longer than four or five minutes.[37] In response to sharp questioning about this and similar incidents, Ordronaux ineptly defended himself. For example, when asked to explain his ignorance of recent events at the notorious Ward's Island Asylum in New York City, he protested, "I can't charge my memory going through so many institutions and taking no copy of the figures I see." Somewhat surprisingly, no one then inquired into the sources of his annual report statistics. No doubt his enemies' allegations that he simply copied them from asylum superintendents' records were correct. He subsequently refused to answer hostile questions about his seeming uninterest in levels of restraint at several New York asylums. Whenever use of mechanical restraints declined, he assumed simply that superintendents' "medical judgement for the day had decided that no restraint was necessary." When one senator then asked caustically if such shifts might not even depend on such factors as the weather, Ordronaux merely replied, "Oh, yes, certainly."[38]

Ordronaux took the witness stand a number of times during these hearings. His testimony offered devastating proof of the ease with which state regulatory agencies could become allies of the regulated, but subsequent events in nineteenth-century New York showed that even those reformers and politicians most critical of Ordronaux were unwilling to draw such a conclusion. Rather than struggle with complex issues relating to the allocation of power, they preferred to focus on Ordronaux's personal failings, just as they attempted to blame Gray's autocratic personality for all flaws in the daily operation of the Utica Asylum. In both cases, they looked for scapegoats rather than for structural flaws in their bureaucratic system. Ordronaux's 1880 testimony also suggested that legislators still felt uneasy about delegating their authority to appointed officials. For example, he complained that lack of staff forced him to "infer good management where I have no evidence to the contrary." Furthermore, despite his frequent complaints, year after year, Ordronaux's annual reports were not printed until well after adjournment of the legislature to which they were addressed. As a result, they were seldom read, let alone acted upon. Although he several times asked for the statutory power to compel asylum managers to correct their failure to supply sufficient food, shelter, clothing, or medical care to the insane under their care, the state legislature still hesitated to delegate substantial powers to an administrative agency.

They wanted Ordronaux to curb the authority of asylum superintendents, but seemingly they themselves were unwilling to give up enough of their own power to permit him to do so.[39] Given such legislative ambivalence, Ordronaux proved a perfect choice for commissioner, for his political ineptitude tended to obscure the structural weaknesses of his office. In 1880 and 1884, reformers within the legislature found satisfying targets for their discontent in Ordronaux and Gray and failed to move substantially beyond criticizing them personally. Although the New York Neurological Society described Ordronaux as "an officer who has more reason to dread an investigation of the asylums in this State than most of the superintendents themselves," its members offered only one remedy for his deficiencies: replacement of a single commissioner with a three-person commission on the English model.[40] The solution was old, the target new: move the locus of power ever higher, by creating a new level of state bureaucracy. Ordronaux fought a valiant but losing battle against this policy. The delegation of supervisory power to the local trustee boards of state asylums was highly appropriate, he argued, for "every charitable institution is, in fact, a domestic forum, needing to adapt itself to local circumstances as well as to rules of government." Appointment of a state commission to oversee local authorities would only create a double-headed monster and lead to dissension and lawsuits. Here, Ordronaux expressed a point of view once considered progressive but now outdated. While acknowledging that he had been criticized for ineffectiveness, he claimed that jurisdiction over most issues relating to care of the insane poor properly belonged to local authorities whose powers derived from a "higher source" than his own.[41]

Eventually, in part as a result of the 1880–1881 hearings, Ordronaux was replaced as commissioner by another doctor, Stephen Smith. Smith proved more conscientious in the execution of his duties, and he supported the campaign for a three-person lunacy commission. Yet Smith's reports differed little from Ordronaux's, except in their detail. He too tended to focus on the blatant problems in county asylums rather than on weaknesses in the powerful state institutions. Also like Ordronaux, he deplored the "unjust censoriousness and distrust" with which the public so often viewed asylum care of the insane. He, the State Board of Charities, and Ordronaux all felt that timely suggestions emanating from an official source, even though without the power of enforcing a single one of them, were more efficacious than legal action. Smith too seldom interfered in cases of alleged attendant abuse "unless circumstances of a peculiarly aggravating character existed which demanded a wider remedy than could be secured by a purely domestic investigation." Smith tried to distinguish himself from Ordronaux by a more energetic execution of his duties, but his efforts produced no dramatically new findings. Like Ordronaux, he felt it was impossible to investigate every petty rumor, and once he started to delve into the tangled relationships among attendants and patients, he too had difficulty distinguishing truths from delusions, half-truths from outright lies. Although he pushed for establishment of a commission in lunacy, a move greatly opposed by Ordronaux and state asylum superintendents, Smith's reports suggested that only the most blatant abusers had much to fear from external regulation, whatever its form.[42]

The other villain at the 1880–1881 hearing was John Gray. While reformers most often pictured Ordronaux as bumbling, inefficient, and somewhat lazy, they conveyed an image of Gray as a malevolent figure, a man of much power consistently abused. He became the embodiment of all that neurologists most disliked about late nineteenth-century institutional psychiatry and often was not even referred to by name but simply alluded to in such terms that his identity as archvillain was clear. In contrast, when Gray finally took the stand himself, his testimony seemed startlingly innocuous. For example, in defense of his purchasing policies, he claimed that competitive bids always determined expenditures (a less than honest statement, it was revealed in 1884). When criticized for the inadequacy of his treatment programs, especially his reluctance to develop work projects, he pointed out that patients were employed whenever such labor was not injurious to their health. He also defended his regulation of patient correspondence (both outgoing and incoming) and the continued use of a minimum of restraint. For the first time faced with hostile legislators, Gray attempted to be conciliatory and to justify his thirty-year reign at Utica. When his defense of Utica's pathology research failed to satisfy his interrogators, he ended the discussion by noting mildly, "It is a pretty difficult thing for anybody to answer this more or less abstruse scientific matter on the spur of the moment." Gray resorted to his usual flamboyant style only once. When questioned about a well-publicized abuse case in which the Utica Asylum finally had been acquitted of criminal negligence, he asserted, "I can hardly recall any patient here who ever received more tender, considerate care than Mr. Brown."[43]

John Chapin, superintendent of the Willard Asylum for the Chronic Insane, also appeared at the same hearings. Without allying himself with the neurologists, he clearly distinguished himself from Gray. He described in a matter-of-fact fashion how he had already eliminated the use of restraints at Willard, initiated active labor programs which involved all of his able-bodied patients, and done away with any regulation of patient correspondence. He spoke highly of the English system of asylum care, arguing that it was better than the American in a number of ways. In part, Chapin's self-conscious divergence from Gray on these key issues originated in disputes between the two men which predated the Civil War. Unlike Gray, Chapin also recognized that most of the most bitterly contested reforms would, in practice, not seriously undercut asylum superintendents' authority nor substantially change asylum life.[44]

1884

Despite the intensity of the debate between pro- and anti-asylum men, state legislators took no action at the end of their investigatory year. Their one-thousand-page report summarized the testimony offered by both sides but drew no conclusions. As the result, frustrated reformers tried again in 1884 to prompt a legislative expose of state asylum care, especially at Utica. The immediate stimulus this time was the death of a Utica patient under suspicious circumstances.

When a fifty-four-year-old farmer, Evan Hughes, was admitted to the New York State Lunatic Asylum at Utica on January 25, 1884, his son reported to the admitting physician that Hughes was violent and had threatened several times to injure himself. Sent to the suicidal ward, Hughes became increasingly agitated, and the next day he was transferred to the ward for the most violent patients. One week later, in a struggle with three ward attendants, Hughes's jaw and seven of his ribs were broken. When one of the broken ribs punctured his lungs, he died. A subsequent coroner's jury investigation concluded that although it could not determine exactly how Hughes's injuries had been received, they had resulted from his fight with the three attendants, who subsequently were discharged from the asylum and indicted for murder.[45]

Hughes certainly was not the first patient to die at the New York State Lunatic Asylum under suspicious circumstances. Yet his alleged homicide sparked a major legislative investigation of the Utica Asylum that lasted for almost two months and led to publication of the fourteen-hundred-page verbatim transcript of the hearings. At its simplest level, the 1884 inquiry reflected public outrage at Hughes's treatment, first aroused by his son and then sustained by the state assemblymen from Hughes's home county. Because of Gray's national reputation, papers outside of New York State also took note of the Hughes incident. According to the *Boston Globe*, Utica attendants had so successfully tried to "calm" a patient by breaking his jaw and most of his ribs that the patient was now dead.[46] Within New York State, the details of Hughes's death appeared in articles under such banner headlines as "Dr. Gray's Butchers" and "The Utica Crime."[47] The former article charged that, while previous efforts to investigate Utica Asylum abuses had been "nipped in the bud . . . by Gray and his clique, who seem to have more power with the Legislature than the people," this time Gray would be brought to justice. The latter gloated that "suave, politic, influential Dr. Gray can not escape this time." A somewhat more balanced but still critical perspective on Gray appeared in the Albany *Evening Journal*. Its editor noted that, while the state was rightfully "proud of his commanding ability and his broad achievements," those same qualities often made his administration appear to the public "an offensive autocracy, subject to no restraints." During the two years preceding Hughes's death, Gray's frequent absences owing to ill health and demands for his presence as an expert witness in insanity trials had weakened his oversight of attendants. The result, an increase in attendant–patient tensions, culminated in Hughes's brutal murder.[48]

Even a strongly pro-asylum paper, the Utica *Observer*, lamented that the Hughes affair "has cast unpleasant suspicion upon the vigilance, good temper and paternal caution which we have had reason to believe characterized the care of patients in the Asylum." (In response, another paper commented acerbically that "unpleasant suspicion" was a mild term to characterize such beatings and called for removal of both Gray and the asylum managers.) In further defense of Gray, the Utica *Observer* published an endorsement of his medical brilliance, along with his "integrity and good management," by a member of the medical faculty at the University of Buffalo.[49]

A similar kind of partisan debate over Gray's character raged in the New York State Assembly, where hostile representatives blamed an "asylum ring" for suppressing the critical recommendations of earlier investigators and called for Gray's temporary suspension. Anti-asylum politicians also insisted that no representative from Oneida County be allowed to serve on the investigatory committee. They feared yet another cover-up of the asylum's weaknesses similar to that engineered the preceding year, when the results of the 1880–1881 Assembly investigation allegedly had been lost before reaching the state printer.[50]

Almost a month before hearings began, state legislators, Democratic newspapers, and even the governor began to call once again for more state power over Gray and his fellow superintendents. Their public debates and press pronouncements lent credence to the charge of Gray's supporters that the goals of the investigation were predetermined; their ferocity also suggested the ease with which the issues involved lent themselves to use by partisan politicians. According to the Albany *Argus*, the Hughes case conveniently reinforced Governor Grover Cleveland's recent call for state-level supervision of insane asylums and his critique of the weak advisory roles played by the state commissioner in lunacy and the State Board of Charities. Other papers used it as an occasion to demand implementation of Apgar's recommendations that business management of all such institutions be unified under state control.[51] By the time a legislative investigating committee began to call witnesses on February 16, 1884, the political atmosphere had become so highly charged that the committee met behind closed doors. Such a strategy, it hoped, would prevent witnesses from influencing each other and give asylum authorities the opportunity to answer allegations before they appeared in print. Its calming effects, however, were immediately offset by the sites chosen for the hearings: the highly charged environs of the asylum itself and the State Capitol in Albany. The list of prospective witnesses was lengthy, although the cast of characters was predictable. From the asylum came Superintendent Gray, his assistant physicians, his steward, members of the board of managers, attendants, and patients. Testimony also was solicited from ex-patients and former attendants across the state. State-level bureaucrats who appeared included Stephen Smith, the commissioner in lunacy, and Edgar Apgar, the state comptroller.

From the first weeks of the hearings, state legislators made clear that they were not interested only in ascertaining the exact circumstances of Hughes's death. They also probed more deeply those issues which had so dominated earlier hearings, including the use (and abuse) of mechanical restraints, the regulation of patient correspondence, the training and pay of attendants, and the interaction of male doctors with female patients. They sought additional information about the Utica Asylum's fiscal management and the relative powers and responsibilities of Gray and his board of managers. They attempted to cut through ambiguous and contradictory evidence by asking the same questions again and again and by confronting witnesses with contradictions, both within their own testimony and between their testimony and that of others.[52]

Although promised in advance what asylum critics considered the generous opportunity to refute all allegations of mismanagement, Gray and his board of managers hired a prominent state senator and lawyer, Alexander Goodwin, to represent them at the hearings. The five-person investigating committee, all of whose members were lawyers, also hired counsel. Such moves accentuated the adversarial nature of the proceedings. Witnesses were first questioned by the legislators and their lawyer, then cross-examined by the asylum counsel as well. Although asylum authorities hoped that hiring a lawyer would protect their interests, the strategy backfired in the end, for it emphasized their defensive posture.[53] For example, during the last two weeks of the investigation, asylum authorities received a complete transcript of the hearings so as to enable them to respond to charges and present witnesses in their own behalf. Goodwin initially tried to paper over the asylum's defensive position by asking that pro-asylum speakers not be treated as witnesses "for the Asylum in any sense."[54] When the committee first rejected this strategy and then objected to his first witness's testimony as irrelevant, Goodwin reversed his tactics, becoming exaggeratedly defensive. He angrily asserted (for the first time) that throughout the investigation he had been treated unfairly by not being allowed to object to testimony or to cross-examine witnesses. His complaints annoyed committee members, who distinctly remembered his cross-examining witnesses, but after a few heated exchanges, the chair brusquely proclaimed, "There is no use wasting time in this discussion" and allowed the controverted witness to proceed with his testimony.[55] Through this interchange, participants implicitly acknowledged the trial like nature of the proceedings, as a result of which courtroom procedures became as important as the testimony offered. Goodwin's defensiveness also suggested that, with the investigation drawing to a close, asylum authorities and their lawyer increasingly feared its outcome.

Because its meetings were closed to the public, the press, whether pro-

or anti-asylum, had few concrete events to discuss during the investigation itself. Hostile papers devoted much energy to sniffing out possible sources of asylum whitewash; for example, they attacked the investigatory committee's lawyer on the grounds that he was a stooge for Gray. They also picked up on the 1883 Apgar Report's hints of financial mismanagement at the asylum and lacerated Gray for his financial extravagance. Most frequently repeated was the allegation that he had used the asylum's supply appropriations to pay for nearly half a million dollars in irresponsible general improvements, but they also charged that he had added greatly to his state salary through a large private practice. Finally, lacking more concrete news, papers across New York repeated the violently anti-Gray rhetoric of preinvestigation editorials. They suggested that one of Gray's strongest defenders within the state medical establishment, Dr. Edward Brush of the Buffalo Asylum, was merely trying to thank Gray for the "fat place" (as an assistant physician) he had once undeservingly held at Utica. More telling were those critics who argued that even if Gray were not personally responsible for Hughes's death (and similar incidents), he still had a responsibility to bring to justice "brutal keepers" who "pound and trample defenseless patients to death."[56] Pro-asylum papers responded by reprinting medical testimonials to Gray, but these hardly had the same news appeal.

Most of the early testimony offered at the 1884 hearings related to the circumstances of Hughes's death. Typically, witnesses claimed to be unable to remember precise details about Hughes's last day. Although frustrated legislators felt certain he had been mistreated, they were unable to elicit testimony sufficient to substantiate criminal charges. Early in the hearings, it became clear that key aspects of the "mystery" of Hughes's death would never be solved. The dramatic momentum of the investigation was somewhat uneven because witnesses appeared in an order more often dictated by their availability than by a coherent investigative strategy. Gray, the public villain of the affair, was the first to testify. As in 1881, his careful, measured remarks belied his colorful image in the popular press, although he also, on almost every point of questioning, reaffirmed his conviction that as superintendent he had final authority over the asylum. Nonmedical persons, whether from his own board of managers or from the State Board of Charities, had no right to question or attempt to modify his decisions.[57]

Next appeared a number of asylum attendants. These men were questioned closely not only about the Hughes's affair but also about the general conditions of their employment and the frequency of patient abuse. Although they denied having discussed their testimony with each other before the hearing, their responses to the most pointed questions were so similar as to suggest the opposite. In general, they claimed that none of the problems asked about by the legislators, ranging from alcoholism among attendants to the rough treatment of difficult patients, existed at the Utica Asylum. In the few situations in which such flat denials were clearly impossible (such as Hughes's stay at the asylum or the frequency with which Gray visited the wards), attendants succumbed to forgetfulness. For example, one supervisor claimed to be unable to remember whether or not any Utica attendants had ever been fired. His evasiveness was so pronounced that an exasperated state senator finally asked, "Is your recollection so very poor about everything?" Doctors, too, suffered convenient lapses of memory; for example, one assistant physician was unable to remember how an ex-patient (testifying the same day) lost his teeth while at the Utica Asylum. A rare exception was the attendant who, when asked how conditions in the institution might be improved, responded, "A man cannot be bright and cheerful when he is confined here like a patient all the time." Only when several ex-attendants and former patients took the stand did the legislators get a clear picture of the circumstances and frequency of attendants' violence toward patients. Then legislators discovered that, contrary to policy, attendants used restraints whenever they pleased and only subsequently got medical approval.[58] In addition to the general issue of patient abuse, legislators showed most interest in the Utica Asylum's fiscal affairs. They questioned Gray, his managers, and his steward about their purchasing and auditing practices. They also unsuccessfully tried to ascertain the truth of allegations that Gray doubled his annual salary through court appearances as an expert witness and through an extensive private practice.[59]

After the 1884 investigation finally ended, it produced no immediate legislative action, and the mildness of the committee's final report startled those who had been following the lurid coverage in the popular press. In self-defense, the investigators, like their predecessors, excused their relative inactivity on the grounds of insufficient time to investigate the many issues presented to them. They also noted the wide differences in expert opinion as to the best way to run asylums and advocated that state supervision replace legislative investigations as a way of checking potential abuse. On the one hand, they exonerated asylum authorities of the charge of having knowingly maltreated patients or detained the sane; on the other hand, they criticized the many irregularities in Utica's business affairs and recommended that the medical superintendent be relieved of all business responsibilities. Assistant physicians should be paid more, they argued, so that they would stay longer, and female physicians should be added to protect female patients from both their own fantasies and the possibility of sexual abuse. All of the institution's doctors, from Gray down to his fourth assistant physician, needed to supervise attendants more closely and to keep firm control of the use of mechanical and chemical restraints.[60]

None of these recommendations was new; all had been debated in both the medical and popular press throughout the preceding decade. In many ways, the 1884 investigation was not an exposé but a recognition by the state's politicians of the importance of the treatment issues so long the concern of reformers. Its interrogations highlighted once again the pro- and anti-asylum positions on issues such as freedom of patient correspondence, the quality and training of attendants, and the limits of asylum superintendents' authority. About none of these issues was it more emphatic than that of mechanical restraint, in part because of Hughes's death in a Utica crib but more importantly because straitjackets, camisoles, and muffs easily served as symbols of that darker side of asylum life so feared by the general public. Thus, the testimony about restraint at the 1884 investigation encapsulated many years of debate and delineated sharply the differences between those inside and outside the asylum on how best to control the institutionalized insane. One indicator of the political sensitivity of the restraint issue in the 1880s, even before Hughes's death, had been the appearance in Utica's annual report of statistics on the small number of people put in restraints. As Gray had noted, in this respect his asylum was much more moderate than the general public, which sent large numbers of insane people to Utica in chains, handcuffs, and even enclosed boxes.[61] Yet Gray, along with his fellow AMSAII superintendents, had refused to emulate British practice in totally abolishing restraint, and he had vigorously attacked those who pressured him to do so.

Although the 1884 legislative investigators seemed generally sympathetic to Utica's critics and suggested that existing rules as to the appropriate supervision of restraint be enforced, their final report offered few firm guidelines for reform in state asylums. The general disregard of their weak conclusions by the popular press, so recently aflame with attacks on Gray, was but one sign of the increasing reorientation of New York's reformers by the mid-1880s away from a number of specific issues having to do with patient treatment toward an almost exclusive focus once more on the question of supervision. The long-standing campaign to replace all county-level care of the insane, begun well before the Civil War, revived with a new intensity, as did efforts to replace the commissioner in lunacy with a purportedly more efficient three-person lunacy commission.

In the midst of the ensuing political turmoil, John Gray died. In many ways, his death marked the passing of an era. During the next five years, New York State legislators approved substantial changes in the administration of state asylums. They established a three-person commission in lunacy. With the passage of the State Care Act in 1890, they finally replaced all county care of the insane poor with mandatory treatment in state institutions, and they centralized fiscal control of the new state system in Albany. Finally, they changed the names of the state asylums to state mental hospitals. While Grob has spelled out in detail the implications of these innovations for twentieth-century mental health care, they signaled a less profound change for patients than for state bureaucracies.[62] By 1890 the benefits of state care had become so firmly accepted, both within lay and medical circles, that it was another half-century before mental health professionals seriously began to reconsider its validity.

The Ideology of State Care

The passage of the State Care Act ended a fifty-year debate about how best to care for the chronically insane in New York State. While its supporters had had to fight hard for their victory, the late nineteenth-century campaign for this new kind of state funding differed from that of the 1830s and 1840s in a number of ways. No longer did anyone challenge the right of acutely ill patients to the best possible therapeutic care. Further, although neurologists and their allies criticized several aspects of New York's state care system in the 1870s, they never attacked the basic notion that institutional care (of some sort) was the best way to treat large numbers of the mentally ill. In the mid-1880s these reformers even joined their long-term enemies, the state asylum superintendents, to lobby for the State Care Act. That union cut off abruptly the lively and diversified discussion of the 1870s about the most appropriate form or forms of institutional care for the insane. By 1890 the only group arguing against state monopoly of mental health care were county superintendents of the poor. Even though they repeated and elaborated upon critical points made earlier by the neurologists, they received no support from reformers, who had decided to close ranks with their other medical colleagues rather than ally with groups primarily interested in the nonmedical care of the insane.[63]

In addition to asylum superintendents and neurologists, the State Care Act was supported by almost all the major newspapers of New York State, the State Medical Society, the State Homeopathic Society, the State Charities Aid Association, and the commissioner in lunacy. These groups finally brought to fruition a half-century campaign to discredit county care. While they relied heavily upon traditional horror stories of inadequate facilities and patient abuse, the urgency of their arguments reflected growing public concern about the increasing number of counties exempted from the Willard Act. As early as 1871, with the permission of the state board of charities, counties were permitted to leave their chronically insane in local asylums. Having more experience with social welfare institutions than their 1850s counterparts, local superintendents of the poor were confident that they could provide for harmless chronically insane paupers more cheaply than could the Willard doctors. With the cost of state care an increasingly large part of the local tax burden, many politicians sought political favor by cutting it. Both asylum doctors and state-level reform groups bitterly opposed the resulting competition with the state asylum system. Superintendents of the poor cared nothing about the welfare of the mentally ill, reformers charged, but only about saving money and getting themselves reelected. In contrast, state hospitals offered well-supervised custodial programs, under medical direction, for those chronically insane paupers who did not require hospitalization or seem to benefit from expensive therapeutic programs. Removed from the turmoil of their daily lives, all were happy and some even recovered (at a cost of only two dollars a week).[64]

This late nineteenth-century campaign succeeded so well that it discredited county care not only in 1890 but for the next fifty years. Yet, despite undeniable problems within many of their asylums, local superintendents of the poor offered a perceptive critique of state-level care. While agreeing that the acutely ill deserved special attention, they argued that many of those whose condition was designated "chronic" did not need expensive hospital treatment. What was wrong, they asked, with the existing "mixed" system of state and county care? Frequent visits from county general practitioners resulted in patients receiving at least as much medical attention as that available on the back wards of a thousand-patient institution. Furthermore, they claimed, more of the "chronically" insane were released each year from local asylums than from state institutions. Housed in their home counties, these men and women kept in touch with relatives, who consequently were more willing to accept them back once the worst symptoms of insanity had diminished.[65] Furthermore, from the perspective of some county officials, the State Care Act offered one last insult to the chronically insane. Although their local situation was far from ideal (many had been taken against their will from their homes to county institutions whose heads aimed primarily to care for them at the lowest possible price), with the passage of the State Care Act, they were told they were no longer welcome even to reside in their native counties.[66]

Superintendents of the poor also tried to portray the conflict over state care as one between the "people" and those who had benefited from the patronage powers of large state asylums, but here their opponents won the rhetorical battle. Despite two decades of criticism of their political power, the so-called asylum ring in 1890 managed to transfer the dread label of special interest from itself to the county officials. As a result, only those state legislators from rural districts most interested in keeping open their local asylums resisted the growing movement for state care. In the heated, mudslinging campaign to get state care, the most persuasive of the county arguments went largely unnoticed. Few politicians or newspapers wanted to hear critiques of the therapeutic inefficiency of large mixed institutions and of the negative implications of relieving counties of all responsibility for their insane citizens. Even less attention was paid to suggestions that larger state administrative structures would not necessarily be better. The progressive conviction that only centralized bureaucracies could solve a wide range of problems increasingly dominated political circles in New York. New York's state government had grown dramatically from its primitive state in the 1840s and 1850s, at which time there was not even a standing committee in the legislature devoted to public health issues, let alone a highly specialized three-person lunacy commission, and the expansion was considered evidence of progress.[67]

The lobbying and political negotiations which preceded the eventual approval of the State Care Act in 1890 (after two unsuccessful attempts to pass similar bills in 1888 and 1889) were lengthy and complex. But the public rhetoric used to support such efforts was quite straightforward, if not always internally consistent. State-level care would be of higher quality than county care, less vulnerable to political and economic pressures, more therapeutic, less custodial—or so its supporters argued. They put less emphasis, in legislative debates, on the anomaly that the intended beneficiaries of enlarged state institutions were the chronically insane, those least likely to benefit from medical treatment. To win taxpayers' support for this group, reformers rearranged somewhat the relative emphases within the traditional economics-of-compassion argument until it more closely resembled a "politics of maintenance." Typical of the new pro–state care arguments was the commissioner in lunacy's explication of the "political economy of insanity": "While humanity demands that kind treatment, proper food, clothing, and shelter be provided for all the insane, justice to the community also requires that in dispensing these bounties, care be taken to discriminate between the mere ideal and the practically useful. . . . Paupers are not justly treated, even if insane, by being given the same surroundings as those belonging to a more refined class of self-supporting lunatics."[68]

Although the State Care Act replaced separate institutions for the chronically insane in New York State with a system of "mixed" institutions, the discussions of the kinds of care to be offered within this enlarged system made it clear that, at best, a heavily segregated dual system of custodial and therapeutic treatment would characterize state mental hospitals in the future. Thus, at the same time that New York's insane asylums all changed their names to hospitals, they moved closer to the custodial image implicit in the term *asylum.* More quickly than even its enemies predicted, the balance of science, humanity, and economics within "the politics of maintenance" shifted strongly to the third. For example, discussions of the therapeutic value of colonies and detached cottages were almost totally replaced by praise of their cheapness.[69] Intended to halt the trend toward custodial care of the insane, in retrospect the State Care Act assured its dominance. Twentieth-century state mental hospitals were to be very different from and, despite scientific advances, less dynamic institutions than their nineteenth-century predecessors.

8

An Unresolved Conclusion

The modern history of madness is characterized by several persistent themes: troubled domestic relationships; inadequate nosologies and unreliable diagnoses; institutional conflicts between therapeutic and custodial goals. Such continuities help to explain why, even though New York's first two insane asylums were established as experiments, their external architecture and internal routines so quickly froze into predictable forms. Yet, it is also important to note that conceptualizations of insanity and its most appropriate treatment have shifted over time in significant, if subtle, ways. Here, too, the stories of the Utica and Willard asylums are illuminating, for the two institutions differed dramatically in mission and clientele. Utica's relatively expensive therapeutic services were made available primarily to those who showed the most promise of recovery and therefore of future productivity. Willard's cheaper services were directed toward many of industrializing New York's weakest members, including epileptics, paretics, and foreign-born domestics.

Within both Utica and Willard, doctors attempted to help patients regain control of their runaway emotions and faltering powers of reason, although at Utica they hoped thereby to assist their charges to leave the asylum, whereas at Willard they aimed to make their patients' indefinite, perhaps permanent, stay as healthy and happy as possible. Strict daily routines were regarded as one of the best ways both to retrain (and restrain) mad minds and to keep an increasingly bureaucratic and complex social world running smoothly. The language of discourse in patient casebook records expressed a dichotomous perspective on the world, with daily life pictured as a continual battle between the forces of order and disorder. Doctors characterized patients as quiet or noisy, clean or filthy, industrious or unable to work, intelligible or incoherent, intelligent or feeble minded, strong in body or physically debilitated. Typically, patients vacillated between these extremes for a time after admission, then either recovered or sank into chronicity. Although doctors did their best to control behavioral and physiological extremes, their powers were limited. They might impose external mechanical restraints, but these did not always diminish internal turmoil. They might bolster patients' diets; dose them with cathartics, tonics, and sedatives; even early in the century bleed them; but problems such as dementia, syphilis, and epilepsy resisted their most heroic efforts.

As a number of historians have pointed out, in their emphasis on segregation, classification, and discipline, asylums resembled a number of other antebellum institutions, including prisons and reform schools. Until late in the century they also shared many features in common with general hospitals, a kinship more often overlooked.[1] Like the heads of these other institutions, asylum superintendents conceptualized their patients as children and their community as surrogate "family." The family metaphor had different implications, however, when applied to delinquent adolescents, insane paupers, and convicted felons. It most quickly lost appeal for reformers dealing with the last group, for many reformers balked at equating murderers and thieves with innocent children and at giving such people even the most minimal privileges of family life.[2] The general nineteenth-century domestic movement to replace rigid discipline with warmth and love only briefly extended to the prison, where its most notable impact was a highly limited one: abolition of the death penalty. By contrast, for most of the century, reform schools and insane asylums tried to rule by reason and religion rather than by fear and punishment, and their frequent failures to do so did not go uncriticized (though they often went unchanged).

Within insane asylums, the more strained the family metaphor became, the more tightly asylum heads clung to it. By the end of the nineteenth century, it was clear that for a substantial number of Utica's and Willard's patients, an institution would be their home for life. For, even if asylum doctors could not cure sick minds, they had learned so to bolster weakened bodies that the chronically mentally ill lived for years and threatened to overwhelm even acute care facilities like Utica. The passage of the State Care Act in 1890 only increased the numbers in state institutions who required primarily custodial care. Its supporters had acted from a variety of motives: humanitarianism, fiscal economy, and a renewed therapeutic optimism. Not surprisingly, the emergent state system could not accomplish all of these goals with equal ease, and the first two tended to overwhelm the third. When New York's state asylums all were formally designated hospitals in 1890, the metaphor of the asylum as a family finally lost its central place in institutional rhetoric. Yet, at least in terms of therapeutics, the appellation of hospital fit their past better than their future. Historians critical of the inflated domestic rhetoric of the nineteenth-century asylum also need to remember that the allegedly scientific world of twentieth-century psychiatry often has been less hospitable to and more detached from the mentally ill than its predecessor. However great may be the distance between father and child, it is usually less than that between scientist and subject.

In addition to describing medical practices, the records of New York's nineteenth-century asylums offer valuable insights into their behavioral ideals: the ways in which clients, their families, and the institutions' staffs felt adults should behave, even if they did not always do so. Here it is important to remember that, although their medical staffs affected the kinds of treatment offered at Utica and Willard, they had to work within the confines of statutory definitions of their missions. While they certainly shared the general values of their society, New York's nineteenth-century state asylum superintendents also manifested a strong element of social criticism in their theoretical writings on mental illness. Many of their patients' problems, they felt, were due to the excitement and stress of life in industrializing America, which nudged those already weakened by hard work, poverty, and poor diets into succumbing to mental illness. Clearly, the earliest superintendents defined their social responsibilities broadly, and they used the prominence of their offices to lend credence to their critiques of society and their involvement with a number of reform movements. While their successors addressed most of their attention to the victims of social change confined within their institutions' walls, they never abandoned the earlier tradition of using annual reports as vehicles for reform as well as self-aggrandizement.

Doctors as well as patients were moved by societal trends outside the asylum walls. In ways too little explored by historians, asylum doctors were expected to act in accordance with sometimes amorphous, often contradictory, and always forceful social dictates, even when they were not given the means with which to satisfy society's complex demands.[3] The latter's influence—and limitations—could be seen most clearly at the several large-scale asylum investigations conducted by New York legislators after the Civil War. While, in their rhetoric, these investigations often took the black-and-white form of morality plays, they more often ended in confusion than in victory for the forces of good. The weaknesses of the villains—abusive attendants and autocratic doctors—were clear, but so few heroes took the stand that little promise of redemption emerged. A number of witnesses proclaimed that good men and women would not abuse patients, yet all with an intimate knowledge of the realities of asylum life admitted the difficulties of ward life. Reformers charged that asylums kept patients well past recovery, but these same critics complained when supposedly recovered patients became social threats after release. The institutionalized insane deserved more freedom and fewer restraints, they argued, but only so long as there was no danger they might misuse it.

Such contradictions permeated popular attitudes toward insane asylums for the entire period covered by this book. They had a medical counterpart in the bitter battles over the relative merits of materialistic, somatic, and moral interpretations of insanity and remind us that, despite their earnest efforts in the name of reason, nineteenth-century asylum doctors never succeeded in dispelling the fundamental mystery of mental illness, either for themselves or for society at large. That mystery continued to envelop not just the insane but all who dealt with them, despite the very real advances in diagnosis and treatment over the century. The unknown and unpredictable behavior of the insane was profoundly unsettling, and it is scarcely surprising that many mistakenly thought those walled-in asylums to be more like enchanted castles than hospitals, their medical staffs more like sinister wizards than plodding, overworked men of science. While the asylums struggled to provide humane care for charges who had lost that most human of qualities, reason, many outside the asylum walls preserved a lingering, ancient fear of those descended into madness and of their keepers, who were attempting to work the miracle of recovery.

An Unresolved Conclusion

In a recent thought-provoking essay, Michael Ignatieff suggests to those seeking to explain nineteenth-century institutional developments, "The real challenge is to find a model of historical explanation which accounts for institutional change without imputing conspiratorial rationality to a ruling class, without reducing institutional development to a formless *ad hoc* adjustment to contingent crisis, and without assuming a hyperidealist, all triumphant humanitarian crusade."[4] The complexity of the sociomedical worlds at the Utica and Willard asylums suggests the wisdom of Ignatieff's observation. While there was a clear hierarchy of authority and power which extended downward from superintendents to assistant physicians, staff, and patients, social interactions involved much more than domination and control. All lived together in institutions which simultaneously served as surrogate families, prisons, refuges, and hospitals. And all were members of and affected by the extra-institutional world as well, sharing its social values and biases, even as they tried to reform it.

Abbreviations

AAS	American Antiquarian Society, Worcester, Massachusetts
AJI	*American Journal of Insanity*
AMSAII	Association of Medical Superintendents of American Institutions for the Insane
AR	*Annual Report*
BHM	*Bulletin of the History of Medicine*
CLMHMS	Countway Library of Medicine, Harvard Medical School, Boston
HLHU	Houghton Library, Harvard University, Cambridge
JNMD	*Journal of Nervous and Mental Disease*
NYSLA	New York State Library Archives, Albany
OCHS	Oneida County Historical Society, Utica, New York
PHMA	Pennsylvania Hospital Medical Archives, Philadelphia
UPCA	Utica Psychiatric Center Archives, Utica, New York
UPCBR	Utica Patient Casebook Record
WPCA	Willard Psychiatric Center Archives, Willard, New York
WPCBR	Willard Patient Casebook Record

Note: The year listed for an annual report in the footnotes refers to the date of publication.

Notes

Preface

1. R. D. Laing, *Sanity, Madness and the Family;* Erving Goffman, *Asylums: Essays on the Social Situation of Mental Patients and Other Inmates;* Joseph P. Morrissey et al., *The Enduring Asylum: Cycles of Institutional Reform at Worchester State Hospital;* Leona Bachrach, "Asylum and Chronically Ill Psychiatric Patients"; H. Richard Lamb, ed., *The Homeless Mentally Ill.*

2. Thomas S. Szasz, *The Myth of Mental Illness;* Michel Foucault, *Madness and Civilization: A History of Insanity in the Age of Reason;* David Rothman, *The Discovery of the Asylum: Social Order and Disorder in the Early Republic;* Goffman, *Asylums.*

3. Bachrach, "Chronically Ill Psychiatric Patients"; Andrew Scull, *Decarceration: Community Treatment and the Deviant—a Radical View;* Walter R. Gove, ed., *Deviance and Mental Illness.*

Introduction

1. Some of the most recent participants in this debate include Anne Digby, *Madness, Morality and Medicine: A Study of the York Retreat, 1796–1914;* Mark Finnane, *Insanity and the Insane in Post-Famine Ireland;* Richard Fox, *"So Far Disordered in Mind": Insanity in California, 1870–1930;* Gerald N. Grob, *Mental Institutions in America: Social Policy to 1875;* idem, *Mental Illness and American Society, 1875–1940;* Michael B. Katz, "Origins of the Institutional State"; idem, *Poverty and Policy in American History;* Michael B. Katz, Michael J. Doucet, and Mark J. Stern, *The Social Organization of Early Industrial Capitalism;* David Rothman, *Conscience and Convenience: The Asylum and Its Alternatives in Progressive America;* Andrew Scull, *Museums of Madness: The Social Organization of Insanity in Nineteenth-Century England;* idem, ed., *Madhouses, Mad-Doctors, and Madmen: The Social History of Psychiatry in the Victorian Era;* Roger Smith, *Trial by Medicine: Insanity and Responsibility in Victorian Trials;* Nancy Tomes, *A Generous Confidence: Thomas Story Kirkbride and the Art of Asylum Keeping, 1840–1883;* Peter Tyor and Jamil S. Zainaldin, "Asylum and Society: An Approach to Institutional Change"; Barbara G. Rosenkrantz and Maris A. Vinovskis, "Caring for the Insane in Ante-Bellum Massachusetts: Family, Community, and State Participation"; idem, "The Invisible Lunatics: Old Age and Insanity in Mid-Nineteenth Century Massachusetts"; idem, "Sustaining the 'Flickering Flame of Life': Accountability and Culpability for Death in Ante-Bellum Massachusetts

Asylums"; and John K. Walton, "Lunacy in the Industrial Revolution: A Study of Asylum Admissions in Lancashire, 1848–1850."

2. Gerald N. Grob, "Reflections on the History of Social Policy in America"; idem. "Public Policy-making and Social Policy"; Scull, *Museums of Madness;* Katz, "Origins of the Institutional State"; idem. *Poverty and Policy.*

1

Life within the Asylum Walls

1. While interest in the internal dynamics of nineteenth-century asylum life is growing, relatively few detailed studies of it have been published. Two exceptions are Digby's *Madness, Morality and Medicine* and Tomes's *A Generous Confidence.* Two earlier works, Gerald N. Grob's *The State and the Mentally Ill: A History of Worcester State Hospital in Massachusetts, 1830–1920* and Rothman's *The Discovery of the Asylum,* offer brief glimpses of life behind nineteenth-century asylum walls. There also is a growing literature on other nineteenth-century institutions of social control; for example, Barbara Brenzel, *Daughters of the State: A Social Portrait of the First Reform School for Girls in North America, 1856–1905,* and Nicole Hahn Rafter, *Partial Jutice: Women in State Prisons, 1800–1935.*

2. Goffman, *Asylums.* See also Howard W. Polsky, Daniel S. Claster, and Carl Goldberg, eds., *Social System Perspectives in Residential Institutions,* and H. Warren Dunham and S. Kirson Weinberg, *The Culture of the State Mental Hospital.*

3. 1835 Assembly *Documents,* no. 167, 16. In 1842, the Utica Asylum Board of Managers asked the well-known architect A. J. Downing to landscape the fifteen acres surrounding the institution so that they would become "as beautiful as the most cultivated and refined taste could desire" (letter from the board of managers to A. J. Downing, September 10, 1842, Uticana Collection, OCHS). Almost forty years later, the commissioners of public charity also argued for the important "symbolic effect" of beautiful public institutions (N.Y. Board of State Commissioners of Public Charities, *Fifth AR* [1872], 13–14). For general descriptions of Utica's physical layout as it changed over the course of the nineteenth century, see N.Y.S. Lunatic Asylum, *First AR* (1844), 40–41; N.Y. Board of State Commissioners of Public Charities, *Second AR* (1869), 8–9; N.Y.S. Board of Charities, *Twelfth AR* (1885), 118–119.

4. N.Y.S. Commissioner in Lunacy, *Sixteenth AR* (1889), 39.

5. Although many suspected that the Utica Asylum had been fenced so as to hide horrors within, its board of managers claimed that the fence was needed to protect both the fruits of the asylum's gardens and its female patients from harassment by neighborhood boys (N.Y.S. Lunatic Asylum, *Eighteenth AR* [1861], 67).

6. For physical descriptions of Willard and how it changed over time, see Willard Asylum for the Chronic Insane (hereafter cited as Willard Asylum), *Third AR* (1872), 16–18; "Willard Asylum," Penn Yan *Vineyardist,* in Willard Scrapbook No. 3, 95–96, WPCA; *Plans and Elevations and a Historical Sketch of the Willard Asylum for the Insane, on Seneca-Lake, New York;* N.Y.S. Board of Charities,

222

First AR (1868); 33; idem, *Third AR* (1870), 37–38; idem, *Sixth AR* (1873), 13–14; idem, *Tenth AR* (1877) 23–24; idem, *Thirteenth AR* (1880), 6–8; and N.Y.S. Commissioner in Lunacy, *Tenth AR* (1883), 80–81. One newspaper captured Willard with its headline "A Village of Insane" (Rochester *Union and Advertiser,* January 23, 1886, Willard Scrapbook No. 2, 2, WPCA). See also "The Willard Asylum," Penn Yan *Democrat,* undated (c. 1869), John B. Chapin Scrapbook, n.p., Department of Manuscripts and University Archives, Cornell University (hereafter cited as Willard Scarpbook No. 1, Cornell).

7. For the characterization of Willard as a New England settlement, see N.Y.S. Commissioner in Lunacy, *Sixteenth AR* (1889), 39. For Willard as a rural paradise where patients sat tranquilly in the sun, see "A Day at Willard," unidentified newspaper clipping in Willard Scrapbook No. 2, 126–17, WPCA. For Willard as a tourist spot, see Willard Asylum, *Eighteenth AR* (1885), 19; "Willard Insane Asylum," Watkins *Democratic-Herald,* January 15, 1887, Willard Scrapbook No. 2, 53, WPCA; and "Amazing Visitors," unidentified newspaper clipping, Willard Scrapbook No. 2, 56, WPCA.

8. For the image of the Utica Asylum as a malevolently enchanted castle, see Orpheus Everts, "The American Style of Public Provision for the Insane, and Despotism in Lunatic Asylums," 129. In response, Gray mockingly declared, "The Magician was the law and the wand was truth and justice" ("Proceedings of the Association of Medical Superintendents," *AJI* 38: 216). There are numerous references to Utica's (as to other asylums') prisonlike qualities. For examples, see "Insanity *vs.* Devilment," 568, and William Trull, *An Inner View of the State Lunatic Asylum at Utica, or How Patients Are Treated in the Model (?) Mad House of New York,* 11. For the imaginative view of Utica's entry hall inscription, see Clarissa Lathrop, *The Secret Institution,* 92.

9. "In the Willard Asylum," *Morning Telegram,* August 4, 1886, in Willard Scrapbook No. 2, 19, WPCA.

10. William Hotchkiss, *Five Months in the New-York State Lunatic Asylum,* 4. For a similar account of a delusion-plagued trip to the Utica Asylum, see "Insanity: My Own Case," 33.

11. WPCBR 1: no. 3259, WPCA.

12. For doctors' complaints, see N.Y.S. Lunatic Asylum, *Forty-seventh AR* (1890), 51; Willard Asylum, *Fifth AR* (1874), 25. Although the Utica and Willard doctors seldom acknowledged it, their counterparts at other state asylums used restraints when transferring chronic patients to Willard just as frequently as did families and county officials. For example, in 1889 a forty-three-year-old housewife was brought in a "camisole" and "mittens" to Willard from the Middletown State Insane Asylum, where she supposedly had spent an entire year confined to her bed by a "protection sheet." Also in 1889 attendants brought a twenty-three-year-old female patient from the Hudson River Hospital in a "camisole," although she required no constraint after admission (WPCBR 13: nos. 4651, 4664, WPCA). For other descriptions of patients brought in restraints, see Willard Asylum, *Fifth AR* (1874), 25; N.Y.S. Lunatic Asylum, *Twentieth AR* (1863), 15; idem, *Twenty-sixth AR* (1869): 9; idem, *Forty-seventh AR* (1890), 51. As Andrew Scull notes, doctors in both England and the United States were fond of describing how once-violent manics were miraculously calmed by the asylum environment; he calls such accounts "quasi-mythical" (Scull, "The Domestication of Madness," 245).

Patients' vivid descriptions of the humiliations they experienced enroute to nineteenth-century asylums suggest that the trip from home to institution might well be characterized as a rite of degradation, intended to separate patients from family and friends and mark them as insane. See Harold Garfinkel, "Conditions of Successful Degradation Ceremonies." As one Utica patient eloquently noted, the commitment process stamped the word *crazy* on the forehead of the person brought to the asylum, leaving "the lune . . . dumb as a sheep before his shearers" ("On the Claims of the Insane to the Respect and Interest of Society").

13. N.Y.S. Lunatic Asylum, *Twentieth AR* (1863), 15.

14. "Life in the Asylum."

15. Hotchkiss, *Five Months in the Asylum*, 6–11.

16. N.Y.S. Commissioner in Lunacy, *Eleventh AR* (1884), 176.

17. "Asylum Life: or, The Advantages of a Disadvantage," 228.

18. N.Y.S. Board of Charities, *Twenty-second AR* (1889), 185; Willard Asylum, *Third AR* (1872), 39, 188; N.Y.S. Commissioner in Lunacy, *Tenth AR* (1883), 83. A contemporary sociologist, James Jacobs, has found that, in prisons, work guards establish the closest relations with inmates because working together engenders comradery (Jacobs, *New Perspectives on Prisons and Imprisonment*, 137). Parole records suggest tht some of the Utica and Willard attendants and patients who shared outdoor labor and skilled craftswork also became friends.

19. N.Y.S. Commissioner in Lunacy, *Twelfth AR* (1885), 100–102. On a few of the back wards, conscientious attendants kept even the most disturbed patients clean and orderly without the use of restraints, but such achievements were unusual. For comments on the range of conditions from front to back wards, see 1884 Assembly *Documents,* vols. 10 and 11, no. 164 (hereafter cited as 1884 Investigation), 484, 1001–1002; N.Y.S. Lunatic Asylum, *Eighth AR* (1851), 44–45. Ex-patients often complained bitterly about the unpleasant, and even threatening, behavior of their back wards fellows. For examples, see Hiram Chase, *Two Years and Four Months in a Lunatic Asylum, from August 20, 1863, to December 20, 1865;* Phoebe B. Davis, *Two Years and Three Months in the New York State Lunatic Asylum at Utica: Together with the Outlines of Twenty Years' Peregrinations in Syracuse;* Hotchkiss, *Five Months in the Asylum;* and Trull, *An Inner View.* One ex-patient fought reinstitutionalization because he feared he would once again be assigned to a violent hall, where abuse, fights, and confusion were daily occurrences (UPCBR 46: no. 32 for the year, UPCA).

20. Chase, *Two Years and Four Months,* 50–57, 77–78, 91–93, 150–151; Hotchkiss, *Five Months in the Asylum,* 29–30, 45; Davis, *Two Years and Three Months,* 4, 56.

21. 1884 Investigation, 423, 428, 523, 586–587, 616, 680, 1008. Patient casebooks record many transfers, but doctors seldom explained them. Such shifts may not have cured, but they certainly facilitated the management of difficult patients. New York State's commissioner in lunacy, Stephen Smith, preferred to think of shifts as "discipline" rather than punishment (1884 Investigation, 797). Chapter 5 contains a more extensive discussion of nineteenth-century views of the therapeutic value of classification.

22. For descriptions of these daily routines, see the Record of the Proceedings of the Board of Managers of the State Lunatic Asylum (hereafter cited as Board of Managers), January 28, 1843, UPCA; N.Y.S. Lunatic Asylum, *First AR*

(1844), 41–43, 47; and Amariah Brigham, "Brief Notice of the New York State Lunatic Asylum, at Utica, and of the Appropriations by the State, for the Benefit of the Insane," 6–7. For one patient's hostility to enforced routines, see Hotchkiss, *Five Months in the Asylum,* 16–18, 28–29. For a description of the daily routine at the Pennsylvania Hospital during this same period, see Tomes, *A Generous Confidence,* 198–210. Superintendent Kirkbride also considered regular schedules a vital therapeutic tool but varied work therapies in response to social class. This happened less often at the Utica Asylum, a state facility, and never at Willard, where all patients were chronic paupers.

23. For complaints that attendants refused to let patients return to their beds during the day, no matter how ill, see Davis, *Two Years and Three Months,* 34–35; Chase, *Two Years and Four Months,* 175–176; Trull, *An Inner Veiw,* 30.

24. This account of a typical day's work was produced by a head attendant on a Willard female ward, for Stephen Smith, the commissioner in lunacy (N.Y.S. Commissioner in Lunacy, *Eleventh AR* [1884], 263–266). Smith's interest in talking to attendants about their experiences was unusual. Other accounts of Willard's routines can be found in Willard Asylum, *Third AR* (1872), 34 and N.Y.S. Board of Charities, *Twenty-second Annual Report* (1889), 186. Rigid routines were not unique to asylums and prisons. At the Boston City Hospital during the later nineteenth century, doctors attempted to control patients' activities rigorously. They forbade patients to leave their wards without permission and allowed them to receive letters and articles only with the superintendent's approval. Like the Utica Asylum, the Boston City Hospital was surrounded by a high brick wall which served to isolate patients from the outside world (Morris J. Vogel, *The Invention of the Modern Hospital: Boston, 1870–1930,* 44).

25. Willard Parole Book, 17–18, 25, 21, WPCA.

26. Ibid., 21, 25. Parole book incidents suggest once again that total control of patients was impossible, even at an isolated insitution like Willard. For example, one group of paroled patients built a shanty in a ravine. There they drank, played cards, and kept a bulldog. When these activities were discovered, their parole activities were promptly revoked (ibid., 66). Although relatively few patients tried to leave Willard without permission, escape was not difficult, even for those locked in their rooms. For example, see the newspaper articles on the patient, a former reporter, who escaped twice, the second time for good ("Hallucinations: An Interview with a Deranged Newspaper Man" and "Insane," *Daily Advertiser,* June 21, 1889, Willard Scrapbook No. 4, 3, WPCA;" "An Escaped Lunatic," Auburn *Dispatch,* June 21, 1889, ibid., 4; "A Crazy Journalist," *Advertiser,* ibid.; "Wilson Made Tracks," Syracuse *Standard,* July 12, 1889, ibid., 5; "Hiram H. Wilson," Albany *Journal,* July 26, 1889, ibid., 7).

27. For a description of how labor market opportunities similarly affected English asylums, see John K. Walton, "The Treatment of Pauper Lunatics in Victorian England: The Case of the Lancaster Asylum," in Scull, *Madhouses, Mad-Doctors, and Madmen,* 180–181.

28. Official descriptions of attendants' duties make clear the demanding nature of their work; for example, see N.Y.S. Lunatic Asylum, *Second AR* (1845), 45–48. Much of the testimony at legislative investigations about patient abuse made the same point, even though Superintendent John Gray of Utica made clear that he felt little sympathy for the stresses of attendants' lives (1884 Investigation,

492–493, 796, 1010–1012, 1111). Isaac Ray eloquently described the impossible demands made on attendants: "They are expected to possess a combination of virtues which, in the ordinary walks of life, would render their possessor one of the shining ornaments of the human race" (Ray, "Popular Feeling towards Hospitals for the Insane," 53).

29. Willard Asylum, *Twelfth AR* (1881), 12.

30. Gray's successor, George Blumer, noted that this innovation greatly improved staff morale (N.Y.S. Lunatic Asylum, *Forty-fifth AR* [1888], 56).

31. For lists of the duties of the Utica assistant physicians, see Board of Managers, 16–17, 42–43; N.Y.S. Lunatic Asylum, *Thirty-seventh AR* (1880), 9; 1884 Investigation, 1154–1155. For the Willard assistant physicians' duties, see *Laws Relating to the Willard Asylum for the Insane and Rules and Regulations of Said Asylum, Adopted July 1, 1869. Revised October 15, 1884,* 26.

32. "The Chronic Insane," *Oswego Daily Times*, April 9, 1889, in Willard Scrapbook No. 3, 129–130, WPCA. Although the doctor–patient ratio was slightly higher at Utica, an ex-patient complained that there were still too few doctors to provide adequate care. How could two doctors adequately care for 700–800 patients, she asked ("Insane Asylums," Auburn *Daily Bulletin*, February 3, 1891, in ibid. No. 4, 117).

33. Complaints about doctors' reliance on attendants for information about patients, as well as about chaotic doctor–patient meetings, appear in Chase, *Two Years and Four Months*, 44, 55, 145–147. He also alleged that one of the assistant physicians had openly proclaimed himself "boss of this shanty" (55). Davis complained about doctors' aloofness from patients and argued that "might makes right" was the therapeutic strategy most popular among Utica doctors (Davis, *Two Years and Three Months*, 23–25, 77, 82). Yet another ex-patient charged that Utica doctors consistently ignored his allegations of attendant abuse, and he called Brigham a "cannibal" (Hotchkiss, *Five Months in the Asylum*, 30–31, 43).

34. "To Dr. ———, On his Return from the Annual Meeting of Superintendents of Asylums"; "To Dr. G——Y"; "To Dr. C—— by a Sick Patient"; To Dr. C——k"; Henry Richardson, "Letters to G. Alder Blumer, from Ward 2 North, Utica, August 11, 1890," vi, UPCA; Chase, *Two Years and Four Months*, 166–167.

35. Particularly noted for his active involvement in patient and staff entertainments was Willard assistant physician Alexander Nellis. When he left Willard for private practice, twenty-three of his attendants gave him a gold-headed cane in gratitude for "the impartial courtesy and urbanity which you have uniformly manifested toward us, in both your official and personal relations with us" (untitled article, *Independent*, February 22, 1889, in Willard Scrapbook No. 3, 88, WPCA). The wedding of Doctor G. A. Blumer of the Utica Asylum to the only daughter of a U.S. congressman was described as "one of the most brilliant social events which has ever occurred in Utica" ("A Brilliant Wedding," Utica *Daily Press*, June 24, 1886, Willard Scrapbook No. 2, 13, WPCA). A Willard assistant physician married the daugher of a state senator in a similar ceremony ("Another Wedding," *Geneva Advertiser*, September 21, 1886, Willard Scrapbook No. 2, 20, WPCA). For descriptions of assistant physicians' trips abroad, see N.Y.S. Lunatic Asylum, *Forty-first AR* (1884), 49; idem, *Forty-second AR* (1885), 71–72; idem, *Forty-Seventh AR* (1890), 65; Board of Managers, July 20, 1882, UPCA.

36. N.Y.S. Lunatic Asylum, *Thirty-sixth AR* (1879), 26. Since the only one

of Gray's assistant physicians to die young did so as a result of contracting typhoid fever during a trip to Naples, Gray was not generalizing from his Utica experience.

37.   For descriptions of assistant physicians taking on extra duties, see Board of Managers, 96, 126, UPCA; 1884 Investigation, 1051. Willard medical staff meetings are described in Willard Asylum, *Eighteenth AR* (1887), 18.

38.   For complaints about chaos on the asylum wards, see Chase, *Two Years and Four Months*, 175–176; N.Y.S. Commissioner in Lunacy, *Tenth AR* (1883), 174–178; UPCBR, 45: No. 33 for year, UPCA. For the knife story, see WPCBR 5: no. 2105, WPCA. One of the two extant volumes of Willard's nineteenth-century clinical records makes clear that patient injuries, especially among males, frequently were inflicted by other patients. For example, one patient thrown down and kicked violently in the left side by another suffered a fractured rib (Willard Clinical Recordbook 1: 43, WPCA).

39.   "Shocking Tragedy at the Asylum" *Sunday Tribune*, June 11, 1882; "An Awful Crime Kept from the Public Four Weeks," Utica *Press*, June 12, 1882. Some papers defended the institution. For example, one praised its decision not to subject friends of the murderer and victim to the annoyance and humiliation or the county to the unnecessary expense of an inquest, especially given the likelihood of such assaults in a large institution, no matter how careful the watch (*Observer*, June 22, 1882). Another commented that the asylum should not be blamed because a criminal patient had been sent to an institution for noncriminals. Nonetheless, it still bore responsibility for agreeing to accept that patient and then trying to conceal a crime committed by him (Auburn *News and Bulletin*, June 17, 1882). (Newsclippings are all part of Poulton's casebook record, UPCBR 56: 113, UPCA.)

40.   For Gray's defense of Utica in the Poulton case and the commissioners' response, see N.Y.S. Lunatic Asylum, *Fortieth AR* (1883), 45–46, plus newspaper clippings in Poulton's casebook (UPCBR 56: 113, UPCA). For a discussion of the large numbers of homicidal and suicidal patients admitted to the Utica Asylum each year, see N.Y.S. Lunatic Asylum, *Fourth AR* (1847), 39, 41–45; idem, *Thirty-ninth AR* (1882), 22–32. For earlier complaints about criminal patients, see idem, *Fifth AR* (1848), 12–14; idem, *Tenth AR* (1853), 5–6, 12; and idem, *Eleventh AR* (1854), 6. The practice continued even after a separate asylum for insane criminals opened at the Auburn prison (N.Y.S. Lunatic Asylum, *Twenty-first AR* [1864], 6, 21; Utica *Daily Press*, March 10, 1889, in UPCBR 76: 99, UPCA).

41.   Clipping from the Utica *Daily Press*, March 10, 1889, in UPCBR 76; 99, UPCA.

42.   Charles A. Lee, "Medico-Legal Suggestions on Insanity," 467–469.

43.   1884 Investigation, 627–631, 721, 1316–1331; UPCBR 45: no. 151 for the year, UPCA; UPCBR 46: no. 359 for the year, UPCA; Chase, *Two Years and Four Months*, 40; Hotchkiss, *Five Months in the Asylum*, 6–11, 26–28.

44.   For example, see "Death of an Asylum Superintendent from a Bite"; "Fatal Assault on Dr. Metcalf"; "Attack on an English Asylum Superintendent." At Utica itself, no deaths resulted from patient attacks, but one patient managed to stab an assistant physician with a penknife (1882 Senate *Documents* [hereafter cited as 1880 Investigation], no. 68, 252). Willard's casebooks document similar incidents. For example, in 1886 one assistant physician was attacked so fiercely by

a delusional patient that several attendants had to come to his rescue (WPCBR 13; no. 4526, WPCA).

45. Willard Asylum, *Eighth AR* (1877), 27; N.Y.S. Commissioner in Lunacy, *Eleventh AR* (1884), 260, 271–289. Even when patient violence at Willard escalated to murder, it attracted relatively little attention. For example, in April of 1891 a demented epileptic first threw two pots at, and then smothered, another patient. The nightwatch found the murderer sitting on the floor in a room splattered with blood. Almost immediately a coroner's jury absolved Willard officials of negligence and responsibility for the death. These events are described in a set of largely local newspapers clippings in Willard Scrapbook No. 2, 133, WPCA, which include the following: "Homocide at the Willard State Hospital," Waterloo *Observer*, April 22, 1891; "Killed by a Lunatic," *Rock Democrat*, April 23, 1891; "One Patient Murders Another," New York *World*, April 23, 1891; "A Lunatic's Crime," Auburn *Bulletin*, April 21, 1891.

46. 1884 Investigation, 324, 462, 527, 1324; Hotchkiss, *Five Months in the Asylum*, 22; Chase, *Two Years and Four Months*, 36–37; 1880 Investigation, 34. For nineteenth-century asylums' heavy reliance on chemical restraints, see the discussion in "Proceedings of the Association of Medical Superintendents," *AJI* 27: 210–223.

47. Utica's patient casebook records are filled with references to the use of physical restraints to control disturbed patients. In abolishing the use of such devices in 1887, Superintendent Blumer described their negative impact on patient–attendant relationships (N.Y.S. Lunatic Asylum, *Forty-fifth AR* [1888], 45–48). See also the newspaper article "Mechanical Restraint: Its Abolition at the State Lunatic Asylum," Utica *Observer*, January 21, 1887, in Willard Scrapbook No. 2, 57–58, WPCA. Chapter 5 has additional discussion of this practice.

48. N.Y.S. Board of Charities, *Twenty-second AR* (1889), 151–160; N.Y.S. Lunatic Asylum, *Forty-fifth AR* (1888), 45–50; Willard Asylum, *Seventeenth AR* (1886), 10.

49. Lathrop, *Secret Institution*, 116; Hotchkiss, *Five Months in the Asylum*, 24–25; "A Few Facts concerning a Patient, by Himself"; S. Weir Mitchell, "Address before the Fiftieth Annual Meeting of the American Medico-Psychological Association, Held in Philadelphia, May 16, 1894," 436.

50. UPCBR 7: no. 89, UPCA. The letter quoted was dated February 29, 1849, only two days after the patient's admission.

51. For a wry description of dinner companions, see "Practical Insanity," 76. For descriptions of patients helping one another, see WPCBR 5: no. 1939, WPCA; 1884 Investigation, 521; "Life in the New York State Lunatic Asylum; or, Extracts from the Diaries of an Inmate," 300.

52. "On the Claims of the Insane," 242; H., "Life at Asylumia," 347.

53. *Laws Relating to the Willard Asylum;* N.Y.S. Lunatic Asylum, *Forty-sixth AR* (1889), 43–44.

54. For a description of school boys frolicking across the asylum grounds, see "The Editor's Table," 6: 95. The humiliation of encountering friends at the asylum is described eloquently by Chase, *Two Years and Four Months*, 75. For the visitation rules at Willard, see Willard Asylum, *Nineteenth AR* (1886), 52. Numerous clippings in the Willard Scrapbooks, WPCA, make clear that its superintendents encouraged inspection visits by county officials, even if they were

unhappy about casual tourists. For example, see "Keuka and Seneca," Watkins *Democrat,* August 4, 1886, Willard Scrapbook No. 2, 37, WPCA; "Supervisors at Willard," Auburn *Morning Dispatch,* November 25, 1886, Willard Scrapbook No. 2, 37, WPCA.

55.   "Editor's Table," 3: 178; 2: 121–122; "The July Days at Asylumia." For a description of similar responses to English asylums, see Scull, "Domestication of Madness," 247–248.

56.   N.Y.S. Commissioner in Lunacy,*Fifth AR* (1878), 5–6; Board of Managers, December 13, 1889, UPCA; N.Y.S. Lunatic Asylum, *Forty-fourth AR* (1887), 52; "The Admission of Visitors to Asylums," 271.

57.   For the traditional English conceptualization of mind-healers as both magicians and doctors, see Michael MacDonald, *Mystical Bedlam: Madness, Anxiety, and Healing in Seventeenth-Century England.*

58.   UPCBR 73: 23, UPCA.

59.   Scull, "Domestication of Madness."

2
The Economics of Compassion

1.   For the early history of state care in New York, see David M. Schneider, *The History of Public Welfare in New York State, 1609–1866;* Amariah Brigham, "Brief Notice of the New York State Lunatic Asylum;" William L. Russell, *The New York Hospital: A History of the Psychiatric Service, 1771–1936.*

2.   Joan Hannon, "Poverty in the Antebellum Northeast: The View from New York State's Poor Relief Rolls." Not only did New York counties differ from one another in the extent of their urbanization and industrialization, but substantial variations sometimes existed within a single county. For example, the sociodemographic characteristics and economic experiences of antebellum Buffalo were strikingly different from those of the rest of Erie Couty (Katz, Doucet, and Stern, *Social Organization,* chap. 1).

3.   The extent of many local communities' early self-interest in state care of the insane was such that, when the Utica Asylum's facilities proved insufficient for the pauper insane, the county superintendents of the poor petitioned the legislature for construction of additional state institutions (1856 Senate *Documents,* no. 17). This report proved a useful tool for Utica's John Gray, who helped the local politicians to frame it (Judson R. Andrews, "Memoirs of John Perdue Gray, M.D., L.L.D.," 23). Such local support for state care faded over the course of the nineteenth century. By the 1870s, many county politicians had reversed their position, arguing that local asylums were both cheaper and better than state institutions (Chapter 7).

4.   For information about Coventry's role,see Pomroy Jones, *Annals and Recollections of Oneida County,* 594–595. In 1841 Coventry was appointed an asylum trustee and in 1842 a manager. Long interested in phrenology, he helped select Amariah Brigham as Utica's first superintendent. In many ways, his concern for the mentally ill continued, on an unpretentious local level, the tradition of "medical patriotism" characteristic of the Revolutionary generation of doctors.

(See Richard Harrison Shyrock, *Medicine and Society in America: 1660–1860*, 118–119. In general, historians have paid little attention to the involvement of local physicians in the antebellum psychiatric movement. (An exception is Samuel B. Thielman's unpublished paper "Community Management of Mental Disorders in Early Nineteenth-Century America, with Special Reference to Southeastern Virginia," delivered at the 1986 meeting of the American Association for the History of Medicine.) Yet the letters of Hartwell Carver, an unsuccessful early applicant for the position of superintendent at Utica, suggest that, like Coventry, this local physician was keenly aware of new ways of treating the insane and had applied them successfully (or so he claimed) to a number of his private patients (letters to Charles Mann from Hartwell Carver, April 2 and April 14, 1842, Uticana Collection, OCHS). For the "Memorial of the Medical Society of the State of New-York, in Relation to Insane Paupers," see 1836 Senate *Documents*, no. 38. Mention of similar earlier petitions can be found in 1834 Assembly *Documents*, no. 347.

5. L. Ray Gunn, "The New York State Legislature: A Developmental Perspective: 1777–1846." Gunn suggests that the legislature's agreement to fund a state asylum in 1836 represented "the accumulations of a number of highly individualized decisions," rather than systematically developed policy (271). Gunn agrees that the rapidity of socioeconomic change in antebellum New York, rather than the vicissitudes of partisan politics, probably accounted for the state's legislative instability. Stanley B. Klein, in "A Study of Social Legislation Affecting Prisons and Institutions for the Mentally Ill in New York State: 1822–1846," notes that the lack of standing committees on the mentally ill also hindered reformers' attempts to get pro-asylum legislation passed (273). See also Gerald N. Grob, "The Political System and Social Policy in the Nineteenth Century: Legacy of the Revolution," for a discussion of how the political instability of antebellum state legislatures made clear formulation of policies difficult. He also suggests that the volatility of legislatures increased the influence of individuals (Grob, "Reflections," 297).

6. For example, see the following Assembly *Documents:* for 1831, no. 305; for 1832, no. 174; for 1834, no. 347; and for 1835, no. 167.

7. Charles Z. Lincoln, ed., *Messages from the Governor* 3: 293–294.

8. The 1830 Assembly report was reprinted in 1835 Assembly *Documents*, no. 167.

9. Lincoln, *Messages* 3: 346–348, 378–379.

10. 1832 Assembly *Documents*, no. 174, 1–9. Interestingly, this same report which castigates the public for its unenlightened views of insanity characterizes the insane as those who have given way to "the basest propensities of human nature" (2).

11. Lincoln, *Messages* 3: 293; 1832 Assembly *Documents*, no. 174, 7–11, 15. Similar early appeals to the "economics of compassion" can be found in 1834 Assembly *Documents*, no. 38, 2. Legislative formulations of the economics-of-compassion argument made surprisingly few explicit references to religious values, but an 1858 restatement of the argument, in a sermon delivered at the Utica Asylum, shows how easily it took on a religious tone. The sermon's author, a local Presbyterian minister, wonderfully mixed political and religious rhetoric. In one sentence, he reminded his listeners of the Bible's humanitarian attitudes toward the physically and mentally deformed; in the next, he added that, because such

unfortunates were "born to the State," it had an obligation to look after them (W. E. Knox, *A Sermon Delivered at the Dedication of the Chapel of the New York State Lunatic Asylum, October 27, 1858,* 8–9).

12.   Such conjoining of appeals to Christian benevolence, the advance of medical science (as measured by high cure rates), fears of the insane, and the savings that would result from the construction of state asylums contined to appear in legislative budget requests, newspaper editorials, and asylum annual reports for the rest of the nineteenth century. Nineteenth century economics-of-compassion arguments for the institutionalization of the insane differed significantly from those used in eighteenth-century Europe, where public concern for the insane primarily reflected fear of them as a physical and moral threat. Eighteenth-century rhetoric lacked the medical component of the economics-of-compassion argument (Colin Jones, "The Treatment of the Insane in Eighteenth- and Early Nineteenth-Century Montpellier," 373–376). By the nineteenth century, a wide range of British and American politicians had adopted it. For Great Britain, see Walton, "The Treatment of Pauper Lunatics," and Scull, *Museums of Madness,* 102–112. In the United States, Dix carried it across the country; for example, see Frederick M. Herrmann, *Dorothea L. Dix and the Politics of Institutional Reform,* 15–17, 26.

13.   1835 Assembly *Documents,* no. 167.

14.   1834 Assembly *Documents,* no. 347.

15.   For a detailed history of the political fortunes of pro-asylum reports, bills, and petitions between 1822 and 1836, see Klein, "Social Legislation," 265–304.

16.   For histories of the early days of the Utica asylum, see N.Y.S. Lunatic Asylum, *Fourth AR* (1847), 59–73; Paul Hoch, "History of the Department of Mental Hygiene"; Lucy Clark, *A Century of Progress at Utica State Hospital,* 4–14.

17.   1837 Senate *Documents,* no. 39.

18.   Ibid. See also 1839 Senate *Documents,* no. 2, for the commissioners' explanation of how they drew up their initial plans after visiting comparable institutions.

19.   Klein, "Social Legislation," 305–355; 1839 Senate *Documents,* no. 2; 1841 Senate *Documents,* nos. 52, 280.

20.   Governor Seward's annual message for 1839 is reprinted in 1847 Senate *Documents,* no. 30, 66–69.

21.   1839 Senate *Documents,* no. 2.

22.   1856 Senate *Documents,* no. 71, 67–68. Many other early state asylums were similarly expensive and, some alleged, extravagant (Ruth B. Caplan and Gerald Caplan, *Psychiatry and the Community in Nineteenth-Century America,* 55). Utica Asylum officials recognized that, despite the legislature's refusal to grant all their requests fully, "hitherto no state or county has been more liberal in providing for its insane" (N.Y.S. Lunatic Asylum, *Third AR* [1846], 41).

23.   1841 Assembly *Documents,* no. 61; Lincoln, *Messages* 4: 279.

24.   Poor fiscal planning was not a weakness only of asylum administrators. At one point, the Utica Asylum was denied already appropriated funds because of the depleted condition of the state treasury (letter to Charles Mann from Governor William Bouck, December 20, 1853, Uticana Collection, OCHS). Such fi-

nancial constraints plagued antebellum asylums outside New York as well and prompted Dorothea Dix's unsuccessful attempt to get federal subsidies for the care of the insane (Caplan and Caplan, *Psychiatry and the Community,* 78–86).

25. The care with which these early legislators investigated the new sciences of asylum administration before formulating their own recommendations is impressive. One early committee not only visited all the institutions for the insane existing in New York, Pennsylvania, Massachusetts, and Connecticut in 1830, but also imported a number of scarce European books on the subject (1835 Assembly *Documents,* no. 167, 3). Perhaps because of the ever-changing composition of the legislature, subsequent committees repeated these investigative trips. Their conscientiousness is remarkable, given that they were not always reimbursed for travel expenses (1841 Assembly *Documents,* nos. 262, 280). The resulting reports offered no original insights into the treatment of the insane, but they effectively summarized the thinking and practice of the leading doctors of the time. Their thoroughness may help to explain the ease with which the first superintendent of Utica was able to run the institution according to guidelines drawn up by the managers before he arrived.

26. 1844 Assembly *Documents,* no. 95, 4–5.

27. For a sample of these letters, see the Uticana Collection, OCHS.

28. N.Y.S. Lunatic Asylum, *First AR* (1844), 1–10.

29. Letter to Thomas Kirkbride from Amariah Brigham, March 3, 1845, Kirkbride Papers, PHMA.

30. 1844 Assembly *Documents,* no. 21, 3–4.

31. Ibid., 8, 12, 13, 23, 30, 32–34.

32. Ibid. For the most part, Dix's memorial emphasized humanitarian reasons to help the insane in county poorhouses, but like several New York legislators, she also argued that state-level care, because of its efficacy and efficiency, ultimately would save money for local communities. From her perspective, the several counties reluctant to send their recent insane to the newly opened Utica Asylum because of the relatively high cost of such state-level care were being shortsighted. Thus, like New York legislators, Dix appealed simultaneously to economic and moral motives. At one point, she did acknowledge the "enormous" financial burden on counties of social welfare programs for New York's poor. She suggested that reformers try to cut back on such expenses, if they could do so without impinging on the "just claims" of the dependent.

33. Ibid., 40. According to Ruth and Gerald Caplan, supporters of nineteenth-century reforms that required state funding had to make highly exaggerated claims for their cause in order to gain even minimal financial support (Caplan and Caplan, *Psychiatry and the Community,* 78–86).

34. 1844 Assembly *Documents,* no. 44.

35. 1855 Senate *Documents,* no.27; 1856 Senate *Documents,* no. 17, 12–13, 16, 18; "The County Superintendents of the Poor."

36. 1856 Senate *Documents,* no. 17, 1, 17–20.

37. L. Ray Gunn, "The Decline of Authority: Public Policy in New York, 1837–1860," 22.

38. 1844 Assembly *Documents,* no. 21, 14–15. See also Willard, *First AR* (1870), 16–17, for similar calculations, although using slightly different numbers and a lower cure rate. The conclusion of both is the same: in the long run, state-level care of the insane saves taxpayers money.

39. Patricia Cline Cohen, *A Calculating People: The Spread of Numeracy in America*, 205–226. For a discussion of the medical profession's similar penchant for statistical evidence, see James H. Cassedy, *American Medicine and Statistical Thinking, 1800–1860*.

40. For example, see Lincoln, *Messages* 3: 290–295, 342–346, 449–454; ibid. 4: 125–128, 276–284, 638–645; ibid 5: 447–450. See also Klein, "Social Legislation," 87–264; W. David Lewis, *From Newgate to Dannemora: The Rise of the Penitentiary in New York, 1796–1848;* Robert S. Pickett, *Houses of Refuge: Origins of Juvenile Reform in New York State, 1815–1857.*

41. Despite this protest, in their annual messages to the legislature, New York's governors continued to lump together all of the state's "charities," including Sing Sing, the Western House of Refuge, and the State Lunatic Asylum. For example, see Hamilton Fish in Lincoln, *Messages* 4: 482–485.

42. 1855 Senate *Documents,* no. 27.

43. 1855 Assembly *Documents,* no. 91.

44. John B. Chapin, "Insanity in the State of New York."

45. Ibid.

46. 1864 *Laws of New York,* chap. 418; "The Willard Asylum Act, and provision for the Insane," 192–194.

47. 1865 *Laws of New York,* chap. 342. The decision to locate the new institution in Ovid resulted from both local and state political machinations. In 1865 the people of Ovid appointed a committee to lobby with the legislature to locate the new institution at the abandoned state agricultural college outside their village, in return for their giving up to Cornell the college's claim to U.S. land grant status ("Historical Sketch of the New State Agricultural College," Ovid *Independent,* October 25, 1887, in Willard Scrapbook No. 2, 33, WPCA). For its Buffalo competitors' complaints about political factors influenced the choice of the Ovid site, see "The Willard Asylum and Why It Was Not Located at Buffalo," unidentified newspaper clipping in Willard Scrapbook No. 1, n.p., Cornell.

48. Robert E. Doran, "History of the Willard Asylum for the Insane and the Willard State Hospital," 1–3, WPCA.

49. Ibid., 2; "The Willard Asylum Act"; "Summary On Separate Asylums for Curables and Incurables"; "Bibliographical Notice."

50. "Proceedings of the AMSAII," 147–249. For a discussion of the same debate in England, see Peter McCandless, "'Build! Build!': The Controversy over the Care of the Chronically Insane in England, 1855–1870."

51. For Gray's attacks on the Willard commissioners' fiscal extravagance and Chapin's self-defense, see "Proceedings of the AMSAII," 240–246, and letters to Dorothea Dix from John C. Chapin of Brigham Hall, February 11 and 23, 1867, Dix Papers, HLHU.

52. John Chapin, "On Provision for the Chronic Insane Poor"; idem, "Report on Provision for the Chronic Insane."

53. "Proceedings of the Association: Provision for the Chronic Insane," 289–294. Such criticism of Gray's efforts to exclude from the *AJI* those with opposing views was not new, and the 1868 rebellion against him was short-lived. In 1869 Gray had the satisfaction of receiving a deferential request from the AMSAII to publish in the *AJI* the official account of the association's annual meetings (Proceedings of the Association of Medical Superintendents," *AJI* 26: 149– 150).

54.   George Cook, "Provision for the Insane Poor in the State of New York," read before the AMSAII on April 24, 1866. Like most annual AMSAII papers, Cook's was subsequently printed in the *AJI*. Cook (or one of his supporters) also had the paper printed privately for independent distribution. The paper seems to have been intended from the start for a broader audience than the AMSAII, for in it Cook made clear that he did not expect support from the clearly partisan organization. In Cook's view, the AMSAII had been too much influenced by the "unfair spirit" and "ill concealed hostility" of *AJI* editorials. His 1866 essay shows Cook's particular skill in using what a contemporary sociolinguist calls "nonmotivated" vocabularies of motive; he relied on appeals to common sense, historical necessity, and a version of positivist empiricism, whose effectiveness depended on their aura of neutrality (Laurie Taylor, "Vocabularies, Rhetoric and Grammar: Problems in the Sociology of Motivation").

55.   Cook, "Provision for the Insane Poor."

56.   "State *versus* County Care"; 1890 Senate- *Documents*, no. 53.

57.   David M. Schneider and Albert Deutsch, *The History of Public Welfare in New York State, 1867–1940,* 90; Gunn, "Decline of Authority," 271.

58.   N.Y.S. Board of Charities, *Fifteenth AR* (1882), 179.

59.   This debate about the relative merits of local versus state care became particularly intense in the late 1880s, right before the State Care Act of 1890 (Chapter 7) mandated state-level care for all the mentally ill, thus doing away with exemptions to the Willard Act.

60.   Additional discussion of the differences in the Utica and Willard budgets can be found in Chapters 5 and 7. My suggestions here about the impact of one version of antebellum reform ideology on public support for state-funded social welfare programs are tentative. I hope that, in the near future, more economic historians will respond to Gerald Grob's 1979 challenge to probe the economics of nineteenth-century social welfare policy so as to determine more precisely the relative levels of support for different dependent groups, the reasons for shifts in those levels, their relationship to prevailing minimal standards of living, and so forth (Grob, "Reflections," 293–294, 303–304).

61.   Almost all antebellum physicians agreed that insanity was most curable in its early stages and, therefore, that beds in the Utica Asylum should be kept for the acutely ill. The letter to Charles A. Mann from A. J. McCall, August 18, 1842, Uticana Collection, OCHS, suggests that lay people caring for the insane agreed. McCall urgently requested help only for the young, recently "deranged" woman in his care, though he also had care of five chronically insane paupers.

3
Medical Men and Medical Power

1.   1834 Senate *Documents*, no. 12, 8. At subsequent managers meetings and in Brigham's annual reports, the superintendent's duties were spelled out in detail. For example, see Board of Managers, January 28, 1843, and N.Y.S. Lunatic Asylum, *Fifth AR* (1848), 48–49. This second formulation eventually was given

statutory authority. According to the 1874 *Laws of New York*, chap. 135, sec. 9, "The superintendent shall be the chief executive officer of the asylum. He shall have the general superintendence of the buildings, grounds, and farm, together with their furniture, fixtures, and stock; and the duration and control of all persons therein, subject to the laws and regulations established by the managers. He shall daily ascertain the condition of all the patients and prescribe their treatment in the manner directed in the by-laws." He also was given the power to nominate his assistant physicians and the responsibility of overseeing them.

2. William A. Hammond, "The Treatment of the Insane," 240. Hammond, a bitter enemy of John Gray, was not the only critic of late nineteenth-century asylum superintendents. Similar remarks can be found in Dorman B. Eaton, "Despotism in Lunatic Asylums," 269–271; S. Weir Mitchell, "Address before the Fiftieth Annual Meeting of the American Medico-Psychological Association, Held in Philadelphia, May 16, 1894," 429. Ye the neurologists were no more realistic in their definition of the superintendent's duties than those they criticized. According to W. W. Godding, "The Superintendent should be a medical man of the highest integrity, with the head to understand the magnitude of the work to which he was called, a heart in sympathy with the afflicted ones confided to his care, the intellect to comprehend what there is to be learned about insanity, a genius for exact management and control . . ." ("The State in the Care of the Insane," 731). E. C. Seguin suggested to investigating New York State legislators in 1880 that asylum superintendents needed to have a good medical education, the ability to read German and French medical literature, and training in logic, psychiatry, the use of a microscope, and modern means of diagnosis (1880 Investigation, 50). Others suggested that the position of superintendent be split into two parts: a business manager and a medical head, a suggestion bitterly opposed by members of the AMSAII and New York asylum doctors (H. B. Wilbur, "Governmental Supervision of the Insane," 84; John Curwen, "On the Propositions of the AMSAII"; and N.Y.S. Commissioner in Lunacy, *Second AR* [1875], 24).

3. "Proceedings of the Association of Medical Superintendents," *AJI* 47: 213.

4. For Brigham's biography, see Charles B. Coventry, "Amariah Brigham, M.D."; E. K. Hunt, "Memoir of Amariah Brigham"; idem, *Biographical Sketch of Amariah Brigham, M.D., Late Superintendent of the New York State Lunatic Asylum, Utica, New York*; Chauncey E. Goodrich, *A Sermon on the Death of Amariah Brigham, M.D., Delivered at the New York State Asylum, October 8, 1849, and Again in the First Presbyterian Church, Utica, November 11, 1849*; Andrew MacFarland, "Reminiscences of the Association and Reflections"; Eric T. Carlson, "Amariah Brigham: I. Life and Works"; idem, Amariah Brigham: II. Psychiatric Thought and Practice"; Henry Hurd, ed., *The Institutional Care of the Insane in the United States and Canada* 4: 360–362.

5. Albany *Evening Journal*, February 13, 1884, 1884 Investigation Scrapbook, UPCA.

6. Letter to Dorothea Dix from John Chapin, September 25, 1884, Dix Papers, HLHU.

7. A typical example of Brigham's family imagery can be found in Brigham, "Brief Notice," 5. According to a friend, Brigham's leadership style at Utica was

much the same as it had been at the Hartford Retreat. There he had treated his staff justly and kindly, without ever permitting "undue license" (Hunt, *Biographical Sketch*, 62–63).

8.　Letter to Judge Sutherland and Charles Mann from S. B. Woodward, April 29, 1842, Uticana Collection, OCHS; letter to C. A. Mann from D. Larrabee, May 14, 1844, Uticana Collection, OCHS. The Uticana Collection also contains letters from other applicants for the superintendent's position.

9.　For their own views, see 1842 Senate *Documents*, no. 12, in which they make clear their adherence to the notion that "mental derangement is the result of some bodily disease which affects the brain." They even quote phrenologist Johann Spurzheim. See also the article on "Physiology of the Brain," subsequently written by one of their most influential members, Charles B. Coventry. Phrenology, with which Brigham was strongly identified, generally had strong adherents in Oneida County. In 1836 they published a local journal, *The Phrenological Magazine, and New York Literary Review*, which noted the officers of the Oneida Phrenological Society and the popularity of its president's lectures on phrenology to the Young Men's Association in Utica. In his letter to the board describing the Hartford Retreat, Brigham tactfully noted the importance of close trustee supervision of asylums. He also pointed out the high cure rates he had achieved using moral treatment but noted that he had dealt with a particularly advantaged patient population (quoted in 1852 Senate *Documents*, no. 3, 155–160).

10.　These include Amariah Brigham, *An Inquiry concerning the Diseases and Functions of the Brain, the Spinal Cord, and the Nerves;* idem, *Observations on the Influence of Religion upon the Health and Physical Welfare of Mankind;* idem, *Remarks on the Influence of Mental Cultivation and Mental Excitement upon Health;* and idem, "Insanity and Insane Hospitals."

11.　Hurd, *Institutional Care* 4: 356; Goodrich, *Sermon*.

12.　Carlson, "Amariah Brigham: I," 911.

13.　Goodrich, *Sermon*, 57.

14.　Brigham, "Insanity and Insane Hospitals," 120. Brigham himself was a fervent Democrat, once accused by a Utica paper of being a "loco-foco democrat." A friend noted that in Hartford, Brigham most often socialized with the well-educated, who preferred a "large freedom of opinion," as well as an occasional glass of wine and a good game of whist (Hunt, *Biographical Sketch*, 59). In a fashion typical of antebellum reformers, Brigham both celebrated and bemoaned the progessive spirit of the day. In a revealing aside, he once commented that progress was as important to the care of the insane as to business ("New Jersey Lunatic Asylum," 384).

15.　Brigham's early ideas about religion are best summarized in Brigham, *Observations,* and idem, *Remarks*. While superintendent at Utica, he continued to emphasize the importance of moderation in his published writings. For example, see idem, "Millerism"; N.Y.S. Lunatic Asylum, *Third AR* (1846), 56. Although he opposed those religious enthusiasms which so often created feelings of unworthiness and suicidal despair in the faithful, he recommended that a minister be attached to every asylum so that its inmates could acquire the self-discipline produced by the study of the proper sort of religion (idem, *An Inquiry*, 299).

16.　Amariah Brigham, "Cases of Insanity," 145.

17.   Brigham, "Insanity and Insane Hospitals," 115.

18.   Johann Christoph Spurzheim, *Observations on the Deranged Mani-festations of the Mind, or Insanity;* Brigham, *Remarks,* table of contents.

19.   Brigham, *An Inquiry.*

20.   Roger Cooter, "Phrenology and British Alienists, ca. 1825–1845," 58–60. See also Eric T. Carlson, "The Influence of Phrenology on Early American Psychiatric Thought," and the debate over the phrenological beliefs of Brigham's first assistant physician at the "Fourth Annual Meeting of the AMSAII," 56–58. At that meeting, Brigham gently disagreed with Butolph and noted that insanity that most commonly seems to be a temporary disease of the brain, resulting from over-action or inaction. Like his colleagues, he agreed with the doctor who quoted one of his patients to the effect that "it was hard to tell what meat is in the smoke house by putting your hand on the roof." In a letter to Pliny Earle, dated March 19, 1845, Brigham said he was not a strong phrenologist, for he did not "feel confidence that the organ of the brain can be ascertained by external examination, but I do not think this case fatal to the doctrine" (Earle Papers, AAS). Despite his rejection of the craniological aspects of phrenology, at his death Brigham was memorialized lovingly in the *Phrenological Journal* (Nelson Sizer, "Death of Dr. Brigham," quoted in the *Water-Cure Journal and Herald of Reform* 8 [November, 1849], 154).

21.   Quoted in Amariah Brigham, *A Letter from Doctor Brigham to David M. Reese, M.D., Author of Phrenology Known by Its Fruits, Etc.,* 9.

22.   For descriptions of attacks on Brigham's attitudes toward religion, see Leonard Eaton, "Eli Todd and the Hartford Retreat," 444, and N.Y.S. Lunatic Asylum, *Fourth AR* (1847), 39.

23.   David Bakan, "The Influence of Phrenology on American Psychology," 212.

24.   Amariah Brigham, "Noble on the Brain."

25.   N.Y.S. Lunatic Asylum, *First AR* (1844), 39.

26.   "Fourth Annual Meeting of the AMSAII," 57.

27.   Goodrich, *Sermon.*

28.   Julius Rubin, "Mental Illness in Early Nineteenth Century New England and the Beginnings of Institutional Psychiatry as Revealed in a Sociological Study of the Hartford Retreat 1824–1843," 343; John A. Pitts, "The Association of Medical Superintendents of American Institutions for the Insane, 1844–1892: A Case Study of Specialism in American Medicine" (hereafter cited as Pitts, "The AMSAII"), 7.

29.   N.Y.S. Lunatic Asylum, *Sixth AR* (1849), 55.

30.   N.Y.S. Lunatic Asylum, *First AR* (1844), 30–34; idem, *Third AR* (1846), 53–57; idem, *Fourth AR* (1847), 25; idem, *Sixth AR* (1849), 36–38; Amariah Brigham, "Sleep, Its Importance in Preventing Insanity."

31.   N.Y.S. Commissioner in Lunacy, *First AR* (1874), 9. Also see Brigham, "Insanity and Insane Hospitals," 101.

32.   Brigham, *An Inquiry,* 289; N.Y.S. Lunatic Asylum, *Sixth AR* (1849), 38–59.

33.   Brigham, *An Inquiry,* 294–297; idem, "The Moral Treatment of Insanity"; idem, "Insanity and Insane Hospitals," 102.

34.   Cooter, "Phrenology."
35.   Brigham, *An Inquiry,* 294–299; idem, "The Medical Treatment of Insanity."
36.   Brigham, "Cases of Insanity—Illustrating the Importance of Early Treatment in Preventing Suicides"; idem, "Schools in Lunatic Asylums"; idem, "The Moral Treatment of Insanity."
37.   Letter to Pliny Earle from Amariah Brigham, May 6, 1845, Earle Papers, AAS; Goodrich, *Sermon,* 66, 75.
38.   Poem by Lydia Sigourney, quoted in Goodrich, *Sermon,* 68.
39.   Letter to Earle from Brigham, May 28, 1844, Earle Papers, AAS.
40.   See Brigham's correspondence with Earle, Earle Papers, AAS, and with Thomas Kirkbride, Kirkbride Papers, PHMA.
41.   Undated draft of a letter by Amariah Brigham, Uticana Collection, OCHS. For descriptions of Brigham's multiple duties, see the following Brigham letters to C. A. Mann, chairman of the board of managers: January 1, 1844 (about political fund raising); September 4, 1844 (about construction problems); August 28, 1845, and January 13, 1846 (about water supply problems); January 13, 1847 (about architectural issues); March 15, 1847 (more about water piping); and to Silas Wright, December 2, 1844 (bringing this influential politician up to date on events at the asylum). All are located in the Uticana Collection, OCHS.
42.   Board of Managers, 1843–1849, UPCA.
43.   Letter to Earle from Brigham, May 28, 1844, Earle Papers, AAS.
44.   Ibid., July 1, 1845.
45.   Ibid., May 5, 1845; November 11, 1846; October 11, 1846.
46.   Ibid., May 6, 1845.
47.   See letter to Kirkbride from Brigham, February 2, 1848, Kirkbride Papers, PHMA, for a description of Brigham's grief and fatigue after the death of his son.
48.   Coventry, "Amariah Brigham, M.D."
49.   "Medical Experts in Cases of Suspected Insanity."
50.   Hurd, *Institutional Care* 4: 356; Board of Managers, November 3, 1849, UPCA; "New York State Lunatic Asylum."
51.   Letters to Thomas Kirkbride from Nathan Benedict, Kirkbride papers, PHMA: June 21, 1850; October 27, 1852; December 24, 1852; December 25, 1852; April 11, 1853.
52.   Letters to Dorothea Dix from Nathan Benedict, Dix Papers, HLHU: July 31, 1850; September 11, 1850; November 3, 1851.
53.   Letter to Dix from Benedict, May 11, 185? (year undecipherable), Dix Papers, HLHU.
54.   N.Y.S. Lunatic Asylum, *Eighth AR* (1851), 14.
55.   Hurd, *Institutional Care* 4: 356; N.Y.S. Lunatic Asylum, *Twelfth AR* (1855), 356; idem, *Twenty-ninth AR* (1872), 9.
56.   N.Y.S. Lunatic Asylum, *Eighth AR* (1851), 14.
57.   See letters to Dix from Benedict, Dix Papers, HLHU: July 31, 1850; February 25, 1851; November 3, 1851.
58.   Letter to A. Munson from Nathan Benedict, October 26, 1853, Uticana Collection, OCHS.

59. Letter to Charles A. Mann from Alonzo Potter of Philadelphia, October 29, 1853, Uticana Collection, OCHS. In a letter to Mann dated June 6, 1854 (Uticana Collection, OCHS), John Gray hinted that some of Benedict's problems stemmed from his inability to control his wife. He attributed Benedict's reluctance to resign to a fear that his reputation thereafter would be tarnished, an apprehension which Gray considered well-founded but for which he had little sympathy. In another letter to Mann, Gray claimed that, if he left, all the other doctors would quit as well. Since he already had tentatively accepted another superintendency, his threat to leave was taken seriously. Benedict, Gray alleged, had been willing to sacrifice everything for the sake of his own comfort. By 1854 he knew fewer than 100 of the 458 patients personally. Gray then emoted, "The magnitude of the object: the best interest of this large collection of sick people comes over my heart like a mighty flood" (letter to Mann from Gray, June 5, 1854, Uticana Collection, OCHS).

60. In a letter to Benedict, Charles Mann, head of the board of managers, claimed that, while the managers much appreciated Benedict's past service, their concern for the welfare of patients, most of whom Benedict no longer knew personally, dictated that he be replaced with someone with better health (letter to Benedict from Mann, November 2, 1853, Uticana Collection, OCHS).

61. For example, see letter to Thomas Kirkbride from D. J. Brown of the Bloomingdale Asylum, September 4, 1854, Kirkbride Papers, PHMA, in which Brown noted that Gray was "regarded as a mutineer in some quarters."

62. In a sad letter to Dorothea Dix, Nathan Benedict, now in Magnolia Lake, Florida, complained that no one answered his letters and he heard little of "the Brethren" (February 26, 1859, Dix Papers, HLHU).

63. See letters to Kirkbride from Benedict, Kirkbride Papers, PHMA: January 31, 1855 and April 7, 1855; Chase, *Two Years and Four Months*, 9–10.

64. Gray's conflicts with neurologists, Utica staff doctors, and attendants thread through the testimony found in both the 1880 Investigation and the 1884 Investigation.

65. M. M. Bagg, ed., *Memorial History of Utica, N.Y., from Its Settlement to the Present Time*, 20–25; "In Memoriam"; Hurd, *Institutional Care* 4: 415–417; "Resolutions of the Oneida Historical Society at Utica in Memory of Dr. John Perdue Gray, L.L.D., December 6, 1886," OCHS, Uticana Collection; J. B. Andrews, "Memoirs of John Gray." Local newspaper obituaries which praise Gray's many accomplishments include the following: "John P. Gray, M.D., LL.D.," Utica *Morning Telegraph*, November 30, 1886, in Willard Scrapbook No. 2, 38–40, WPCA; "Dr. John P. Gray," *Observer*, November 30, 1886, in ibid., 40–41; "Dr. Gray Dead!" unidentified newspaper, n.d., in ibid., 42; "The Late John P. Gray," *Observer*, December 12, 1886, in ibid., 45.

66. John P. Gray, "The Dependence of Insanity on Physical Disease"; N.Y.S. Lunatic Asylum, *Twenty-seventh AR* (1870), 15; John P. Gray, "Insanity, and Its Relation to Medicine"; idem, "Pathology of Insanity"; idem, "Thoughts on the Causation of Insanity."

67. John P. Gray, "General View of Insanity, Lecture Delivered before the Bellevue Hospital Medical College, Session of 1874–1875."

68. "In Memoriam," 154.

69. Charles E. Rosenberg, *The Trial of the Assassin Guiteau: Psychiatry and Law in the Gilded Age*, 190–197. Rosenberg describes Gray as "a strong controversialist and an enduring hater" (73).

70. N.Y.S. Lunatic Asylum, *Sixteenth AR* (1859), 18, 22–23.

71. S. P. Fullinwider, "Insanity as the Loss of Self: The Moral Insanity Controversy Revisited."

72. For legislative exposes, see 1880 Investigation and 1884 Investigation. For his views on pathology, see Gray, "General View of Insanity"; idem, "Pathology of Insanity"; Andrews, "Memoirs of John Gray."

73. Robert J. Waldinger, "Sleep of Reason: John P. Gray and the Challenge of Moral Insanity," 179.

74. N.Y.S. Commissiner in Lunacy, *Eleventh AR* (1884), 363.

75. Edward N. Brush, "Obituary: John B. Chapin, M.D., L.L.D."

76. Ibid., 696–701.

77. Willard Asylum, *Ninth AR* (1878), 39–40; idem, *Twelfth AR* (1881), 30. In contrast to Brigham and Gray, John B. Chapin wrote little about his work except for brief summaries in his annual reports. He produced several articles on the importance of institutional care of the chronically insane poor in the 1850s (see Chapter 2), and in 1898, *A Compendium of Insanity* for the use of students and general practitioners.

78. Mitchell, "Fiftieth Annual Meeting," 429.

79. Ibid.; see also Hammond, "Treatment of the Insane," 240.

80. 1884 Investigation, 1047.

81. See also N.Y.S. Commissioner in Lunacy, *Second AR* (1875), 24; 1884 Investigation, 792–794, 797–803.

82. Willard Asylum, *Twelfth AR* (1881), 6.

83. N.Y.S. Lunatic Asylum, *Forty-fifth AR* (1888), 89.

84. "The *AJI*." For Blumer's biography, see "Dr. Blumer Appointed," *Observer*, December 14, 1886, Willard Scrapbook No. 2, 50, WPCA; "Dr. G. Alder Blumer," unidentified newspaper clipping, undated (c. December 1886), ibid.

85. "Dr. Blumer's Lecture: Music's Impression on the Mind," Utica *Daily Press*, March 27, 1890, Willard Scrapbook No. 3, 63, WPCA. For other changes introduced after Gray's death, see "State Lunatic Asylum, Business Methods to be Changed," Utica *Daily Press*, November 12, 1886, Willard Scrapbook No. 2, 32, WPCA.

86. "The State Asylum," unidentified newspaper clipping, undated (c. March 1887), Willard Scrapbook No. 2, 78, WPCA.

87. For Wise's biography, see "Dr. P. M. Wise," which appeared in the Ogdensberg *Daily Journal*, September 16, 1889, Willard Scrapbook No. 4, 17, WPCA, when Wise left Willard for the superintendency of the St. Lawrence State Asylum, a mixed institution which gave him "the opportunity for progressive work not available in the older institutions." For examples of his published writings, see P. M. Wise, "The Barber Case: The Legal Responsibility of Epileptics"; idem, "Case of Sexual Perversion"; idem, "Recovery of the Chronic Insane"; idem, "The Care of the Chronic Insane"; and idem, "Vaginal Hernia and Uterine Fibroids, with Delusions of Pregnancy."

88. "A Remarkable Cure," *Seneca County Courier*, November 11, 1886, in Willard Scrapbook No. 2, 29, WPCA.

89. "Experts on Insanity: The National Convention Well under Way," Detroit *Tribune*, June 15, 1887, in ibid., 96–97.
90. This was a national phenomenon; see Pitts, "The AMSAII," 66.
91. Board of Managers, 16–17, UPCA.
92. N.Y.S. Lunatic Asylum, *Fifth AR* (1848), 42–43; Board of Managers, 42–43. See similar lists in N.Y.S. Lunatic Asylum, *Thirty-seventh AR* (1880), 9; 1884 Investigation, 1154–1155; Willard Asylum, *Sixth AR* (1875), 30; *Laws Relating to the Willard Asylum*, 26.
93. Letter to Edward Jarvis from C. B. Coventry of Utica, June 13, 1842, Uticana Collection, OCHS.
94. N.Y.S. Commissioner in Lunacy, *Twelfth AR* (1885), 14–15.
95. E. C. Seguin, "Lunacy Reform, I: Historical Considerations," 196–197.
96. N.Y.S. Lunatic Asylum, *Thirty-seventh AR* (1880), 46.
97. Idem, *Twenty-seventh AR* (1870), 15.
98. A sample of the applicant letters received by Chapin can be found at the WPCA.
99. N.Y.S. Lunatic Asylum, *Forty-sixth AR* (1889), 59; idem, *Forty-third AR* (1886), 72.
100. Letter to Dorothea Dix from John P. Gray, January 10, 1869, Dix Papers, HLHU.
101. Letter to John B. Chapin from E. Wirt Lamoureau, March 25, 1880, WPCA.
102. Letters to Chapin from A. Vause, November 26, 1873, and James L. Babcock, November 27, 1873, WPCA.
103. Letter to Chapin from Harvey Jewett, March 1, 1883, WPCA; letters to Chapin from James Bristol: December 30, 1882; February 21, 1883; March 24, 1883, WPCA.
104. Rough draft of letter to the N.Y.S. Senate from Chapin, n.d., except for 187–, WPCA.
105. Letter to Chapin from "Superintendent XXX," n.d., WPCA.
106. Letter to Chapin from "Superintendent XXXX," ibid.
107. Letter to Hon. D. O. Ogden from G. E. Weeks, February 11, 1880, UPCA.
108. 1884 Investigation, 91–268, 777–779. See also 1880 Investigation, 10–12, and "Review of *Second Annual Report of the State Commissioner in Lunacy, for the State of New York, for 1874*, 466–470, for a statement of Utica's objections. For arguments in favor, see N.Y.S. Commissioner in Lunacy, *Second AR* (1875), 15; idem, *Tenth AR* (1883), 172–174; idem, *Fifteenth AR* (1888), 46–47; untitled newspaper editorial, Utica *Sunday Tribune*, January 30, 1887, Willard Scrapbook No. 2, 59, WPCA; "Female Physicians," Rochester *Democrat and Chronicle*, February 6, 1890, Willard Scrapbook No. 3, 30, WPCA.
109. N.Y.S. Board of Charities, *Twenty-third AR* (1890), 207.
110. N.Y.S. Lunatic Asylum, *Forty-eight AR* (1891), 56.
111. "To Women Physicians," unidentified newspaper clipping, March 16, 1889, Willard Scrapbook No. 3, 103, WPCA.
112. "Proceedings of the Association of Medical Superintendents," *AJI* 47: 228.
113. "Discussion," 443.
114. The issue of female doctors continued to be debated well into the

1890s. It was a frequent topic for discussion at national meetings of the Conference of Charities and Corrections, at one of which Dr. Margaret Cleaves of the Harrisburg (Pennsylvania) Asylum called for separate hospitals for women, run by women. She also noted that, in 1880, only eight hospitals in the country had female physicians on their staffs ("The Debate on Insanity," 27–28). Another female participant argued that, although she was "not a Woman's Rights woman," women had a right to demand female doctors for those state institutions in which more than half of the inmates were women (Clara Leonard, "Women as Hospital Physicians"). Both continued to use arguments about "female delicacy" to justify the care of female patients by female doctors. Not until the 1890s was the possibility of using female physicians to treat male patients, as well, mentioned at one of these meetings ("Minutes and Discussion," 44). For further discussion of these issues, see G. C. Paoli and James G. Kiernan, "Female Physicians in Insane Hospitals, Their Advantages and Disadvantages," and Constance M. McGovern, "Doctors or Ladies? Women Physicians in Psychiatric Institutions, 1872–1900."

115. Alice May Farnham, "Uterine Disease as a Factor in the Production of Insanity." Farnham stayed at Willard for almost three years and then seems to have taken a comparable position in a New York City asylum (N.Y.S. Board of Charities, *Twenty-second AR* [1889], 267).

116. Examples of the kinds of research published by nineteenth-century assistant physicians at Utica and Willard include H. A. Butolph, "The Relation between Phrenology and Insanity"; John B. Chapin, "Cases Illustrating the Pathology of Mental Disease Arising from Syphilitic Infection"; A. O. Kellogg, "Imbecility and Insanity"; Charles W. Pilgrim, "A Visit to Gheel"; C. E. Atwood, "Three Cases of Multiple Neuritis Associated with Insanity"; H. E. Allison, "Mental Changes, Resulting from Separate Fractures of Both Thighs"; idem, "The Moral and Industrial Management of the Insane"; Willis Ford, "Clinical Cases: Syphilitic Insanity"; Judson B. Andrews, "Exophthalmic Goitre with Insanity"; William Mabon, "Clinical Observations on the Action of Sulfonal in Insanity."

117. Albert Deutsch, *The Mentally Ill in America*, 275.

118. Willard Asylum, *Eleventh AR* (1880), 39.

119. E. C. Seguin, "Lunacy Reform: II. Insufficiency of the Medical Staff of Asylums," 314; see also Traill Green, "Functions of the Medical Staff of an Insane Hospital," 277.

120. For a description of the working seminars held at Willard twice a month, see "Notes and Comments." Paper topics in 1886 included the gross anatomy and convolutions of the brain, the moral and industrial management of the insane, and masked phthisis. See also Willard Asylum, *Eighteenth AR* (1887), 18. As the end of the century approached, however, the Willard medical staff had increasingly little time for such intellectual exercises. In 1890, the Willard superintendent complained that, with one doctor for every three hundred patients, his assistant physicians had little opportunity for research, even when interested in it (Willard Asylum, *Twenty-second AR* [1891], 27).

121. Willard Asylum, *Thirteenth AR* (1882), 31–36; N.Y.S. Lunatic Asylum, *Forty-second AR* (1885), 49; idem, *Forty-third AR* (1886), 71.

122. Letter to Judge Hadley from John B. Chapin, January 19, 1883, WPCA.

123. Pitts, "The AMSAII," 44–45; N.Y.S. Lunatic Asylum, *Thirty-first AR* (1874), 10.

124.　Pitts, "The AMSAII," 44–45; 1884 Investigation, 1104; N.Y.S. Lunatic Asylum, *Twenty-fifth AR* (1868), 30.

125.　Willard Asylum, *Eleventh AR* (1880), 16.

126.　Pitts, "The AMSAII," 66.

127.　Seguin, "Lunacy Reform: I," 314; Green, "Functions of a Medical Staff," 277.

128.　N.Y.S. Lunatic Asylum, *Forty-sixth AR* (1889), 18.

129.　N.Y.S. Lunatic Asylum, *Thirtieth AR* (1873), 8.

130.　Tomes, "A Generous Confidence," 139.

131.　N.Y.S. Lunatic Asylum, *Second AR* (1845), 51.

132.　N.Y.S. Lunatic Asylum, *Forty-fifth AR* (1888), 54.

4
A Distanced Relative

1.　Letters to the Superintendent of the State Lunatic Asylum, from J. M. of Catteraugus, New York, May 1 and May 30, 1842; letter (on behalf of his widowed sister) to the Overseer of the Insane Hospital from W. D. of Chenango Point, New York, October 20, 1843. Even the editor of a large New York City newspaper found himself in need of the asylum's services for a partially insane relative who lived near Utica. The woman had no kin who could care for her and few financial resources, although she did not qualify as a pauper (letter to Charles Mann from A. C. of New York City, May 30, 1842). These and similar letters from the families of the insane are part of the Uticana Collection, OCHS.

2.　1842 *Laws of New York*, chap. 135; 1850 *Laws of New York*, chap. 282, sec. 2; John Ordronaux, *Commentaries on the Lunacy Laws of New York and on the Judicial Aspects of Insanity at Common Law and In Equity, including Procedure, as Expounded in England and the United States.* Several patients at the Utica Asylum complained that private patients could be retained indefinitely, if families continued to pay for their care (Chase, *Two Years and Four Months*, 26–29; Henry Richardson, "A Letter to Dr. G. Alder Blumer, from Ward 2 North, Utica, August 11, 1890," 17, UPCA).

3.　For families' reluctance to institutionalize, see "Early Indications of Insanity" by Utica assistant physician Judson H. Andrews. Andrews noted that families seldom recognized the early symptoms of insanity, largely because they were convinced that such a misfortune could not happen to them. He warned families to be on the outlook for such premonitory symptoms as morbid dreams, sleep impairments, constant headaches, emotional exaggerations, excessive religious scruples, and changes in habits of dress and cleanliness. Yet he himself admitted the frequent difficulty of distinguishing changes produced by disease from eccentricity or capriciousness. For a description of what they consider to be the barely concealed hostility of many nineteenth-century asylums toward patients' families, see Rosenkrantz and Vinovskis, "Caring for the Insane," 192–194.

4.　Since about one-third of Utica's patients were private until the end of the nineteenth century, the Utica Asylum served as a refuge for families of all classes rather than being reserved for the insane poor (its legal responsibility). For a similar discussion of nineteenth-century families' unwillingness to institutionalize, see Tomes, *A Generous Confidence,* 108–113. This reluctance persists into the twentieth century; for a summary of recent research on families' resistance to recognizing mental illness in members, see Allan V. Horwitz, *The Social Control of Mental Illness,* 36–44.

5. UPCBR 6: nos. 1910, 1862, UPCA.

6. According to Norman Dain, physicians began to distinguish between the exciting and predisposing causes of insanity in the eighteenth century (Dain, *Concepts of Insanity in the United States, 1789–1865,* 7–8). For the perspective of a Utica physician on this issue, see John P. Gray, "Thoughts on the Causation of Insanity," 282–283.

7. UPCBR 6: no. 1820, UPCA.

8. Brigham, "Insanity and Insane Hospitals." Even before Brigham was hired, New York State legislators stressed the value of collecting insanity statistics on the assumption that, once enough statistical information had been collected, the mystery of insanity would unfold (1842 *Laws of New York,* chap. 135). In this respect, they shared the fascination of many nineteenth-century Americans with statistical evidence (P. Cohen, *A Calculating People;* Cassedy, *American Medicine*).

9. For doctors' struggles to make casebook histories more reliable, see N.Y.S. Commissioner in Lunacy, *Tenth AR* (1883), 82; "Proceedings of the Association," *AJI* 37, 167–168; Walter Channing, "A Consideration of the Causes of Insanity."

10. Unfortunately, casebooks do not give admitting doctors' names.

11. For a description of English commitment decisions during this same period, see John K. Walton, "Lunacy in the Industrial Revolution," 1–3. According to Walton, in nineteenth-century Lancashire, three key variables affected the social definition of mental illness: migration patterns, family structure and economy, and the scale of urban living. Those living in middle-rank textile towns were least likely to institutionalize family members because they had access to more social supports than were available in the country or large cities. In contrast to Great Britain, New York State had both state and local institutions for the insane; the former attracted patients from all over the state, rather than from a single district, for most of the nineteenth century. As a result, I cannot test Walton's interesting hypotheses in New York, using only Utica and Willard data. Yet it seems likely to me that many of the social forces he observes in Lancashire also operated in New York. For example, in both places, large numbers of patients were between the ages of thirty-five and forty-five at admission, the point at which (Walton observes) the pressures of poverty were most acute, for children had just begun to contribute to the family income, and living accommodations for laborers were extremely crowded.

12. For a description of this "normalization" process, see Horwitz, *Social Control,* 36–42.

13. UPCBR 6: no. 1903, UPCA.

14. WPCBR 5: no. 2125, WPCA.

15. ˙ WPCBR 13: no. 4423, WPCA.

16. Charles W. Pilgrim, "Pyromania (So-Called), with Case."

17. UPCBR 6: no. 890, UPCA. For a description of the same patterns in familial decisions to institutionalize the mentally retarded, see Mark Freedberger,

"The Decision to Institutionalize: Families with Exceptional Children in 1900"; see also UPCBR 73: no. 175 for year, UPCA.

18.　For cases in which, after many years, families no longer could cope with epileptic members, see Chase, *Two Years and Four Months*, 89–90; WPCBR 5: nos. 1897, 1924, WPCA; WPCBR 13: no. 4476, WPCA. In the last case, the epileptic patient (a female) had been cared for at home for forty-five years.

19.　For Gray's attitudes toward alcoholics, see "Dipsomania"; N.Y.S. Lunatic Asylum, *Eighteenth AR* (1861), 81–82; "Asylum for Inebriates," 353.

20.　Rosenkrantz and Vinovskis suggest that the old were underrepresented in nineteenth-century asylums because communities hesitated to subsidize relatively expensive state-level care for them (Rosenkrantz and Vinovskis, "The Invisible Lunatics").

21.　Rosenkrantz and Vinovskis, "Caring for the Insane," 204. For a similar situation in New York State, see Walter R. Gardinier, Jr., "Pauperism and Insanity: Aspects of Social Welfare in Nineteenth Century Chatauqua County."

22.　1844 Assembly *Documents*, no. 21, 3–4.

23.　Paul Starr, "Medicine, Economy, and Society in Nineteenth-Century America," 588–596.

24.　Gray, "Dependence on Physical Disease." UPCBR 76: no. 96, UPCA.

25.　UPCBR 2: nos. 685 and 686, UPCA; UPCBR 3: no. 869, UPCA; UPCBR 4: no. 1174, UPCA; UPCBR 5: nos. 869, 1556, UPCA; UPCBR 18: no. 6380, UPCA; UPCBR 62: no. 214 for year, UPCA.

26.　UPCBR 77: no. 119 for year, UPCA; see also UPCBR 76: no. 210 for year, UPCA.

27.　Joan Jacobs Brumberg, "(Ruined Girls): Changing Family and Community Responses to Illegitimacy in Upstate New York, 1890–1920," 247.

28.　UPCBR 13: no. 122 for year, UPCA.

29.　Lathrop, *Secret Institution;* Richardson, "Letter to G. Alder Blumer," UPCA; UPCBR 79: no. 220 for year, UPCA; UPCBR 3: no. 658, UPCA; UPCBR 78: no. 90 for year, UPCA; UPCBR 26: no. 3821, UPCA.

30.　"Proceedings of the Association," *AJI* 37: 151; William C. Krauss, "The Hypnotic State of Hysteria," 526; "The Alleged Increase of Insanity"; Channing, "Consideration of the Causes," 70; A. O. Wright, "The Increase of Insanity," 229; "Increase of Insanity," *New-York Daily Tribune*, January 19, 1882.

31.　Elaine Showalter, "Victorian Women and Insanity," 159. See also Myra Himmelhoch with Arthur Shaffer, "Elizabeth Packard: Nineteenth Century Crusader for the Rights of Mental Patients."

32.　WPCBR 13: no. 4591, WPCA; "What Can Be Done?" Indianapolis *Locomotive*, June 15, 1850, 3.

33.　Case of Emily M., October 6, 1871, Albany County Court Commitment Papers, NYSLA.

34.　Willard Asylum, *Fourth AR* (1873), 13.

35.　Eric H. Monkkonen, "A Disorderly People? Urban Order in the Nineteenth and Twentieth Centuries."

36.　UPCBR 14: no. 209, UPCA.

37.　"Statistics of Insanity"; "Proceedings of the Association," *AJI* 37: 167.

38.　For a discussion of nineteenth-century notions about masturbation, see Vieda Skultans, *English Madness, Ideas on Insanity, 1580–1890;* Vern L.

Bullough and Martha Vogt, "Homosexuality and Its Confusion with the Secret Sin in Pre-Freudian America."

39. WPCBR 5: no. 1919, WPCA.

40. Wise, "Case of Sexual Perversion"; WPCBR 7: no. 2680, WPCA. Newspapers clippings pasted into her casebook record refer to Lobdell as "the Hunter of Long Eddy" and mention a published account of her life. At the time of institutionalization, she was described as "obscene, insists on wearing men's attire, threatens lives and does herself violence."

41. WPCBR 4: no. 1992, WPCA; Peter Tyor, "Denied the Power to Choose the Good: Sexuality and Mental Defect in American Medical Practice, 1850–1920." See also Nicolas F. Hahn, "Too Dumb to Know Better: Cacogenic Family Studies and the Criminology of Women."

42. John P. Gray, "Heredity."

43. For a general review of the nineteenth-century medical literature on sex roles and psychopathology, see Ellen Dwyer, "A Historical Perspective."

44. The sample includes 1,666 Utica patients for the years 1843–1868 and 1,868 for the years 1869–1890. There are 974 patients in the Willard sample, which exists only for the second period because Willard did not open until 1869.

45. Unfortunately, I cannot ascertain the characteristics of the population at risk to be sent to the N.Y.S. Lunatic Asylum before 1890. The institution accepted acutely ill patients from all sections of the state except New York City, although most of its patients came from upstate New York. As other state asylums opened in the 1870s and 1880s, Utica's catchment area narrowed, but until the state established formal asylum districts in 1890, it continued to lack precise geographical boundaries. Two sociologists interested in the impact of economic events on admission patterns to New York's twentieth-century mental hospitals warn that relying on state-level economic and patient data may lead one to overlook the impact on admission patterns of hospital-specific policy decisions and of regional economic trends in different parts of New York State (James B. Marshall and George W. Dowdall, "Employment and Mental Hospitalization: The Case of Buffalo, New York, 1914–1955").

46. The major differences at admission between my sample of Willard's Irish ($N = 655$) and of other foreign-born patients ($N = 488$) were as follows: the Irish were 57.4 percent female, while the others were 48.4 percent; the Irish were 43.3 percent single, while the others were 27.6 percent; 71.7 percent of the Irish were unskilled laborers or domestics in comparison with 49.5 percent of the others; 86 percent of the Irish were Catholic in comparison with 20.5 percent of the others; only 46.3 percent of the Irish had had a common school education in comparison with 74.9 percent of the others. Clearly, all institutionalized insane immigrants were not alike.

47. 1844 Assembly *Documents,* no. 21; WPCBR 13: no. 4423, WPCA; Channing, "Consideration of the Causes," 89.

48. N.Y.S. Lunatic Asylum, *First AR* (1844), 27.

49. Katz, *Poverty and Policy,* 130–134.

50. Almost 1 percent of the nineteenth-century Utica patient population was black. Black patients generally resembled whites in sociodemographic profiles, diagnoses, and treatments.

51. UPCBR 17: no. 6088, UPCA.

52. UPCBR 18: no. 6263, UPCA.

53. John Gray was particularly sympathetic to the plight of overworked mothers and attempted to start a maternity fund in Utica to ensure postpartum women proper help. See John P. Gray, "Insanity: Its Frequency: and Some of Its Preventable Causes"; "John P. Gray, M.D., L.L.D.," Utica *Morning Herald*, November 30, 1886, in Willard Scrapbook No. 2, 38–40. WPCA. He also published a moving essay on the psychological impact of hard work and isolation on newly married farm women (E. H. Van Deusen, "Observations on a Form of Nervous Prostration [Neurasthenia], Culminating in Insanity").

54. In addition, in the nineteenth century (as in the twentieth), women may have been more willing to acknowledge the onset of psychological problems than men (Ronald C. Kessler, Roger L. Brown, and Clifford L. Broman, "Sex Differences in Psychiatric Help-keeping: Evidence from Four Large-Scale Studies"). A study of nineteenth-century patients at the Trenton (New Jersey) State Asylum found that the lower a person's income and status, the more quickly deviant behavior was noticed and commitment proceedings begun (Joel Schwartz, "Women and the Mental Hospital in Nineteenth Century America: The Case of the Trenton State Asylum," 14).

55. Families experienced much difficulty in dating the onset of illness. Not uncommon were descriptions such as the following: has been insane "for one year decidedly" but has had symptoms for four to five years, and "has been insane for one year but not been entirely sane for ten to twelve years" (UPCBR 6: nos. 2048 and 2148, UPCA). Willard's records are even more confusing. Large numbers of patients are simply characterized as "chronic"; others have one calculation under the entry "date when insanity commenced" and a different one under "duration of insanity," with no explanation of the inconsistency (WPCBR 5: nos. 1914, 1902, WPCA). Yet, despite these problems, the magnitude of the difference between duration data for men and women is so large as to suggest that families more quickly found themselves unable to deal with anomalous behavior in women (perhaps because women were the major caretakers). For examples of duration of insanity charts in annual reports, see N.Y.S. Lunatic Asylum, *Twentieth AR* (1863), 24; idem, *Twenty-third AR* (1866), 43; idem, *Twenty-Eighth AR* (1871), 75; idem, *Thirty-eighth AR* (1881), 40; idem, *Forty-Third AR* (1886), 38–39; idem, *Forty-eighth AR* (1891), 26.

56. Willard Asylum, *Twenty-third AR* (1890).

57. N.Y.S. Lunatic Asylum, *Fourth AR* (1847), 21.

58. 1842 *Laws of New York*, chap. 135.

59. Draft of a letter to Brigham from C. A. Mann, November 27, 1843, Uticana Collection, OCHS.

60. N.Y.S. Lunatic Asylum, *Tenth AR* (1853), 33.

61. 1850 *Laws of New York*, chap. 282.

62. N.Y.S. Lunatic Asylum, *Sixth AR* (1849), 8.

63. 1850 *Laws of New York*, chap. 282.

64. Ordronaux, *Commentaries*, 53.

65. Governor Butler, quoted in Clark Bell, "The Rights of the Insane and Their Enforcement," 12. For patients' criticisms of commitment laws, see "On the Claims of the Insane to the Respect and Interest of Society"; Chase, *Two Years and Four Months*, 26–29; UPCBR 24: no. 8266, UPCA; Lathrop, *Secret Institu-*

tion, 105. For the English controversy, see Peter McCandless, "Liberty and Lunacy: The Victorians and Wrongful Commitment."

66. For a discussion of the conflict between neurologists and asylum superintendents, see Bonnie Ellen Bluestein, "'A Hollow Square of Psychological Science': American Neurologists and Psychiatrists in Conflict"; and idem, "New York Neurologists and the Specialization of American Medicine."

67. 1874 *Laws of New York,* chap. 446.

68. Ordronaux, *Commentaries,* 53.

69. Ibid., 52–59.

70. 1874 Senate *Documents,* no. 86, 4.

71. 1882 Senate *Documents,* no. 96, 431.

72. "Fortieth Annual Report of the Managers of the State Lunatic Asylum, Utica, New York, for the Year 1882," 111–112.

73. A. B. Richardson, "The Restriction of Personal Liberty in the Care of the Insane," 270.

74. For an account of the trial and the three Supreme Court judges' arguments, see "Medical Jurisprudence," 508–523.

75. A. E. MacDonald, "The Examination and Commitment of the Insane."

76. Prudden Letters, N.Y.S. Board of Charities Correspondence, NYSLA; UPCBR 18: no. 285 for year, UPCA.

77. "A Few Facts concerning a Patient, by Himself"; UPCBR 73: 67, UPCA; Davis, *Two Years and Three Months,* 29. Chase, *Two Years and Four Months,* 26–29; "Memorial to the President."

78. UPCBR 24: no. 8194, UPCA.

79. UPCBR 16: 258, UPCA; Chase, *Two Years and Four Months,* 7, 124; Lathrop, *The Secret Institution,* 129; UPCBR 46: no. 36 for year, UPCA.

80. For examples, see UPCBR 26: no. 8834, UPCA; UPCBR 16: 254, UPCA; Lathrop, *The Secret Institution,* 111–114, 127–128.

81. M. MacDonald, *Mystical Bedlam,* 73–105; Marian Radke Yarrow, Charlotte Green Schwartz, Harriet S. Murphy, and Leila Calhoun Deasy, "The Psychological Meaning of Mental Illness in the Family"; E. S. Paykel, "Life Stress and Psychiatric Disorders: Applications of the Clinical Approach"; S. Henderson, P. Duncan-Jones, H. McAuley, and K. Ritchie, "The Patient's Primary Group."

82. Willard Asylum, *Fifth AR* (1874), 10. See also Ellen Dwyer, "'The Weaker Vessel': The Law versus Social Realities in the Commitment of Women to Nineteenth-Century New York Asylums," 85–106. In 1873 the New York Medico-Legal Society suggested to the legislature that every person responsible for institutionalizing an alleged insane person be required by law to visit that person at least twice a year ("The Proposed Law Submitted by the Committee of the Medico-Legal Society to the Legislature of the State of New York, Session of 1873," 135); for negative comments, see also N.Y.S. Commissioner in Lunacy, *Fifth AR* [1878], 6; idem, *Eleventh AR* [1884], 20.

83. George Beard, "Why We Need a National Association for the Protection of the Insane," 149; R. S. Dewey, "Present and Prospective Management of the Insane," 85.

84. Tyor and Zainaldin, "Asylum and Society," 41; Grob, *Mental Illness and American Society;* Katz, *Poverty and Policy,* 198.

85. UPCBR 73: 13, UPCA; Christopher Lasch, *A Haven in a Heartless World.*

5
Destiny in a Name

1.   Utica's doctors never themselves described in detail either their admission procedures or the diagnostic process. Both must be reconstituted from casebook records and patient memoirs. Some insight into the Willard process can be gleaned from a newspaper article which described the arrival of new patients. After their admission orders had been made out, new patients were given numbers; cards with names and numbers were pinned on their backs; and they were taken to their wards ("A Trip to Ovid," unidentified newspaper clipping, undated [c. 1869], Willard Scrapbook No. 1, n.p., Cornell).

2.   Although a greater rift has developed between lay and professional views of mental illness, families still most frequently initiate the institutionalization process for the mentally ill. For the nineteenth century, see Skultans, *English Madness*, 141; Finnane, *Insanity and the Insane*, 161–174; Tomes, *A Generous Confidence*, 108–128. For the twentieth century, see Atwood D. Gaines, "Definitions and Diagnoses: Cultural Implications of Psychiatric Help-seeking and Psychiatrists' Definition of the Situation in Psychiatric Emergencies." In this respect, the diagnostic process seems to have changed remarkably little over the past three centuries. Colin Jones describes a similar situation in eighteenth-century France, where the medical certificates required to commit insane persons seldom offered an independent check on their insanity (C. Jones, "Treatment of the Insane," 377). Today, Erving Goffman argues, psychiatrists primarily "interpose a technical perspective" on the community's recognition of certain behavior as deviant. By so doing, they hope to persuade offended members of society to treat the mentally ill with understanding (just as did their nineteenth-century medical brethren) (Erving Goffman, *Interaction Ritual: Essays on Face-to-Face Behavior*, 137–138).

3.   Sample descriptions of how classification at the N.Y.S. Lunatic Asylum at Utica worked as a therapeutic stategy can be found in the following annual reports: *First AR* (1844), 12–13; *Seventeenth AR* (1860), 19; *Thirty-fourth AR* (1877), 18; *Thirty-Seventh AR* (1880), 19–20; *Forty-first AR* (1884), 52. For John Chapin's views on the role of classification at Willard, see his "Report on Provision for the Chronic Insane," 196.

4.   A. O. Kellogg, "Notes on a Visit to Some of the Principal Hospitals for the Insane in Great Britain, France, and Germany, with Observations on the Use of Mechanical Restraint in the Treatment of the Insane"; J. Parigot, "General Medical Therapeutics," 397.

5.   For example, see Grob, *Mental Institutions*, 224–229. Several Utica patients also complained that ward transfers were used more often as rewards or punishments than for therapeutic purposes. See Davis, *Two Years and Three Months*, 84; Chase, *Two Years and Four Months*, 91; 1884 Investigation, 423, 428, 523, 616, 680, 1008–1009.

6.   Amariah Brigham, "Definition of Insanity: Nature of the Disease," 97–116.

7.   N.Y.S. Lunatic Asylum, *First AR* (1844), 36–88.

8.   Amariah Brigham, "The Medical Treatment of Insanity."

9.   Amariah Brigham, "The Moral Treatment of Insanity."

10.   N.Y.S. Lunatic Asylum, *Fourth AR* (1847), 34–35.

11. J. Gray, "Dependence on Physical Disease"; N.Y.S. Lunatic Asylum, *Twenty-first AR* (1864), 20–21, 35–38; idem., *Twenty-third AR* (1866), 25–29; "The Willard Asylum Act," 203; "Proceedings of the Fourteenth Annual Meeting of the AMSAII," 71.

12. Charles E. Rosenberg, "The Practice of Medicine in New York a Century Ago," 243.

13. Doctors casebook comments often did not fully document their prescriptions. For example, not uncommon are notes ordering the discontinuation of a form of restraint or a particular drug in case histories where the initial prescription had never been noted. Similarly, they frequently noted starting patients on a particular drug and never mentioned taking them off of it. In addition, although at the thirteenth annual meeting of the AMSAII, Utica's doctors discussed their frequent use of chloroform to quiet the violent insane, relatively few references to such use of chloroform appear in casebook records ("Proceedings of the Thirteenth Annual Meeting of the AMSAII," 91).

14. For example, see Daniel H. Kitchen, "Conium in the Treatment of Insanity"; idem, "Ergot in the Treatment of Nervous Diseases"; idem, "Nitrate of Amyl in the Treatment of Spasmodic Asthma and Acute Bronchitis"; Willis E. Ford, "Phosphorus in Insanity"; William Mabon, "Clinical Cases: Chloralamid as a Hypnotic for the Insane"; idem, "Clinical Observations on the Action of Sulfonal in Insanity." For an overview of drug use in nineteenth-century insane asylums, see Garfield Tourney, "A History of Therapeutic Fashions in Psychiatry, 1800–1966," 97; Edward Cowles, "Progress in the Care and Treatment of the Insane during the Half-Century;" 122–35; Finnane, *Insanity and the Insane,* 205–208; Eric T. Carlson, "Cannabis Indica in Nineteenth-Century Psychiatry"; Grob, *The State and the Mentally Ill,* 136, 249; Cheryl L. Krasnick, "'In Charge of the Loons': A Portrait of the London, Ontario, Asylum for the Insane in the Nineteenth Century."

15. John P. Gray, "Hyoscyamia in Insanity." For a general description of medical treatments at Gray's Utica, see N.Y.S. Lunatic Asylum, *Twenty-third AR* (1866), 26–29. "The Use of Sedatives in Insanity" describes the patient conditions for which these popular late nineteenth-century asylum drugs were prescribed. At the Pennsylvania Hospital during the same period, Thomas Kirkbride used the same drugs, but in a somewhat different fashion. He continued to rely on morphine after Gray had abandoned it and, especially after several unexpected patient deaths, used chloral only with great caution (Tomes, *A Generous Confidence,* 188–191).

16. For descriptions of addicted patients at Utica and the problems entailed by their care, see UPCBR 6: no. 54 for the year, UPCA; N.Y.S. Lunatic Asylum, *Twenty-seventh AR* (1870), 61; idem, *Thirtieth AR* (1873), 68–75; idem, *Forty-fifth AR* (1888), 21; idem, *Forty-sixth AR* (1889), 56. See also David T. Courtwright, "Opiate Addiction as a Consequence of the Civil War," and idem, "The Female Opiate Addict in Nineteenth-Century America."

17. "Poisonous Dose of Chloral." See also "Action of Chloral" and "Psychological Retrospect." At the 1874 meeting of the AMSAII, Doctor Judson Andrews again defended the Utica Asylum's heavy reliance on chloral on the grounds that he had not observed the ill effects noted in medical journals. He cited the case of a melancholic patient who took sixty grams a night for eighteen months so that he might sleep and subsequently was released as cured ("Proceedings of the AM-

SAII," *AJI* 31: 213–214). For criticism of the heavy use of chloral at the Utica Asylum, allegedly without careful attention to its potential ill effects, see "Proceedings of the Twenty-fourth Meeting of the AMSAII," 210–223.

18. Carlos F. MacDonald, "Hydrate of Chloral"; "Action of Chloral."

19. "Proceedings of the Fourteenth AMSAII," 81–83. Although American doctors were aware of the dangers involved in overusing drugs (see "Reports from American Asylums—July 1873," 123, for a discussion of the problems associated with prolonged use of bromides), in general they were more likely to overuse both chemical and physical restraints than their English and Irish counterparts. See Finnane, *Insanity and the Insane*, 205–206, for a summary of English alienists' doubts about drugs. John Gray, in particular, embraced drug therapies with enthusiasm. For example, see Carlson, "Cannabis Indica," 1005–1006.

20. For descriptions of patients' physical problems, see N.Y.S. Lunatic Asylum, *Seventeenth AR* (1860), 25; idem, *Twenty-first AR* (1864), 22; idem, *Twenty-second AR* (1865), 13; idem, *Twenty-third AR* (1866), 26–27; 1884 Investigation, 588. Epidemic threats are described in N.Y.S. Lunatic Asylum, *Seventh AR* (1850), 16; idem, *Twenty-third AR* (1866) 15; idem, *Twenty-fifth AR* (1868), 36; and idem, *Thirtieth AR* (1873), 29. Utica's death rates and the most common causes of death are described in N.Y.S. Lunatic Asylum, *Eighteenth AR* (1861), 34–36; idem, *Twenty-second AR* (1865), 18–19; idem, *Twenty-seventh AR* (1870), 79; idem, *Twenty-eighth AR* (1871), 29–64; idem, *Twenty-ninth AR* (1872), 15.

21. N.Y.S. Lunatic Asylum, *Thirtieth AR* (1873), 26; John P. Gray "Pathological Researches"; idem, "Pathology of Insanity."

22. For Gray's attacks on asylum schools, see "Proceedings of the Association of Medical Superintendents," *AJI* 31: 183; N.Y.S. Lunatic Asylum, *Twenty-fifth AR* (1868), 15; idem, *Thirty-fourth AR* (1877), 65; and 1884 Investigation, 124–142. For Gray's policies on patient labor, see N.Y.S. Lunatic Asylum, *Seventeenth AR* (1860), 34.

23. For typical entertainments offered at Gray's Utica, see N.Y.S. Lunatic Asylum, *Sixteenth AR* (1859), 25; idem, *Twenty-first AR* (1864), 56; idem, *Twenty-ninth AR* (1872), 81–82; idem, *Thirty-second AR* (1877), 66; idem, *Thirty-third AR* (1876), 63; idem, *Thirty-sixth AR* (1879), 22; idem, *Fortieth AR* (1883), 70–71, 94–95; idem, *Forty-third AR* (1886), 16; N.Y.S. Board of Charities, *Second AR* (1869), 15. For Gray's evaluation of the secondary importance of moral treatment, see N.Y.S. Lunatic Asylum, *Twenty-seventh AR* (1870), 16–17. For a description of his combined use of medical and moral treatments, see "Case of Mania with the Delusions and Phenomena of Spiritualism." Gray preferred diversions like gymnastics, which strengthened as well as amused, to simple entertainments. In 1860 Dio Lewis introduced his well-known gymnastics system to Utica's patients (N.Y.S. Lunatic Asylum, *Eighteenth AR* [1861], 52). Such exercises were considered particularly beneficial for melancholics. As Lloyd Sederer points out, the "potent, albeit largely unsatisfied, promise of other therapeutic modalities inspired by scientism" weakened the effectiveness of moral treatment, even among its supporters, by undermining the sense of personal responsibility for behavior, which was one of its basic tenets (Sederer, "Moral Therapy," 271). Private institutions like the Pennsylvania Hospital continued to offer elaborate programs of moral treatment well into the late nineteenth century (Tomes, *A Generous Confidence*, 193–197).

24. For Blumer's constant references to Brigham to justify the many changes

he instituted after Gray's death, see N.Y.S. Lunatic Asylum, *Forty-fourth AR* (1888), 48; idem, *Forty-fifth AR* (1885), 48–50. Although many praised the self-control taught at the patients' school, the commissioner in lunacy was more condescending. He, too, saw the school as successful and noted that "although boys will be boys the boys in this school seem to take more of an interest in their studies than those in other schools." His tone is particularly offensive, given that one of the "boys" had been a school commissioner and two of the "girls," school teachers (N.Y.S. Commissioner in Lunacy, *Fifteenth AR* [1888], 45). For other examples of moral treatments reintroduced by Blumer, see N.Y.S. Lunatic Asylum, *Forty-fourth AR* (1887), 39; idem, *Forty-fifth AR* (1888), 10–14, 43–52; idem, *Forty-sixth AR* (1889), 39; idem, *Forty-seventh AR* (1890), 53, 56–57; idem, *Forty-eighth AR* (1891), 55; "The State's Insane Wards," *New York Times*, July 4, 1887.

25. N.Y.S. Lunatic Asylum, *Forty-fifth AR* (1888), 45; idem, *Forty-sixth AR* (1889), 43–45.

26. Letters to Dorothea Dix from Nathan Benedict, July 31, 1850, and September 11, 1850, Dix Papers, HLHU.

27. N.Y.S. Lunatic Asylum, *Twenty-first AR* (1864), 22. See WBCBR 13: no. 4631, WPCA, for the story of a mother who took an attendant's job in order to reside at Willard with her suicidal and somewhat feeble-minded daughter.

28. "To My Mother."

29. For William Hammond's testimony at the 1880 Senate investigation, see 1880 Investigation, 58; for the advice to a distraught mother, see UPCBR 73: 54, UPCA.

30. UPCBR 73: 20, UPCA.

31. UPCBR 73: 48, UPCA.

32. N.Y.S. Commissioner in Lunacy, *Sixteenth AR* (1889), 11.

33. "Editor's Table," 6: 21. More obviously satirical was an earlier editor who compared the Utica Asylum to a "city set on a hill" and asked whether "this noble temple of humanity, should not be converted into a grand theater . . . the rooms into literary lounges—that everyone can come hither and rest under this wonderful shade of humanity—and Governor and Cabinet make this a retreat from the world's cares during the dog days" ("Editor's Table" 2: 317).

34. "Life in the N.Y. State Lunatic Asylum."

35. Hotchkiss, *Five Months in the Asylum*.

36. UPCBR 5: no. 392, UPCA.

37. Hotchkiss, *Five Months in the Asylum*, 58.

38. Despite Davis's complaints about Benedict's elitism, she clearly shared his values. She repeatedly noted with distaste her enforced association with lower-class patients and Irish attendants on the wards (Davis, *Two Years and Three Months*, 24–25).

39. Chase, *Two Years and Four Months*, 25–26, 36–37, 76.

40. 1884 Investigation, 526–527, 1324, 1206–1216. See also Lathrop, *Secret Institution*, 209–219. In further confirmation of patient allegations that the use of drugs was less careful than suggested by *AJI* reports, casebook histories reveal that patients who failed to respond quickly to one sort of medicine were switched rapidly to another, and then to a third, if necessary. For example, see UPCBR 45: no. 286 for the year, UPCA.

41. For positive patient testimonials, see "Asylum Life: or, The Advantage of a Disadvantage," 228; "A Few Words by an Old Patient"; UPCBR 73: no. 64,

UPCA. Nineteenth-century asylum superintendents frequently warned of the unreliability of descriptions of asylum life written by ex-patients who had never fully recovered from their illnesses. The general public, they admonished, should view these memoirs with the same skepticism accorded such patients' paranoic complaints against the family members and friends who had institutionalized them (N.Y.S. Lunatic Asylum, *Twenty-first AR* [1864]: 5; idem, *Twenty-sixth AR* [1869], 43; 1884 Investigation, 680–681, 1078–1079; E. H. Van Deusen, "Provision for the Care and Treatment of the Insane," 526–527). Ex-patients were aware of these criticisms and often included third-party testimonials to their respectability (Davis, *Two Years and Three Months*, frontispiece; Chase, *Two Years and Four Months*, 6–9, 183–184; Hotchkiss, *Five Months in the Asylum*, iii.) For a twentieth-century discussion of mental patients' perspective on institutionalization, see Raymond M. Weinstein, "The Mental Hospital from the Patient's Point of View." Weinstein suggests that patients' motives for seeking institutionalization strongly influence their views of the subsequent experience. Those who perceive the mental hospital as a refuge usually feel positively toward it. The same situation seemed to prevail at nineteenth-century Utica.

42. My discussion of Willard's therapeutic practices is slightly longer than that of Utica's because historians have paid relatively little attention to treatment programs for the chronically insane.

43. Cook, "Provision for the Insane Poor." Willard's supporters' arguments that the chronic poor needed only inexpensive custodial care were more successful with state legislators than they had intended. For example, when the superintendent later requested funds to acquire a library for those many patients who enjoyed reading, the legislature turned him down, finding it hard to imagine that chronically insane paupers might enjoy reading (Willard Asylum, *Tenth AR* [1879], 22). Also rejected were requests for funds to improve the grounds. The doctors argued that even the poor, intellectually disordered insane could appreciate the beautiful and had a right to minimal ornamentation of their "life abode" (Willard, *Sixth AR* [1875], 11).

44. Statistics on asylum budgets and patient work were an invariable part of the Utica and Willard annual reports. For Willard Superintendent John B. Chapin's views on the therapeutic value of labor, see Chapin, "Lunatic Asylum Reform," 754.

45. Chapin, "Report," 198–199; idem, "Lunatic Asylum Reform," 754. One of Willard's assistant physicians also argued that if one hemisphere of an insane patient's brain had become incapacitated, work and education programs might permit the other hemisphere to assume the functions of the diseased section of the brain (H. E. Allison, "The Moral and Industrial Management of the Insane," 289).

46. Cook, "Provision for the Insane Poor," 71–72.

47. Chapin, "On Provision," 29–31; idem, "Report," 193.

48. Willard Asylum, *Seventeenth AR* (1886), 39.

49. WPCBR 13: nos. 4406, 4651, WPCA.

50. See also Willard Asylum, *Thirteenth AR* (1882), 11; idem, *Sixteenth AR* (1885), 25; idem, *Seventeenth AR* (1886), 23; Allison, "Moral and Industrial Management," 293; N.Y.S. Commissioner in Lunacy, *First AR* (1874), 20–21; idem, *Sixth AR* (1879), 18.

51. 1880 Investigation, 550.

52. Willard Asylum, *Fourteenth AR* (1883), 26.
53. Willard Asylum, *Second AR* (1871), 28; "The Insane Kept at Work," *New York Daily Tribune,* March 20, 1882; "A Home for the Insane," ibid., December 23, 1882; "Care of the City Insane," ibid., August 19, 1883.
54. WPCBR 5: no. 2027, WPCA; see also ibid., nos. 1944, 2002, WPCA; WPCBR 13: nos. 4406, 4531, WPCA; WPCBR 1: no. 201, WPCA.
55. Willard Asylum, *Fifteenth AR* (1884), 15–16.
56. Willard Asylum, *Twentieth AR* (1889), 14–15; N.Y.S. Board of Charities, *Twenty-second AR* (1889), 12, 183; "Discussion of the Papers on Insanity," 109–110.
57. WPCBR 1: nos. 5, 196, WPCA.
58. N.Y.S. Board of Charities, *Twentieth AR* (1887), 144; Willard Asylum, *Fifteenth AR* (1884), 31; idem, *Sixth AR* (1875), 7; idem, *Fourteenth AR* (1883), 2.
59. Willard Asylum, *Seventeenth AR* (1886), 19.
60. 1880 Investigation, 60–61, 36.
61. For example, see Edward Jarvis, "Mechanical and Other Employments for Patients in the British Lunatic Asylums"; Willard Asylum, *Fourteenth AR* (1883), 28. In a review of Willard's *Twelfth AR,* an *AJI* editor noted that, while English asylums offered a greater number of "mechanical trades" programs, at admission their patients had more diversified skills than did Willard's ("Bibliographical").
62. N.Y.S. Commissioner in Lunacy, *Tenth AR* (1883), 156–168; Willard Asylum, *Sixteenth AR* (1885), 25.
63. For example, see "The Willard Asylum Act," 211; Willard Asylum, *Thirteenth AR* (1882), 48; Dewey, "Present and Prospective Management," 62–65.
64. N.Y.S. Commissioner in Lunacy, *Thirteenth AR* (1886), 50; Stephen Smith, "Compensation of Insane Labor, Suggestions in Reference to the Better Organization of a System of Labor for the Chronic Insane," 225.
65. Willard Asylum, *Twentieth AR* (1889), 21.
66. Willard Asylum, *Sixteenth AR* (1885), 20; idem, *Eighteenth AR* (1887), 18; idem, *Nineteenth AR* (1888), 22.
67. Willard Asylum, *Eighteenth AR* (1887), 13.
68. For example, see Seguin's testimony at the 1880 Investigation, 52.
69. Chapin, "Report," 106.
70. WPCBR 1: no. 111, WPCA; see also WPCBR 1: nos. 136, 196, WPCA.
71. Willard Clinical Recordbook 1: 27, WPCA.
72. Ibid.: 57, WPCA.
73. WPCBR 1: no. 26, WPCA.
74. WPCBR 1: no. 5, WPCA. See also WPCBR 5: no. 2027, WPCA, for an almost identical case.
75. Willard Asylum, *Seventeenth AR* (1886), 18, 21; idem, *Eighteenth AR* (1887), 13; idem, *Twenty-first AR* (1890), 15–16; N.Y.S. Commissioner in Lunacy, *Thirteenth AR* (1886), 21. John Walton describes a similar situation in the Lancaster (England) Asylum for the pauper insane, where, he argues, "The problem of chronic and congenital cases was probably less serious and more soluble than the problems associated with size, organization, and the tyranny of monotonous routines" (Walton, "Treatment of Pauper Lunatics," 190). I suspect that at Lancaster, as at Willard, the first exacerbated the second.

76. WPCBR 1: no. 161, WPCA. The first time he returned voluntarily, and the second time he was found in a nearby town by asylum attendants.

77. WPCBR 13: no. 4566, WPCA. See also ibid., nos. 1897, 1054, 1949, WPCA.

78. Willard Asylum, *Seventeenth AR* (1876), 12–13; Stephen Smith, "Care of the Filthy Insane."

79. Willard Asylum, *Nineteenth AR* (1888), 23.

80. N.Y.S. Board of Charities, *Eighteenth AR* (1885), 121; N.Y.S. Commissioner in Lunacy, *Eleventh AR* (1884), 271; idem, *Twelfth AR* (1885), 16–20.

81. WPCBR 5: no. 2115, WPCA.

82. S. Smith, "Care of the Filthy Insane," 149–150; N.Y.S. Commissioner in Lunacy, *Eleventh AR* (1884), 176.

83. Chapin listed the causes and numbers of deaths in every annual report. At Willard, and elsewhere, the most frequent cause of death was "exhaustion from chronic mental disease." As Jacques Quen notes, without more details historians cannot determine if such deaths were due to manic excitement, severe depression, anorexia nervosa, or organic brain disease (Jacques Quen, "Early Nineteenth Century Observations on the Insane in the Boston Almshouse," 81). Other common causes of death included old age, tuberculosis, epilepsy, paresis, and enteric fever (Willard Asylum, *Ninth AR* [1878], 35–37; idem, *Thirteenth AR* [1882], 28).

84. Letter to Dr. Russell from John Chapin, October 16, 1901, NYSLA; N.Y.S. Commissioner in Lunacy, *Tenth AR* (1883), 139. How often and for how long patients were kept in restraints before Chapin's reforms cannot be determined from individual casebooks, filled as they are with comments such as the following: "not worn restraints during the last year" (WPCBR 1, no. 61, WPCA). Frequent notes that some patients "never require restraints" suggests that others did (WPCBR 76: no. 86 for year, WPCA).

85. Willard Asylum, *Seventeenth AR* (1886), 11, 23; idem, *Eighteenth AR* (1887), 14–15; N.Y.S. Commissioner in Lunacy, *Fourteenth AR* (1887), 60; N.Y.S. Board of Charities, *Eighteenth AR* (1885), 49.

86. For descriptions of the moral treatments available at Willard, see the following annual reports: Willard Asylum, *Sixth AR* (1875), 11; idem, *Eighth AR* (1877), 27; idem, *Ninth AR* (1878), 32–33; idem, *Tenth AR* (1879), 22; idem, *Seventeenth AR* (1886), 23; idem, *Eighteenth AR* (1887), 19; idem, *Nineteenth AR* (1888), 22; idem, *Twenty-first AR* (1890), 23; idem, *Twenty-second AR* (1891), 24; N.Y.S. Commissioner in Lunacy, *Fourteenth AR* (1887), 173–174; Allison, "Moral and Industrial Management," 294–295. Willard's reintroduction of schools was a reform strongly supported by critics of John Gray. Somatic diseases do not require only somatic treatments, they argued; by reintroducing "healthy conceptions" to disordered minds, schools contribute to recoveries (James G. Kiernan, "School Training of the Insane").

87. For a description of the Willard school, see Willard Asylum, *Nineteenth AR* (1888), 22. In 1890, when Willard doctors treated 2,255 patients, a daily average of 33 students attended school during the winter and spring months (Willard Asylum, *Twenty-second AR* [1891], 24).

88. Willard Asylum, *Fourteenth AR* (1883), 26. See Chapter 1 for an extended description of Willard's parole policies. According to a visiting English doctor, few American asylums offered their patients much outdoor exercise (John

Charles Bucknill, "Notes on Asylums for the Insane in America," 26). See also "Report of Mr. Ross from the Committee Appointed by the Cayuga County Board of Supervisors, to Visit the Willard Asylum for the Insane," Auburn, November 30, 1886, in Willard Scrapbook No. 2: 47, WPCA.

89. Willard Asylum, *Fifth AR* (1874), 29.

90. Willard Asylum, *Tenth AR* (1879), 22; idem, *Sixth AR* (1875), 11.

91. N.Y.S. Board of Charities, *Eighteenth AR* (1885), 53. Similarly, while the so-called "detached cottages" were supposed to suggest a more homelike atmosphere than that offered by institutions which kept hundreds of patients in large central buildings, their fifty- to one hundred–patient capacity resembled few homes.

92. Willard Asylum, *Third AR* (1872), 39.

93. Willard Asylum, *Tenth AR* (1879), 22; idem, *Third AR* (1872), 39; idem, *Sixth AR* (1875), 11; idem, *Seventeenth AR* (1886), 23; idem, *Eighteenth AR* (1887), 18.

94. "Christmas at the Willard Asylum," *Independent*, January 1, 1889, in Willard Scrapbook No. 3, 86, WPCA; "Christmas at the Asylum," *Orange County Press*, December 28, 1888, in ibid.

95. WPCBR 1: nos. 16, 21, 45, 216, WPCA. When a twenty-five-year-old English woman was admitted in 1869, she seemed to respond well to moral treatment. By 1881, however, she was described as sitting quietly on the floor, except for an occasional shriek. By 1887 she had further deteriorated, sitting "stupidly about the hall" and drooling from the mouth (WPCBR 1: 66, WPCA).

96. J. A. L., "A Day at Willard," Palmyra *Democrat*, n.d. (c. 1887), in Willard Scrapbook No. 2, 126–127, WPCA.

97. "In the Willard Asylum," *Morning Telegram*, n.d. (c. September 1886), in Willard Scrapbook No. 2, 19, WPCA.

98. Allison, "Moral and Industrial Management of the Insane," 286.

99. WPCBR 1: no. 216, WPCA.

100. Two extant volumes of Willard's clinical recordbook, which focus on patients' physical problems, offer startlingly different descriptions of male and female health problems. The women's records focus almost exclusively on the findings of gynecologic examinations, although few treatments were prescribed for such common problems as irritated vulva and prolapsed uteri (Clinical Recordbook 8, WPCA). The male records are both lengthier and more diverse. They deal with problems ranging from epilepsy and paresis to physical injuries inflicted by other patients (such as an inflammation of the left hand caused by a human bite) and contagious infections like erysipelas (Clinical Recordbook 1, WPCA).

101. WPCBR 1: nos. 1, 16, 66, WPCA; WPCBR 5: nos. 1944, 1974, WPCA; WPCBR 13: no. 4506, WPCA; Willard Asylum, *Fifth AR* (1874), 24; idem, *Seventeenth AR* (1886), 19; idem, *Twenty-first AR* (1890), 17.

102. For example, see WPCBR 1: nos. 51, 56, WPCA; WPCBR 13: no. 4501, WPCA; WPCBR 5: no. 2057. New York's doctors were not unique in their concern to keep death rates low. See Barbara Rosenkrantz and Maris Vinovskis, "Sustaining 'The Flickering Flame of Life,'" 155–182.

103. WPCBR 1: no. 92, WPCA.

104. See Willard Asylum, *Third AR* (1872), 29; idem, *Thirteenth AR* (1882), 42.

105. Willard Asylum, *Third AR* (1872), 29; idem, *Fourth AR* (1873), 28; idem, *Fourteenth AR* (1883), 29; N.Y.S. Commissioner in Lunacy, *First AR* (1874), 32.

106. See "1880 Investigation," 52; "Proceedings of the AMSAII," *AJI* 47: 187.

107. For example, see WPCBR 1: nos. 1, 31, 106, WPCA; WPCBR 5: no. 1978, WPCA.

108. WPCBR 5: nos. 982, 1015, WPCA.

109. Eric T. Carlson and Maribeth M. Simpson, "Opium as a Tranquilizer," 114.

110. WPCBR 13: nos. 4556, WPCA. This patient was subsequently discharged improved and then returned a year later when neighbors complained that he refused to mind his mother.

111. Hurd, "The Minor Treatment of Insane Patients"; WPCBR 5: no. 1912, WPCA.

112. WPCBR 5: no. 1919, WPCA.

113. Vieda Skultans, *English Madness: Ideas on Insanity, 1580–1890*, 1.

114. WPCBR 13: no. 4611, WPCA.

115. WPCBR 5: no. 1992, WPCA.

116. Willard Clinical Recordbook 8, WPCA.

117. WPCBR 5: no. 1887, WPCA.

118. "The Insane Asylums of the States," *Peekskill Democrat*, November 5, 1887, in Willard Scrapbook No. 3, 1, WPCA.

119. Allison, "Moral and Industrial Management," 288–289.

120. Hurd, "A Plea for Systematic Therapeutical, Clinical and Statistical Study," 28. For the nineteenth-century debate about curability statistics and their meaning, see Pliny Earle, *The Curability of Insanity: A Series of Studies;* Isaaac Ray, "Recoveries from Mental Diseases"; "Review: Twenty-fifth Report of the State Lunatic Asylum at Northampton"; "Review: Annual Report of the State Lunatic Asylum, Northampton." For a wonderful satirization of the practice of relying on official recovery statistics to assess an asylum's success or failure, see Daniel Clark, "Wrinkles in Ancient Asylum Reports."

121. For Judge Lawrence's ruling that discharged lunatics must be absolutely harmless, see "Judge Lawrence on the Release of Lunatics." For a discussion of nineteenth-century discharge laws, see Horatio Pollock, "The Development and Extension of the Parole System in New York State," 53. See also "Rights of the Insane"; 1842 *Laws of New York*, chap. 135; 1865 *Laws of New York*, chap. 353. See Davis, *Two Years and Three Months*, 63–64; Hotchkiss, *Five Months in the Asylum*, 41–42; and "The Commitment and Detention of the Insane," 177. Doctors at both Utica and Willard campaigned for almost half a century for statutory approval of provisional releases, but nineteenth-century legislators were reluctant to grant their request.

122. N.Y.S. Lunatic Asylum, *Second AR* (1845), 16.

123. N.Y.S. Lunatic Asylum, *Ninth AR* (1852), 18. For evidence of the institution's century-long struggle with this problem, see idem, *Second AR* (1845), 16; idem, *Third AR* (1846), 22; idem, *Tenth AR* (1853), 13; idem, *Eleventh AR* (1854), 16; idem, *Fifteenth AR* (1858), 25; idem, *Seventeenth AR* (1860), 16; idem, *Fortieth AR* (1883), 52–69; 1884 Investigation, 1309–1310; N.Y.S. Commissioner

in Lunacy, *Thirteenth AR* (1886), 10–11. Patients were more cynical about the need to treat doctors politely and to dissemble in order to be released as cured. For example, see Davis, *Two Years and Three Months,* 63–64; Hotchkiss, *Five Months in the Asylum,* 41–42.

124. N.Y.S. Lunatic Asylum, *Eleventh AR* (1854), 16.

125. N.Y.S. Lunatic Asylum, *Fifteenth AR* (1858), 25–26.

126. Richard Hunter and Ida Macalpine, *Psychiatry for the Poor, 1851 Colney Hatch Asylum-Friern Hospital 1973: A Medical and Social History,* 178.

127. N.Y.S. Lunatic Asylum, *Second AR* (1845), 17; idem, *Forty-seventh AR* (1890), 45–46; idem, *Eighteenth AR* (1861), 18.

128. N.Y.S. Lunatic Asylum, *Eighteenth AR* (1861), 19; Brigham, "Insanity Illustrated by Cases, and by the Conversation and Manners of the Insane," 55. In one report, Gray argued that insanity's tendency to recur only proved its susceptibility to treatment (N.Y.S. Lunatic Asylum, *Twenty-first AR* [1864], 16). For readmission statistics, see idem, *Eighth AR* (1851), 25; idem, *Ninth AR* (1852), 17. The second report argued that only 206 of the 1,300 patients released as recovered during the preceding nine years had been readmitted. Of course, such calculations did not take into account ex-patients who may have ended up in other institutions, including jails and local poorhouses.

129. For comments which span the century on the need to find suitable homes for convalescent patients, see N.Y.S. Lunatic Asylum, *Second AR* (1845), 49; idem, *Sixteenth AR* (1859), 13; idem, *Forty-first AR* (1884), 33. For discussions of release circumstances, see UPCBR 46: no. 32 for the year, UPCA; Chase, *Two Years and Four Months,* 72–73; Lathrop, *The Secret Institution,* 203–204; 1880 Investigation, 282. For a discussion of discharge bonds, see N.Y.S. Lunatic Asylum, *Thirty-second AR* (1875), 14, 48; "Rights of the Insane," 422. For advice to ex-patients on how to preserve their newly regained health, see Brigham, *The Asylum Souvenir;* N.Y.S. Lunatic Asylum, *Seventeenth AR* (1860), 17–18; idem, *Twenty-fifth AR* (1869), 12–13; idem, *Thirty-sixth AR* (1879): 20. For one of John Gray's many scathing attacks on those who accused him of detaining recovered patients deliberately, see N.Y.S. Lunatic Asylum, *Fortieth AR* (1883), 12–14. For testimony about public fear of ex-patients who unexpectedly turned violent, see UPCBR 44: no. 404 for the year, UPCA; "The Unfortunate Woman," Utica *Observer,* January 24, 1889, UPCA; "Escaped Lunatic Arrested," Utica *Morning Herald,* May 14, 1882, UPCA; "Editorial," Utica *Press,* July 15, 1889, UPCA; "Practical Insanity: A Lecture"; N.Y.S. Lunatic Asylum, *Twenty-second AR* (1865), 7. The asylum's (and home communities') preference for releasing patients who looked economically self-sufficient may help explain the slightly more frequent discharge of men. In general, however, it is hard to interpret discharge and readmission data because many ex-asylum patients ended up in county almshouses and local jails rather than back in a state asylum.

130. N.Y.S. Lunatic Asylum, *Fourth AR* (1847), 18.

131. N.Y.S. Lunatic Asylum, *Seventh AR* (1850), 28; idem, *Eleventh AR* (1854), 9, 17; idem, *Fifteenth AR* (1858), 25; idem, *Sixteenth AR* (1859), 32; idem, *Twenty-fourth AR* (1867), 16–17; Board of Managers, 362, UPCA.

132. Board of Managers, 376, 391, UPCA; N.Y.S. Lunatic Asylum, *Thirty-second AR* (1875), 14.

133. N.Y.S. Lunatic Asylum, *Eighteenth AR* (1861), 18; idem, *Thirty-third AR* (1876), 14; "Persons Discharged from Asylums as Not Insane."

134.   Charles Pilgrim, "Report of a Case of Epileptic Insanity, with the 'Echo Sign' Well Marked," 411.

135.   N.Y.S. Lunatic Asylum, *Fourth AR* (1847), 18.

136.   Chase, *Two Years and Four Months*, 44, 116; Richardson, "Letter to G. Alder Blumer," 14, UPCA. For accounts of successful habeas corpus cases, see 1884 Investigation, 1004, 1996–1997; N.Y.S. Lunatic Asylum, *Fortieth AR* (1883), 11, 44, 55; idem, *Forty-first AR* (1884), 5, 53–55; idem, *Forty-second AR* (1885), 32–33; "Death of James B. Silkman," *New York Evening Post*, n.d. (c. 1888), in Willard Scrapbook No. 3: 20, WPCA; Board of Managers, 223–224, 254, UPCA. For New York asylum doctors' hostility to patients' use of the habeas corpus plea, see N.Y.S. Lunatic Asylum, *Thirtieth AR* (1873), 9–15; idem, *Thirty-third AR* (1876), 58; "The Writ of Habeas Corpus and Insane Asylums"; John B. Chapin, "Public Complaints against Asylums for the Insane and the Commitment of the Insane."

137.   N.Y.S. Lunatic Asylum, *Twenty-ninth AR* (1872), 19–20; idem, *Fortieth AR* (1883), 32–39. Too often twentieth-century critics of the discharge policies of nineteenth-century asylums assume that, because we now recognize the tendency of such institutions to turn into custodial warehouses, the medical staffs of the time also should have done so and, on those grounds, restricted their admission and liberalized their discharge policies.

138.   Willard Asylum, *Fifth AR* (1874), 27; idem, *Eleventh AR* (1880), 16; idem, *Fourteenth AR* (1883), 28; idem, *Fifteenth AR* (1884), 13; idem, *Eighteenth AR* (1887), 6, 14.

139.   WPCBR 13: no. 4416, WPCA. See also WPCBR 5: no. 4416, WPCA; WPCBR 1: nos. 221, 296, WPCA; N.Y.S. Commissioner in Lunacy, *Thirteenth AR* (1886), 27.

140.   WPCBR 13: no. 4597, WPCA. For an eloquent plea to doctors and attendants not to abandon their efforts to cure chronic patients, see J. A. Campbell, "On Three Cases of Recovery after a Lengthened Duration of Insanity, with Remarks."

141.   For accounts of the Willard medical staffs' therapeutic pessimism, see Willard Asylum, *Fourth AR* (1873), 5; idem, *Fifth AR* (1874), 28; idem, *Eighth AR* (1877), 29; idem, *Ninth AR* (1878), 32; idem, *Twelfth AR* (1881), 31; WPCBR 13: no. 4597, WPCA.

142.   For example, see UPCBR 16: no. 253 for the year, UPCA; UPCBR 26: no. 8834, UPCA. According to a twentieth-century official, nineteenth-century asylum superintendents also sometimes bypassed the official discharge process by paroling patients and then "forgetting" to recall them. In 1890 the Commission in Lunacy attempted to eliminate this legal loophole by restricting the kinds of patients eligible for parole and limiting parole periods to thirty days (Pollock, "The Parole System," 53–54).

143.   N.Y.S. Lunatic Asylum, *Twenty-sixth AR* (1869), 9; UPCBR 16: no. 115 for the year, UPCA.

144.   "Practical Insanity," 82; C. A. H., "A Token of Remembrance"; "Editor's Table" 7: 164.

145.   N.Y.S. Commissioner in Lunacy, *Eleventh AR* (1884), 356–357.

146.   Allison, "Moral and Industrial Management," 289–290.

147.   Willard Asylum, *Fourth AR* (1873), 29; idem, *Fifth AR* (1874), 24; idem, *Seventeenth AR* (1886), 19, 30; idem, *Nineteenth AR* (1888), 6.

148. For a contemporary discussion of this phenomenon, see Erving Goffman, *Relations in Public: Microstudies of the Public Order*, 335–357.
149. UPCBR 18: no. 285 for the year, UPCA; see also N.Y.S. Commissioner in Lunacy, *Tenth AR* (1883), 53.
150. Board of Managers, 102–104, UPCA.
151. Grob, *Mental Illness and American Society*, 179–200.
152. WPCBR 56: 113, WPCA.

6
Attendants and Their World of Work

1. Both published and unpublished sources contain many references to the asylum population as constituting a family and to the institution as a home. For examples, see N.Y.S. Lunatic Asylum, *Eighth AR* (1851), 44; idem, *Eighteenth AR* (1861), 31; idem, *Forty-first AR* (1884), 52; idem, *Forty-sixth AR* (1889), 45; 1884 Investigation, 1111, 1269; Willard Asylum, *Third AR* (1872), 31; idem, *Sixth AR* (1875), 13; N.Y.S. Board of Charities, *Eighteenth AR* (1885), 53. By and large, there have been few historical studies of asylum attendants or nurses. Three exceptions, all about the English experience, are Mick Carpenter, "Asylum Nursing before 1914: A Chapter in the History of Labour"; Alexander Walk, "The History of Mental Nursing"; and Digby, *Madness, Morality and Medicine*, 140–170. Recently Olga Moranjian Church completed a dissertation which looks at the nineteenth-century development of schools for asylum nurses (Church, "That Noble Reform: The Emergence of Psychiatric Nursing in the United States, 1882–1963").
2. 1884 Investigation, 1111–1112; N.Y.S. Commissioner in Lunacy, *First AR* (1874), 25. Such attitudes were not unique to New York State; see Ray, "Popular Feeling toward Hospitals for the Insane," 52–55, for a similar description of the characteristics needed by attendants.
3. Board of Managers, 17–26, 47–53, UPCA. For similar published statements of attendants' duties at Utica (which varied little over time), see N.Y.S. Lunatic Asylum, *Second AR* (1845), 45–46; idem, *Thirty-seventh AR* (1880), 10.
4. Board of Managers, 17–22, UPCA; Willard Asylum, *First AR* (1870), 48–57.
5. Willard Employee Recordbook, 8, 35, WPCA. The Willard Employee Recordbook consists of brief entries on all members of the nonprofessional staff hired between 1869 and 1890. Although the specific details collected on individuals vary over time, the records offer unusually rich information about the conditions of work and job mobility for nineteenth-century insane asylum attendants. In 1883 ninety-two attendants left Willard, of whom twenty had been fired. Four of these lost their jobs because of patient abuse, but a more frequent reason for discharge was "inherent vice and depravity," which usually meant alcoholism (Willard Asylum, *Fifteenth AR* [1884], 15). Several attendants were fired for leaving their assigned work places without permission (Willard Employee Recordbook, 47, 51, 84, 95, 109) or for negligence, especially for allowing patients to escape (ibid., 36, 58, 75, 89, 112, 122, 130, 145). A female with four-and-one-half

years' service was discharged for allowing a drunken attendant to remain in her room for "some time" and then failing to report the incident (ibid., 124).

6. For the brain/hands quote, see "Minutes and Discussion," 442; for Gray's comments, see 1884 Investigation, 1109–1110. Similar sentiments can be found in N.Y.S. Commissioner in Lunacy, *Eleventh AR* (1884), 366. Gray's attitude was shared by many of his fellow superintendents. For example, at an AMSAII annual meeting, the head of the Illinois state insane asylum noted that total obedience to superiors was an essential quality for attendants. "What might be servility in other departments of hired service," he added, "is only a just and proper requirement in an employment so responsible as this." Obedience needs to be as prompt as in military service ("Proceedings of the Fifteenth Annual Meeting of the AMSAII, 56).

7. 1884 Investigation, 451; N.Y.S. Board of Charities, *Twenty-third AR* (1890), 160.

8. N.Y.S. Commissioner in Lunacy, *Second AR* (1875), 25; Willard Asylum, *Seventeenth AR* (1886), 21; N.Y.S. Board of Charities, *Twenty-second AR* (1889) 186; idem, *Eighteenth AR* (1885), 121.

9. N.Y.S. Commissioner in Lunacy, *Eleventh AR* (1884), 176; Willard Asylum, *Third AR* (1872), 40; idem, *Nineteenth AR* (1888), 23; N.Y.S. Lunatic Asylum, *Forty-seventh AR* (1890), 60–61.

10. For Chapin's discussion of the need for a hall, see Willard Asylum, *Twelfth AR* (1881), 12. For programs from Willard entertainments, see Willard Scrapbook No. 2, 141–149, WPCA; Willard Scrapbook No. 3: 133–151, WPCA.

11. For example, in a two-year period beginning in August 1888, a dozen entries were made in Willard's Employee Recordbook, WPCA, regarding new employees' musical skills. These included "no musical abilities" (141), "plays violin some" (146), "plays flute" (131), and "plays violin and sings" (146). See also ibid., 106, 114, 116, 117, 124, 128, 140, 144. At the London (Ontario) Asylum for the Insane during this period, all job applicants for attendants' jobs also were asked if they played musical instruments. Because music was considered a vital part of moral therapy, those who did not were not hired (Krasnick, "'In Charge of the Loons,'" 166).

12. Willard Scrapbook No. 3, 146, WPCA.

13. Willard Asylum, *Twenty-first AR* (1890), 11. According to a newspaper report, when in 1887 Governor Hill vetoed a bill prohibiting the sale of alcohol within fifteen miles of the Willard Asylum, the Willard superintendent was very displeased. Wise had written the legislature that, since liquor licenses had been permitted near the asylum, the number of staff members discharged for intemperance had increased greatly ("The Willard Asylum Bill," *Seneca County Courier* [April 14, 1887], in Willard Scrapbook No. 2, 79, WPCA).

14. See Willard Employee Recordbook, 103, 116, 122, WPCA, for the three ward attendants' cases. For the history of the attendant who left her hall, see ibid., 87, and ibid., 59.

15. In 1886 a kitchen worker with six years' service led a strike against doing extra work; after evincing "evidence of repentance," she was allowed to remain as an attendant at a five-dollar reduction in her monthly pay (Willard Employee Recordbook, 31, WPCA). For other firings, see ibid., 43, 78, 84, 100, 137, 154.

16. 1884 Investigation, 442–443, 490, 552, 585, 671–673, 692. No comparable direct testimony exists for Willard's hiring practices. In theory, selection was based on four factors: personal fitness, morality, good habits, and a willingness to subscribe (in writing) to the institution's rules and regulations (Willard Asylum, *Tenth AR* [1879], 22). Yet, the perfunctoriness of the steward's notes about new employees in his Employee Recordbook suggests that youthfulness, good health, and an "honest appearance" usually sufficed.

17. N.Y.S. Lunatic Asylum, *Forty-first AR* (1884), 26–27. See also 1884 Investigation, 1099–1108, and N.Y.S. Lunatic Asylum, *Forty-second AR* (1885): 21. For the application of the 1883 civil service regulations by Willard, see Wise, "To Applicants for Positions in the Willard Asylum for the Insane," in Willard Scrapbook No. 3, 103, WPCA.

18. 1884 Investigation, 7–9. In an effort to pacify critics, in 1884 the Utica board of managers appointed a subcommittee of its members to investigate hiring practices. Subsequent board minutes suggest that the subcommittee never met, mute testimony to the board's indifference to hiring procedures (1884 Investigation, 552; Board of Managers, 1885–1890, UPCA).

19. For discussions of the phenomenon of "asylum tramps" whose incompetence plagued superintendents for the entire nineteenth century, see letter to Dorothea Dix from Nathan Benedict, May 11, 185?, Dix Papers, HLHU; letter to Edward Jarvis from John Gray, November 10, 1862, CLMHMS; "Proceedings of the Association of Medical Superintendents," *AJI* 45: 146.

20. Letter to Thomas Kirkbride from John Gray, August 16, 1859, Kirkbride Papers, PHMA. Only 8 percent of those hired at Willard between 1869 and 1890 left because of poor health. Even fewer of Utica's attendants left because of health-related problems (2 percent of those between 1867 and 1882). Of course, most attendants were young men and women in their twenties (N.Y.S. Commissioner in Lunacy, *Eleventh AR* [1884], 364). For comments on physical size of new female employees, see Willard Employee Recordbook, 76, 77, 94, 105, 113, 119, 121, WPCA.

21. For a discussion of domestic servants' ethnicity, see David Katzman, *Seven Days a Week: Women and Domestic Service in Industrializing America*, 304. That the Utica Asylum was willing to hire attendants who could speak only Welsh came to light during a legal investigation into the mysterious death of a patient, Thaddeus Leonard. When one key attendant appeared to testify, he had to speak through an interpreter ("Who Was to Blame?" Utica *Daily Observer* [April 19, 1889], in Willard Scrapbook No. 3, 116, WPCA). Reference to Willard's Danish-speaking painter/attendant can be found in the Willard Employee Recordbook, 111, WPCA. Although the absolute number of Irish attendants at Willard increased in the mid-1880s, only 38 percent of those hired at Willard between 1886 and 1890 were foreign born. Of the female attendants, most were young women from the neighboring towns (N.Y.S. Commissioner in Lunacy, *Tenth AR* [1883], 84). Utica's patients, in particular, often expressed resentment at having to deal with uncouth, foreign-born attendants, a phenomenon discussed in Chapter 1. Patients' disdain for attendants whom they considered inferior to them was effectively expressed in a patient mural which portrayed attendants as monkeys. Although the attending physician reported this incident with much amusement, it is unlikely he would have shown the same equanimity if the medical staff had been

so portrayed (N.Y.S. Commissioner in Lunacy, *Fifteenth AR* [1888]: 37). Several nineteenth-century asylum superintendents blamed poor care on the increasing number of foreign-born employees "mixed up with our own people," but Gray felt that attendants' ethnicity did not affect the quality of their work ("Proceedings of the Association of Medical Superintendents," *AJI* 28: 323). Twentieth-century American historians have paid relatively little attention to the sociodemographic characteristics of asylum attendants. An exception is Nancy Tomes, who describes the Pennsylvania Hospital attendants as young and often Irish men and women, many of whom had had previous asylum work experience. Here, too, women tended to work longer than men, although both generally considered their attendants' positions short-term work rather than lifetime careers (Tomes, *A Generous Confidence*, 179–181).

22. N.Y.S. Lunatic Asylum, *Twenty-first AR* (1864), 55; Katzman, *Seven Days a Week*, 139; N.Y.S. Lunatic Asylum, *Fortieth AR* (1883), 95; Chase, *Two Years and Four Months*, 69; 1884 Investigation, 1101, 1110–1112. For a discussion of how local economic conditions affected attendants' quality at a nineteenth-century English asylum, see Walton, "Treatment of Pauper Lunatics," 180–181.

23. Willard Asylum, *Ninth AR* (1878), 38; 1880 Investigation, 566–567; N.Y.S. Commissioner in Lunacy, *First AR* (1874), 26. In 1889 turnover greatly increased at Willard when attendants were allowed to leave without notice during a one- to four-month trial period. Once permanently engaged, they had to stay a year and after that give thirty days' notice (Willard Scrapbook No. 3, 103, WPCA). Willard's greater ease in attracting and retaining attendants contradicted the *AJI* argument that only big cities offered the diversions and "frequent contact with healthy minds" needed by attendants ("An Asylum for the Insane Should Be Near a Large City").

24. N.Y.S. Commissioner in Lunacy, *Tenth AR* (1883), 176; Letter to the Commissioners of Public Charities from Lewis Prudden, January 9, 1868, N.Y.S. Board of Charities Correspondence, NYSLA; Katzman, *Seven Days a Week*, 146–183. Concerning Mary Ryan's career, see the Willard Employee Recordbook, 27, WPCA. For a rare firsthand account by an early twentieth-century attendant at several Indiana state hospitals, see Carrie E. Lively, "Reminiscences of a State Mental Hospital Attendant." Lively describes the great variations in working conditions from ward to ward, as well as the employment opportunities for women at state mental hospitals. Obviously, domestics' and attendants' work was not perfectly comparable, but their similarities were well recognized in the nineteenth century. According to one reformer, most attendants were unmarried young men and women looking for an alternative to manual labor or "more menial" household employment. As a result, they often defined their work solely in terms of the provision of material needs, ignoring its psychological (or "moral") dimensions (Dewey, "Present and Prospective Management," 86).

25. For instance, in the 1880s the steward demoted a conscientious and hard-working laundry supervisor because he "lacked certain qualities which have been considered quite important for a head laundry man to have" (Willard Employee Recordbook, 53, WPCA; see also ibid., 22, 49, 69). The Willard Employee Recordbook offers much evidence of the tendency to promote from within. For a discussion of Utica's similar policy, see *Forty-fifth AR* (1888), 55–56.

26. Some husband-and-wife teams were hired together, while others mar-

ried after joining the Willard work force (Willard Employee Recordbook, 128, 142, WPCA). The recordbook offers several examples of women rehired after leaving to have children (for example, ibid., 30, 55). A particuarly coveted position for women was that of matron. Willard's first matron, Sarah Bell, came from New York City, where she had held a similar position at the New York Hospital. Bell was an energetic, self-confident widow who, in her letter of application, assured Chapin, "If it is a post a woman can fill—why should I fail to fill the position with credit to myself" (letter to John C. Chapin from Mrs. Sarah H. Bell, May 19, 1869, WPCA). One of Willard's trustees who interviewed Bell in New York reported, "Her appearance and manners are pleasing and those of a lady—she seems to possess a good deal of force and decision" (letter to John Chapin from C. C. Wells, May 18, 1869, WPCA). Bell served for several years. After resigning, she was replaced with a more typical matron: the steward's wife.

27.   Willard Asylum, *Fifteenth AR* (1884), 15.

28.   Since the steward did not consistently record salaries, a complete statistical analysis of Willard's salary structure is impossible. The examples given of entry-level salaries in the 1880s, however, offer overwhelming evidence of sex-based wage differentials.

29.   The first discussion of attendants' wages in the Utica board of managers' minutes did not appear until March 7, 1866, some twenty-three years after the asylum had opened, although the managers frequently discussed the need to raise the wages of the medical and skilled labor staffs (Board of Managers, 136, UPCA). The second discussion took place almost twenty years later, when the board referred to its auditing committee the written request of thirty-seven attendants for higher wages but took no further action (ibid., 231). For information about threatened strikes, see N.Y.S. Lunatic Asylum, *Twenty-first AR* (1864): 55; idem, *Twenty-second AR* (1865), 27.

30.   These reforms were mentioned in several annual reports before they were finally implemented. See N.Y.S. Lunatic Asylum, *Forty-fifth AR* (1888), 56; idem, *Forty-sixth AR* (1889), 22; 1880 Investigation, 457; 1884 Investigation, 796; Willard Asylum, *Twenty-first AR* (1890): 22.

31.   See N.Y.S. Lunatic Asylum, *Forty-third AR* (1886): 53–54; idem, *Forty-fifth AR* (1888), 53–54; idem, *Forty-seventh AR* (1890), 60; Board of Managers, 328, UPCA.

32.   1884 Investigation, 15, 687. For another comment on the difficulty of selecting good attendants, see "Apropos of Recent Insane Asylum Investigations." For criticism of Gray's farm purchases, see 1884 Investigation, 15.

33.   When the Utica Asylum was still relatively small, Amariah Brigham tried to make the asylum not just a place of work but the home and principal focus of life for his employees. He claimed that the level of entertainment available at the institution was so high that most of its workers had little desire to seek relaxation elsewhere. Several particularly devoted attendants, refusing to take even their allotted free hours, did not leave the asylum for four to five months at a time. He clearly did not consider that his attendants might benefit from a break in their demanding work routines. A medical journal article expressed the condescension implicit in many late nineteenth-century reformers' attitudes toward attendants. "The more ignorant an attendant is," the editor proclaimed, "the more self-conceited and opinionated he is likely to be regarding how to control the . . . insane" ("Apropos of Recent Asylum Investigations," 491–492). On the other hand,

asylum administrators themselves recognized the tensions involved in the daily care of insane patients. According to an *AJI* editorial, "Irritability and ennui are the natural effects of constant association with the insane and the thousand petty annoyances which beset and the wearisome duties which devolve upon such attendance" ("An Asylum for the Insane Should be Near a Large City"). W. W. Godding noted that, although families brought members to mental hospitals because they could no longer bear the strain of their care, they unrealistically expected attendants "never to grow weary, nor to bear the oath or the obscene word" ("Reports of American Asylums," *AJI* 30: 364). See also the recent literature on family violence, including Murray A. Straus, Richard J. Gelles, and Suzanne K. Steinmetz, *Behind Closed Doors: Violence in the American Family;* Ruth S. Kempe and Henry C. Kempe, *Child Abuse.*

34. 1884 Investigation, 261, 280, 796; Isaac Ray, "Popular Feeling towards Hospitals for the Insane," 40; "Review of the *Tenth Annual Report of the New York State Commissioner in Lunacy, for the Year 1882,*" 496–497; "Proceedings of the Association," *AJI* 43: 165. For comments on the mechanical and perfunctory fashion in which attendants often performed their duties, see N.Y.S. Commissioner in Lunacy, *Fourth AR* (1877), 43–44.

35. Willard Employee Recordbook, 19, 117, 132, WPCA; Willard Asylum, *Seventh AR* (1876), 26; idem. *Eighth AR* (1877), 27; idem, *Eleventh AR* (1886), 34; idem, *Twelfth AR* (1881), 11. Even harsher was the editor of the *Alienist and Neurologist,* who advocated that abusive attendants be sent to state penitentiaries ("How the Jealous Public Protect the Insane," 329). In contrast, at Utica one matron never investigated the frequent patient charges about attendant Ann Burns. She also claimed to have no idea if the male night watch had passkeys to the female wards (1884 Investigation, 671–672). Patients frequently complained that superintendents always accepted attendants' stories rather than patients' (Chase, *Two Years and Four Months,* 43). For a formal warning to attendants to control their tempers when assaulted, see N.Y.S. Commissioner in Lunacy, *Third AR* (1876), 53. At both Willard and Utica, the number of employees actually fired was relatively small. For example, 127 (or 15.9 percent) of Willard's 798 employees during this period were fired. The largest group (31.5 percent) of those who did not stay were described as having "left on their own accord" or because their agreed-upon term of service was over. Some of these included attendants who had been demoted for disciplinary reasons. Comparable statistics do not exist for Utica, but in his 1883 report to the commission in lunacy, Gray noted that, of the 287 attendants employed during the past fifteen years, most had left with good records, having completed their terms of service or gained permission to take other jobs. Of the 89 who left in unfavorable circumstances (some of whom were not actually fired), the reasons included the following: 24 for staying out at night or leaving their wards without permission; 20 for "non-adaptability to service"; 19 for inefficiency or negligence; 9 for patient abuse; 4 for lying; 3 for intoxication; 3 for profanity and rough speech; 3 for immorality while away from the asylum; 2 for wearing patients' clothing; and 2 for quarreling with other attendants (N.Y.S. Commissioner in Lunacy, *Eleventh AR* [1884], 369).

36. N.Y.S. Commissioner in Lunacy, *Eleventh AR* (1884), 368; 1884 Investigation, 7⁺8; N.Y.S. *Fifth AR* (1848), 45. For a similar comparison of attendants' work with service, see N.Y.S. Commissioner in Lunacy, *First AR* (1874), 26.

37. N.Y.S. Commissioner in Lunacy, *Tenth AR* (1883), 157–158; N.Y.S.

Board of Charities, *Eighteenth AR* (1885), 21. Even a male attendant who dealt only with quiet patients noted that, if patients "gave some slang back" when asked to sit down, attendants would kick their feet out from under them (1884 Investigation, 586). A good argument for attendant training schools was offered by a female attendant at the New York City Ward's Island Asylum. She claimed that, as a rule, attendants were not willfully neglectful, but they had never been taught how to treat the insane. They quickly became so accustomed to patient violence that they did not even try to quiet patients, and few realized that to protect patients from outbursts of excitement and violence was part of their duty (1880 Investigation, 87).

38. "Proceedings of the Association of Medical Superintendents," *AJI* 47: 228–229.

39. N.Y.S. Lunatic Asylum, *Forty-sixth AR* (1889): 56; idem, *Forty-first AR* (1884), 56; "Quarterly Summary: New Jersey."

40. Willard Asylum, *Nineteenth AR* (1888), 24–25; idem, *Twenty-first AR* (1890), 22. For newspaper accounts of graduations, see "The Willard Training School," in Willard Scrapbook No. 3, 82, WPCA; "Willard Asylum for the Insane: The Graduation of a Class of Trained Nurses," *Union and Advertiser,* December 12, 1888, in Willard Scrapbook No. 3, 82, WPCA; "Commencement Exercises at the Willard State Hospital Training School for Nurses and Attendants," Ovid *Independent,* May 12, 1891, in Willard Scrapbook No. 4, 137–138, WPCA. The last listed the names of the graduating class: ten of the twelve had Irish surnames. For references to Utica's erratic training efforts in the 1880s, see N.Y.S. Lunatic Asylum, *Forty-first AR* (1884), 56–57; idem, *Forty-sixth AR* (1889), 56; N.Y.S. Commissioner in Lunacy, *Eleventh AR* (1884), 178. For a description of the first such school in New York, see "The Commencement Exercises of the Training School for Attendants at the Buffalo Asylum." This article published sample examination questions and examples of student essays. The physician in charge at Buffalo also wrote an attendants' manual for use in training classes. It offered three chapters of somewhat diluted medical theorizing about insanity (e.g., "The Nervous System and Some of Its More Important Functions") plus seven chapters on patient care ("Review"). Training schools for psychiatric nurses in the United States were started about a decade after those for general nurses (Elvin H. Santos and Edward Stainbrook, "A History of Psychiatric Nursing in the Nineteenth Century").

41. Willard Asylum, *Twenty-second AR* (1891), 24. At the 1890 AMSAII meeting, Wise expressed similar sentiments. Nurses must understand, he declaimed, that their duties were to observe and record facts and nothing else; interpretation was medical staff's prerogative (*Proceedings of the American Medico-Psychological Association, at the Fifty-First Annual Meeting Held in Denver, June 11–13, 1895,* 90). A more pragmatic rationale for limiting attendants' education was offered by Richard Dewey of the Kankakee (Illinois) Asylum. Dewey argued that insane asylums should hire trained nurses to care for the physically ill inmates instead of trying to turn attendants into nurses. Attendants needed a specialized training, which included instruction in ward housework. Because most attendants had poor educational backgrounds, their instruction had to be "of the most direct, plain, and simple character" (Richard Dewey, "Training Schools for Attendants in Asylums for the Insane.").

42. A. Campbell Clark, "The Special Training of Asylum Attendants."

43. N.Y.S. Lunatic Asylum, *Twenty-fifth AR* (1868), 61. Gray himself did little to improve attendants' status beyond offering them formulaic thanks for their assistance at the end of his annual reports.

44. WPCBR 5: no. 1909, WPCA; N.Y.S. Lunatic Asylum, *Thirty-seventh AR* (1880), 10.

45. 1884 Investigation, 504, 516, 658, 663, 666, 1505. By the late nineteenth century, Utica's supervisors tried to discourage reports from their staff about patient mistreatment. They then pleaded ignorance when abuse charges were brought. For example, at the 1884 investigation, Utica's matron testified that she seldom looked into patients' complaints about attendants (1884 Investigation, 674–675). Thomas J. Scheff notes that attendants, by withholding information about patients from doctors, gain at least partial control of ward policies (Scheff, "Control over Policy by Attendants in a Mental Hospital," 94–95).

46. N.Y.S. Commissioner in Lunacy, *Ninth AR* (1882), 12–46.

47. 1884 Investigation, 653–662.

48. Chase, *Two Years and Four Months*, 135.

49. Ibid., 72–73; 1884 Investigation, 410–411; Davis, *Two Years and Three Months*, 49, 67.

50. Goffman, *Interaction Ritual*, 78–81. For the use of female physicians to oversee bathing, see N.Y.S. Board of Charities, *Twenty-second AR* (1889), 207. Injuries to patients during bathing happened at many asylums. For example, see John C. Bucknill and Daniel H. Tuke, *A Manual of Psychological Medicine: Containing the History, Nosology, Description, Statistics, Diagnosis, Pathology, and Treatment of Insanity*, 477–481; "Asylum Mismanagement," New York *Medical Journal*, December 1883, 608. One Utica patient advised his fellows to grow beards to avoid being shaved by attendants, which he characterized as "skinning" because of the dullness of the razors (Chase, *Two Years and Four Months*, 78–79).

51. UPCBR 15: no. 145 for the year, UPCA; 1884 Investigation, 720.

52. N.Y.S. Lunatic Asylum, *Forty-fifth AR* (1888), 55; letter to William Russell from John C. Chapin, November 16, 1901, NYSLA; N.Y.S. Lunatic Asylum, *Thirtieth AR* (1873), 29; Willard Asylum, *Third AR* (1872), 29; idem, *Eleventh AR* (1880), 13. Ex-patients, too, praised individual attendants for their kindness and humanity, although they tended to regard them as atypical. See 1884 Investigation, 417, 429–430; Lathrop, *Secret Institution*, 166–182. For other defenses of attendants, see Willard Asylum, *Eighth AR* (1877), 25–26; N.Y.S. Lunatic Asylum, *Twenty-fifth AR* (1867), 61; idem, *Thirty-seventh AR* (1880), 47; idem, *Fortieth AR* (1883), 95; 1884 Investigation, 1106–1107. In more than one situation, attendants and other unskilled asylum workers demonstrated the closeness of their ties with patients and helped them evade institutional restrictions. For example, at Utica, a female drug addict obtained illicit laudanum first from an ironing girl, and then from a dining room girl (UPCBR 6: no. 292 for the year, UPCA).

53. N.Y.S. Lunatic Asylum, *Second AR* (1845): 51; idem, *Tenth AR* (1853), 22; idem, *Thirty-seventh AR* (1880), 47; idem, *Twenty-fifth AR* (1868), 61; 1884 Investigation, 1106–1107; Willard Asylum, *Eighth AR* (1877), 25–26; idem, *Eleventh AR* (1880), 13.

54. Isaac Ray described the temptation to abuse as an inevitable part of the attendant's "almost unlimited authority over those under his control" (Ray, "Ameri-

can Hospitals for the Insane," 54). For a similar description of asylum attendants' tendency to treat undemanding patients well and more difficult ones harshly, see Russell Hollander, "Life at the Washington Asylum for the Insane, 1871–1880," 239–240.

55.   For examples of the use of military and industrial metaphors, see N.Y.S. Lunatic Asylum, *Forty-third AR* (1886), 54; idem, *Forty-sixth AR* (1889), 49; idem, *Forty-seventh AR* (1890), 60; N.Y.S. Board of Charities, *Twenty-second AR* (1889), 53. Many of Donald Cressey's observations about prison guards apply to asylum attendants: "They do not use inmates productively any more than they themselves are used productively by prison managers. Guards manage, and are managed, in organizations where management is an end, not a means" (Cressey, "Prison Organization," 1024). That asylum attendants often were described as guards in late nineteenth-century asylum literature suggests the frequency with which their therapeutic role was subordinated to a custodial one. The result was not surprising: a further decline in the quality of the attendant–patient relationship. As the commissioner in lunacy noted, to preserve order and discipline in wards, attendants frequently had to act in ways considered arbitrary and oppressive by patients. To ease this conflict, he suggested a further specialization of duties, so that some attendants would serve only as companions, while others would keep the wards clean and orderly (N.Y.S. Commissioner in Lunacy, *Tenth AR* [1883], 176). Brigham had thus used teachers many years before, but Gray felt that the establishment of two distinct classes of attendants would demoralize those assigned only menial work ("Review of Tenth Annual Report of the N.Y.S. Commissioner in Lunacy").

56.   Much of the drive to persuade attendants to wear uniforms reflected doctors' desires to "follow the habits of general hospitals" (N.Y.S. Lunatic Asylum, *Forty-third AR* [1886], 53; see also idem, *Forty-fifth AR* [1888], 53–54). For an account of how the English psychiatric establishment finally recognized that its staff no longer accepted "the fiction of the common line of interest between Doctors and Attendants," see Francis R. Adams, "From Association to Union: Professional Organization of Asylum Attendants, 1869–1919." For the situation of nurses in general hospitals, see Susan Reverby, "The Search for the Hospital Yardstick: Nursing and the Rationalization of Hospital Work." The failure of these efforts to give attendants the status of regular nurses is described by Carpenter in "Asylum Nursing before 1915."

57.   Many of these nineteenth-century problems have not been solved by the twentieth-century psychiatric establishment (Pearl Yaruss Adelson, "The Back Ward Dilemma"). In many contemporary hospitals, attendants are still expected to meet nineteenth-century ideals: "to possess a combination of virtues which, in the ordinary walks of life, would render their possessor one of the shining ornaments of the race" (Ray, "Popular Feeling," 53).

7
The Politics of Maintenance

1.   *New York Times*, September 19, 1869.
2.   Schneider and Deutsch, *History of Public Welfare*, chap. 6.

3. Ibid.

4. 1869 Senate *Documents,* no. 80; 1882 *Governor's Messages,* no. 2; 1873 Senate *Documents,* no. 40; 1880 Investigation; 1884 Investigation.

5. For numerous newspaper clippings which detail this battle, see Willard Scrapbook No. 4, WPCA.

6. 1890 *Laws of New York,* chap. 273.

7. 1867 *Laws of New York,* 951; Schneider and Deutsch, *History of Public Welfare,* 13–33; Paul Hoch, "History of the Department of Mental Hygiene," 3.

8. Grob, "Political System and Social Policy," 13. See also William R. Brock, *Investigation and Responsibility: Public Responsibility in the United States, 1865–1900.*

9. Pitts, "The AMSAII," 116–117.

10. N.Y.S. Board of Charities, *Fifth AR* (1872), 5; idem, *Sixth AR* (1873), 76–77, 96; Schneider and Deutsch, *History of Public Welfare,* 19. As Chapter 2 notes, this approach to problem solving had time-honored historical roots in New York State, although Hoyt's was by far the most ambitious survey undertaken. By the 1864 *Laws of New York,* chap. 418, the State Medical Society had been authorized to investigate the condition of the insane in local facilities, but their efforts had been impeded by the Civil War. In 1874–1875 Hoyt conducted a similar but even more probing examination of paupers in New York State. As Michael Katz points out, this survey was so structured as to support charity reformers' arguments that most paupers were personally responsible for their condition (Katz, *Poverty and Policy,* 92–93). Perhaps because of the frequency with which John Gray and his friends argued that most insane people had been hard-working, productive citizens before their affliction had made them paupers, Hoyt did not accuse the insane of causing their own financial ruin.

11. See N.Y.S. Board of Public Charities, *Annual Reports,* 1–24, for repeated statements of this theme.

12. For differing interpretations of the close cooperation of the two groups, see Schneider and Deutsch, *The History of Public Welfare,* 20–21; Katz, *Poverty and Policy,* 188–189. Their conflicts, which mainly involved issues of internal authority and of reform style (the Charities Aid Association being the more radical) rather than of basic social welfare policies are noted in the *Address from the State Charities Aid Association to Its Local Visiting Committee throughout the State of New York, July 1886.*

13. Pitts, "The AMSAII," 119. Typical of the post–Civil War exposés of asylum care were the following *New York Times* series: "A Horrible Tragedy," September 15, 1872; "The Ward's Island Inquiry," September 19, 1872; "Cruelty on Ward's Island," October 31, 1872; "Ward's Island," November 3, 1872; "Ward's Island Horrors," November 8, 1872; "The Ward's Island Lunatic Asylum Homicide," December 25, 1872.

14. Lee, "Medico-Legal Suggestions," 467.

15. 1873 *Laws of New York,* chap. 571, sec. 14.

16. David B. Wexler, "The Structure of Civil Commitment: Patterns, Pressures and Interactions in Mental Health Legislation," 3.

17. Gabriel Kolko has suggested that early twentieth-century regulatory agencies were easily manipulated by the groups they oversaw (Kolko, *The Triumph of the Conservatives: A Re-interpretation of American History, 1900–1916*). Initially, New York politicians clearly were uncertain what sort of creature

they had created with this new position of commissioner in lunacy. According to Ordronaux, right after his appointment, he visited the governor to ask about his responsibilities. The governor responded that he did not know the scope of the office because it was a "new jurisdiction which seemed to hardly have a foothold in any proper field as yet" (1882 Senate *Documents*, no. 96, 437).

18.   D. J. Mellett, "Bureaucracy and Mental Illness: The Commissioners in Lunacy, 1845–1890."

19.   Hurd, *Institutional Care* 4: 467–469.

20.   1874 Senate *Documents*, no. 86; 1874 *Laws of New York*, chap. 446.

21.   Mellett, "Bureaucracy and Mental Illness," 245.

22.   "Rights of the Insane," 429.

23.   See Andrews's testimony during the "Discussion on Provisions for the Insane," 389.

24.   For criticism of the jury trial notion, see "Rights of the Insane," 415; "The Commitment and Detention of the Insane," 177; N.Y.S. Commissioner in Lunacy, *Twelfth AR* (1885), 20–21; and L.A.T., "Lunacy Legislation," Utica *Daily Press*, February 9, 1889, Willard Scrapbook No. 3, WPCA.

25.   Pitts, "The AMSAII," 119.

26.   M. B. Anderson and J. C. Devereux, *Extract from the Sixth Annual Report of the State Board of Charities of the State of New York, Relating to Hospitals for the Sick and Insane, to Which Is Appended a Report Relating to the Management of the Insane in Great Britain by H. B. Wilbur, M.D.*; H. B. Wilbur, "Governmental Supervision of the Insane," 72–81; idem, "Buildings for the Management and Treatment of the Insane," 134–158.

27.   Several historians have chronicled this debate, including Bonnie J. Blustein, "Hollow Square"; Grob, *Mental Illness and Society*, 46–107; David J. Rothman, *Conscience and Convenience: The Asylum and Its Alternatives in Progressive America*, 290–302; and Barbara Sicherman, *The Quest for Mental Health in America, 1880–1917*, 12–77.

28.   1869 Senate *Documents*, no. 80 (hereafter referred to as 1869 Investigation).

29.   1873 Senate *Documents*, no. 40 (hereafter referred to as 1873 Investigation); 1873 *Laws of New York*, chap. 571. Even before neurologists and the State Board of Charities began to campaign for a commissioner in lunacy, local and state medical societies lobbied for the appointment of a doctor to investigate the condition of the insane in poorhouses and jails (Lincoln, *Messages* 5: 447). Ironically, the State Board of Charities in 1873 had opposed a bill proposed by the Medico-Legal Society to appoint a five-person lunacy commission ("The Proposed Law Submitted by the Committee of the Medico-Legal Society to the Legislature of the State of New York, Session of 1873," 128–133). In its place, they substituted one calling for the appointment of a single commissioner in lunacy to be selected by them and subject to their direction. When Ordronaux succeeded in gaining independence of the board in 1874, one of its members commented angrily that, instead of "abolishing" the board and giving its duties to a single officer, the legislature should increase its powers and provide adequate funds for its support (letter to C. S. Hoyt from Howard Potter, April 18, 1874, State Board of Charities Correspondence, NYSLA). His letter suggests that at least one of the legislature's motives in granting Ordronaux independence was fear of the excessive concentration of administrative authority in a single agency.

30. 1879 Senate *Documents*, no. 77 (hereafter referred to as the 1879 Apgar Report). Utica was not the only state asylum to be accused of fiscal extravagance, but it became the most popular target in New York. According to an 1873 Senate report, the initial construction of the Hudson River State Hospital for the Insane was conducted "on a scale of extravagance that has no parallel" (1873 Senate *Documents*, no. 107, 2).

31. 1882 Senate *Documents*, no. 68.

32. 1880 Investigation, 2, 6, 30, 45, 48, 50, 67, 265–270.

33. 1880 Investigation, 332–337, 509–531. See also Pitts, "The AMSAII," 155.

34. John Ordronaux, *Commentaries of the Lunacy Laws of New York and on the Judicial Aspects of Insanity at Common Law and in Equity, including Procedure, as Expounded in England and the United States; 1874 Laws of New York*, chap. 446.

35. 1880 Investigation, 263. For discussions of the board's hostility to Ordronaux's independence of it, achieved after his first year in office, see "Discussion of the Papers on Insanity," 106–107. Ordronaux's annual reports seldom criticized state asylums and often praised them fulsomely. He even defended the use of the controversial "protection bed" at Utica (N.Y.S. Commissioner in Lunacy, *Fourth AR* [1877], 8–11; idem, *Tenth AR* [1883], 137).

36. 1879 Senate *Documents*, no. 60, 414–441. A less charitable interpretation of Ordroneaux's ineffectiveness was offered by L. A. Tourtellot, who charged that Ordronaux once had been employed by the Utica asylum as a writer and had obtained his commissioner's position through Gray's influence (Tourtellot, "The Senate Committee on the Insane Asylums of New York," 351). E. C. Spitzka also alleged that Ordronaux was a personal friend of Gray and other asylum superintendents (Spitzka, "Merits and Motives of the Movement for Asylum Reform," 705). The truth of these accusations is impossible to ascertain, although Tourtellot certainly hated John Gray (who had fired him at Utica). At the 1872 AMSAII meeting, Gray expressed doubts about need for a commissioner in lunacy, but he supported Ordronaux after his appointment.

37. Letter to Charles J. Hoyt from Nicholas Devereux, May 2, 1878, N.Y.S. Board of Charities Correspondence, NYSLA.

38. 1880 Investigation, 428.

39. For examples of Ordronaux's limited powers, see N.Y.S. Commissioner in Lunacy, *First AR* (1874), 7; idem, *Sixth AR* (1879), 9–10. New York legislators' reluctance to give administrative power to a commissioner in lunacy partially may have come from their general inexperience with administrative agencies (James Leiby, *A History of Social Welfare and Social Work in the United States*, 99).

40. 1880 Investigation, 442, 531, 700.

41. N.Y.S. Commissioner in Lunacy, *Fourth AR* (1877), 8–10; idem, *Second AR* (1875), 10, 25–55; idem, *Third AR* (1876), 16. For an example of Gray's opposition, see "Reports of American Asylums," *AJI* 30: 488.

42. 1880 Investigation, 45–50; "Proceedings of the Association," *AJI* 32: 346–348; N.Y.S. Commissioner in Lunacy, *Thirteenth AR* (1886), 9–10. Long-time editor of the New York *Journal of Medicine*, Smith had been a professor of clinical surgery at New York University and a member of the State Board of Charities for several years. He served as commissioner in lunacy from 1882 to 1888. During this period, he too failed to get his annual reports to the legislature before it ad-

journed (N.Y.S. Commissioner in Lunacy, *Sixteenth AR* [1889], 5–6).

43. 1880 Investigation, 480–488. Although Gray restrained himself on the witness stand, he reverted to a more aggressive stance in an *AJI* review of the investigation. There he claimed that, despite their lengthy testimony, his opponents had failed to offer a single new idea about asylum management. Since their criticisms never rose "above the grade of misrepresentation, cavil, and quibble," he concluded that it was hardly surprising that the investigating legislators failed to make any final recommendations ("Review: Lunacy Investigation").

44. 1880 Investigation, 556–570.

45. N.Y.S. Lunatic Asylum, *Forty-second AR* (1885), 31–32; 1884 Investigation, 1–7.

46. Quoted in Buffalo *News* February 12, 1884. This and all subsequent newspaper clippings can be found in a special scrapbook on the 1884 investigation available at UPCA.

47. Ibid.; Buffalo *Commercial Advertiser,* February 9, 1884, UPCA.

48. Albany *Evening Journal,* February 13, 1884, UPCA.

49. Utica *Observer,* February 8, 1884, 5, UPCA; Albany *Morning Express,* February 13, 1884, UPCA; Attica *Observer,* February 28, 1884, UPCA.

50. *Evening Star,* February 22, 1884, UPCA; Albany *Evening Journal,* February 22, 1884, UPCA; Utica *Daily Press,* February 25, 1884, UPCA. Hughes's death also revived allegations of earlier asylum cover-ups of patient abuse. Particular attention was refocused on the notorious case of Norris Tarbell, who had died under suspicious circumstances in December 1859, only twenty-one days after admission. Although the asylum was never convicted officially of responsibility for his death (which, like Hughes's, allegedly resulted from injuries inflicted by brutal attendants), the incident aroused much public suspicion. Its investigation also revealed that attendants afraid of Tarbell kept him locked up in a crib for most of his asylum stay (L.A.T. Tourtellot, "The Senate Committee on the Insane Asylums of New York," 353–355; UPCBR 16: no. 5704; UPCA; N.Y.S. Lunatic Asylum, *Eighteenth AR* [1861], 10–12; "Reports of American Asylums," *AJI* 18: 269–271; Board of Managers, 120–123, UPCA).

51. Albany *Argus,* February 12, 1884, UPCA; 1879 Apgar Report, 13; Albany *Evening Journal,* February 13, 1884, UPCA.

52. 1884 Investigation.

53. Ibid.

54. Ibid., 728.

55. Ibid., 729–730.

56. Utica *Daily Press,* February 25, 1884, UPCA; Utica *Observer,* February 28, 1884, UPCA; ibid., March 1, 1884, UPCA; Buffalo *Courier,* February 15, 1884, UPCA; Utica *Daily Press,* March 15, 1884, UPCA; Utica *Morning Herald and Daily Gazette,* February 14, 1884, UPCA; Utica *Morning Herald,* March 5, 1884, UPCA.

57. 1884 Investigation, 40–46.

58. Ibid., 55–139, 221, 241–258, 410, 441–446, 498, 502–507, 722, 795–797, 805, 993, 1279–1299, 1347.

59. Ibid., 238, 263–278, 284–287.

60. Utica *Morning Herald and Daily Gazette,* February 23, 1884, UPCA; 1884 Investigation, 4–30.

61. N.Y.S. Lunatic Asylum, *Thirty-eighth AR* (1881), 43–65.

62. Grob, *Mental Illness and American Society.*

63. See Willard Scrapbook No. 4, WPCA, for rare clippings of county officials defending local care with vigor and credibility.

64. The attacks on county care filled late nineteenth-century New York newspapers, including the *New York Times* and the *New York Tribune.* For typical criticisms, see N.Y.S. Commissioner in Lunacy, *Second AR* (1875), 21–22, 29–34; idem, *Third AR* (1876), 23; idem, *Sixth AR* (1879), 11–14; N.Y.S. Board of Charities, *Second AR* (1869), xix–lxxiv; idem, *Twenty-third AR* (1890), 26–27. For typical praise of state care, see P. M. Wise, "The Care of the Chronic Insane"; idem, "Recovery of the Chronic Insane."

65. "Conference of Superintendents of the Poor," Elizabethtown (N.J.) *Post and Gazette,* November 14, 1889, in Willard Scrapbook No. 4, 20, WPCA; "State or County Care of the Insane," *Western New Yorker,* August 29, 1889, in Willard Scrapbook No. 4, 13–14, WPCA; "Care of the Insane in State Institutions: Rural Members Object," *New York Herald,* March 21, 1890, in Willard Scrapbook No. 4, 55, WPCA.

66. Gordinier, "Pauperism and Insanity," 85; A. A. Holmes, "Care of the Indigent Insane: A Plea for the System of County Supervisors," *New York Times,* December 13, 1889.

67. For a description of this progressive ideology, see Robert Wiebe, *The Search for Order, 1877–1920.* For a rare contemporary defense of the county position, see Katz, *Poverty and Policy,* 213–215.

68. N.Y.S. Commissioner in Lunacy, *Sixth AR* (1879), 6. For similar arguments, see "Caring for the Insane," *New York Daily Tribune,* March 6, 1885; "State Care of the Insane," ibid., April 1, 1889; "The Burdens of Society: Caring for the Pauper and the Lunatic," *New York Times,* December 10, 1880; "Costly Insane Asylums," ibid., February 25, 1878.

69. "Proceedings of the Association of Medical Superintendents," *AJI* 28: 324–327; Frederick H. Wines, "Hospital Building for the Insane," 143–150; Allison, "Moral and Industrial Management," 29; Winthrop B. Hallock, "Accommodations for the Insane on the Cottage Plan"; Francis Wells, "Hospital Building," 114–119.

8
An Unresolved Conclusion

1. Brenzel, *Daughters of the State;* Estelle Freedman, *Their Sister's Keepers: Women's Prison Reform in America, 1831–1930;* W. David Lewis, *From Newgate to Dannemora: The Rise of the Penitentiary in New York, 1796–1848;* Christopher Lasch, *The World of Nations: Reflections on American History, Politics and Culture,* 3–17; Blake McKelvey, *American Prisons: A History of Good Intentions;* Pickett, *House of Refuge;* Rothman, *Discovery of the Asylum;* Stephen Schlossman, *Love and the American Delinquent: The Theory and Practice of "Progressive" Juvenile Justice, 1825–1920;* Morris J. Vogel, *The Invention of the Modern Hospital, Boston, 1870–1930.*

2. Compare Lewis and McKelvey with Brenzel, Pickett, and the material presented in this book (see n. 1).

3. An exception is Tomes's study of the Pennsylvania Hospital, *A Generous Confidence*.

4. Michael Ignatieff, "State, Civil Society and Total Institutions: A Critique of Recent Social Histories of Punishment," 185. See also idem, *The Needs of Strangers*.

Bibliography

Primary Sources

Manuscripts

Albany County Court. Commitment Papers, 1843–1875. New York State Library Archives, Albany.
Chapin, John B. Scrapbook. Division of Manuscripts and University Archives, Cornell University, Ithaca.
Dix, Dorothea. Papers. Houghton Library, Harvard University, Cambridge.
Earle, Pliny. Papers. American Antiquarian Society, Worcester.
Jarvis, Edward. Papers. Countway Library of Medicine, Harvard Medical School, Boston.
Kirkbride, Thomas S. Papers. Pennsylvania Hospital Medical Archives, Philadelphia.
New York State Board of Charities. Correspondence. New York State Library Archives, Albany.
New York State Lunatic Asylum. Records. Utica Psychiatric Center, Utica.
Uticana Collection. Oneida County Historical Society, Utica.
Willard Asylum. Records. Willard Psychiatric Center, Willard.

Published Annual Reports

New York Board of State Commissioners of Public Charities. *Annual Reports*, 1–6, 1868–1873.
New York State Board of Charities. *Annual Reports*, 7–24, 1874–1891.
New York State Commissioner in Lunacy. *Annual Reports*, 1–16, 1874–1889.
New York State Commission in Lunacy. *Annual Reports*, 1–2, 1890–1891.
New York State Lunatic Asylum. *Annual Reports*, 1–49, 1844–1892.
Willard Asylum for the Chronic Insane. *Annual Reports*, 1–22, 1870–1891.

Selected New York State Legislative Documents (in chronological order)

"Recommendation to Establish a System of Relief for the Insane Poor." 1832 *Governors' Messages*, no. 11.
"Report of the Select Committee, on So Much of the Governor's Message, as Relates to Insane Paupers, with Comparative Statistics of New York and Other State Asylums." 1832 Assembly *Documents*, no. 174.
"Report on So Much of the Governor's Message as Relates to the Insane Poor." 1834 Assembly *Documents*, no. 347.
"Report of the Select Committee on So Much of the Governor's Message as Relates to the Insane Poor." 1835 Assembly *Documents*, no. 167.
"Memorial of the Medical Society of the State of New York, in Relation to Insane Paupers." 1836 Senate *Documents*, no. 38.

"Report of the Commissioners Appointed to Locate the New York State Lunatic Asylum." 1837 Senate *Documents,* no. 39.

"Documents Accompanying the Governor's Message: Statement of the Commissioners for Building the Lunatic Asylum." 1839 Senate *Documents,* no. 2.

"Liberal Appropriation Recommended for the Building of the State Lunatic Asylum." 1839 *Governors' Messages.*

"Report on the Governor's Message Regarding the State Lunatic Asylum." 1839 Senate *Documents,* no. 39.

"Report on So Much of the Governor's Message as Relates to the State Lunatic Asylum." 1840 Senate *Documents,* no. 105.

"Communication from the Commissioners of State Lunatic Asylums Regarding the Amounts Necessary to Complete Building." 1841 Senate *Documents,* no. 52.

"Message from the Governor, Transmitting a Communication Relative to the Erection of the Asylum for the Insane." 1841 Assembly *Documents,* no. 280.

"Report in Part of the Select Committee on So Much of the Governor's Message as Relates to the Lunatic Asylum." 1841 Assembly *Documents,* no. 61.

"An Act to Organize the State Lunatic Asylum, and More Effectually to Provide for the Care, Treatment, and Recovery of the Insane." 1842 *Laws of New York,* chap. 135.

"Report of the Trustees of the State Lunatic Asylum, with Documents Accompanying the Same, Pursuant to the Act of the Legislature Passed May 26, 1841." 1842 Senate *Documents,* no. 12.

"An Act in Relation to the State Lunatic Asylum." 1843 *Laws of New York,* chap. 224.

"Message from the Governor to the Senate and Assembly." 1844 Assembly *Documents,* no. 2.

"Memorial of Dorothea Dix to the Honorable the Legislature of the State of New York." 1844 Assembly *Documents,* no. 21.

"An Act in Relation to the State Lunatic Asylum." 1844 *Laws of New York,* chap. 337.

"Report of the Minority of the Select Committee on So Much of the Governor's Message as Relates to the State Lunatic Asylum." 1844 Assembly *Documents,* no. 94.

"Report of the Select Committee on So Much of the Governor's Message as Relates to the State Lunatic Asylum." 1844 Assembly *Documents,* no. 95.

"Report of the Committee on Medical Societies and Colleges, to Whom was Referred the Subject of the State Lunatic Asylum at Utica, Etc." 1846 Senate *Documents,* no. 12.

"An Act in Relation to the State Lunatic Asylum." 1850 *Laws of New York,* chap. 282.

"An Act to Amend the Act Entitled, 'An Act to Organize the State Lunatic Asylum, and More Effectually to Provide for the Care, Treatment, and Recovery of the Insane.'" 1851 *Laws of New York,* chap. 446.

"Report on the Appointment of Commissioners to Locate the Second State Lunatic Asylum." 1855 Assembly *Documents,* no. 91.

"Report of the Committee on Medical Societies and Colleges, Relative to a Commission to Examine into Lunatic Asylums, Workhouses, Jails, Etc." 1855 Senate *Documents,* no. 27.

"Report regarding the Commission to Examine into Lunatic Asylums, Workhouses, Jails, Etc." 1855 Senate *Documents*, no. 27.

"Report and Memorial of the County Superintendents of the Poor of This State on Lunacy and Its Relation to Pauperism, and for the Relief of the Insane Poor." 1856 Senate *Documents*, no. 17.

"Report of the Select Committee on the Report and Memorial of the County Superintendents of the Poor, on Lunacy and Its Relation to Pauperism." 1856 Senate *Documents*, no. 71.

"Report of the Senate Select Committee to Visit the Charitable and Penal Institutions of the State." 1857 Senate *Documents*, no. 8.

"Report of the Select Committee on So Much of the Governor's Message as Relates to the State Lunatic Asylum." 1858 Senate *Documents*, no. 26.

"Report of the Select Committee, to Which Was Referred the Memorial of Dr. Saunders, and Others, Asking for an Investigation of the Death of Norris Tarbell, at the State Lunatic Asylum, at Utica." 1860 Senate *Documents*, no. 43.

"An Act in Relation to Insane Persons in Poor Houses, Almshouses, Insane Asylums, and Other Institutions, in the State of New York." 1864 *Laws of New York*, chap. 418.

"Enactment of a Law Authorizing the Appointment of a Member of the Medical Profession as Commissioner in Lunacy; His Duty to Examine the Condition of the Insane Now Confined in Almshouses, Jails, and Private Lunatic Asylums." 1864 *Governors' Messages*, no. 2.

"Recommendation regarding the Appointment of Commissioners for Supervision of Various Public Charities." 1864 *Governors' Messages*, nos. 14–15.

Report on the Condition of the Insane Poor in the County Poor Houses of New York. 1865 Assembly *Documents*, no. 19.

"An Act to Amend the Acts in Relation to the State Lunatic Asylum." 1865 *Laws of New York*, chap. 353.

"An Act to Authorize the Establishment of a State Asylum for the Chronic Insane, and for the Better Care of the Insane Poor, to Be Known as 'The Willard Asylum for the Insane.'" 1865 *Laws of New York*, chap. 342.

"Report on the Condition of the Insane Poor in the County Poor Houses of New York." 1865 Assembly *Documents*, no. 19.

"Report of the Joint Committee of the Senate and Assembly to Examine into the Management and Affairs of the State Lunatic Asylum at Utica." 1869 Senate *Documents*, no. 80.

"An Act in Relation to the Chronic Pauper Insane." 1871 *Laws of New York*, chap. 282.

"Preamble and Resolution Adopted by the Eclectic Medical Society of New York State regarding the Illegal Incarceration of Lunatics." 1871 Senate *Documents*, no. 25.

"An Act Further to Define the Powers and Duties of the Board of State Commissioners of Public Charities, and to Change the Name of the Board to the State Board of Charities." 1873 *Laws of New York*, chap. 571.

"Report of Commissioners Appointed to Investigate Charges against Lunatic Asylums in the State; Also an Act Accompanying the Same." 1873 Senate *Documents*, no. 40.

"Report on a Codification of the Laws Relating to the Insane." 1874 Senate *Documents*, no. 86.

"An Act to Revise and Consolidate the Laws of the State Relative to the Care and Custody of the Insane; the Management of the Asylums for Their Treatment, and Safeguarding; and the Duties of the State Commissioner in Lunacy." 1874 *Laws of New York*, chap. 446.

"An Act Further to Amend Chapter 476 of the Laws of 1874." 1876 *Laws of New York*, chap. 267.

"An Act in Relation to the Powers and Duties of the State Commissioner in Lunacy." 1878 *Laws of New York*, chap. 47.

"Communication from the Comptroller, Submitting to the Senate the Report of the Agent Appointed to Examine the Charitable Institutions of the State of New York." 1879 Senate *Documents*, no. 77.

"Memorial of the State Board of Charities Relative to Insane Poor of the State." 1879 Assembly *Documents*, no. 119.

"Report of a Committee of the State Board of Charities, regarding the Insane Asylum of the Onondaga County Poor-House." 1879 Senate *Documents*, no. 60.

"Report of the Committee on Public Health Relative to Lunatic Asylums." 1879 Senate *Documents*, no. 64.

"Minutes of the Binghamton Insane Asylum Investigation." 1880 Senate *Documents*, no. 57.

"An Act in Relation to the Officers and Medical Staff of Willard Asylum for the Insane, and to Provide for the Appointment of a Committee for the Discharge of Patients in Said Asylum." 1881 *Laws of New York*, chap. 190.

"Report of the Select Committee Appointed by the Senate of 1880 and 1881 to Investigate the Condition of the Insane Asylums." 1882 Senate *Documents*, no. 68.

"Reproof to the Managers of the N.Y.S. Lunatic Asylum for Neglecting to Report a Detailed and Classified Statement of Expenditures." 1882 *Governors' Messages*, no. 2.

"Testimony before the Select Committee of the Senate Appointed May 25, 1880, to Investigate Abuses in the Management of Insane Asylums." 1882 Senate *Documents*, no. 96.

"Report of the Committee of State Charitable Institutions in the Matter of the Asylum Investigation." 1883 Assembly *Documents*, no. 175.

"Report of the Special Committee of the Assembly, Appointed to Investigate the Affairs and Management of the State Lunatic Asylum at Utica." 1884 Assembly *Documents*, vols. 10 and 11, no. 164.

"An Act in Relation to the Discharge of Patients from the Willard Asylum for the Insane." 1885 *Laws of New York*, chap. 178.

"An Act to Establish and Organize the State Commission in Lunacy, and to Define Its Duties." 1889 *Laws of New York*, chap. 283.

"An Act Changing the Name of the Several State Asylums for the Insane." 1890 *Laws of New York*, chap. 132.

"An Act to Amend, Revise, and Consolidate Certain Acts and Parts of Acts Relating to the State Commission in Lunacy, and the Care and Custody of the Insane, the Management of the Asylums for Their Treatment and Safekeeping, as Provided in Chap. 446 of the Laws of 1874 and Chap. 283 of the Laws of 1889, and Chap. 713 of the Laws of 1871." 1890 *Laws of New York*, chap. 273.

"An Act Changing the Name of the Several State Asylums for the Insane." 1890 *Laws of New York*, chap. 182.

"An Act to Promote the Care and Curative Treatment of the Pauper and Indigent Insane in the Counties of this State, except New York, Kings, and Monroe Counties, and to Permit Said Exempted Counties or Either of Them, in Accordance with the Action of Their Respective Local Authorities, to Avail Themselves or Any One or More of Them, of the Provisions of This Act." 1890. *Laws of New York*, chap. 126.

"An Act to Provide for the Employment of a Woman Physician in the State Asylums and Hospitals." 1890 *Laws of New York*, chap. 243.

"Communication from the State Commission in Lunacy regarding the Establishment of State Insane Asylum Districts." 1890 Senate *Documents*.

Articles and Books

"An Act for the Appointment of a Commissioner of Lunacy for the State of New York." *AJI* 19 (1863): 479–480.

"Action of Chloral." *AJI* 31 (1875): 395–396.

"Action of Narcotic Medicines in Insanity." *AJI* 28 (1871): 114–117.

Address from the State Charities Aid Association to Its Local Visiting Committees throughout the State of New York, July, 1886. New York: State Charities Aid Association, 1886.

"Address of the President-General R. Brinkerhoff, of Mansfield, Ohio." In *Proceedings of the Seventh Annual Conference of Charities and Corrections, Held at Cleveland, June and July, 1880*, edited by F. B. Sanborn, 1–36. Boston: Williams, 1880.

"Address to Our Patrons." *AJI* 3 (1853): frontispiece.

"The Admission of Visitors to Asylums." *AJI* 42 (1885): 271.

"The Age of Melancholy." *AJI* 41 (1885): 467–469.

"The Alleged Increase of Insanity." *AJI* 42 (1886): 540.

Allison, H. E. "Mental Changes Resulting from Separate Fractures of Both Thighs." *AJI* 43 (1886): 104–109.

———. "The Moral and Industrial Management of the Insane." *Alienist and Neurologist* 7 (1886): 286–297.

———. "Notes in a Case of Chronic Insanity." *AJI* 43 (1887): 481–484.

"American Journal of Insanity, Dr. Gray, and Clark Bell, Esq." *American Psychological Journal* 1 (1883): 306–310.

Anderson, M. B., and Deveraux, J. C. *Extract from the Sixth Annual Report of the State Board of Charities of the State of New York, Relating to Hospitals for the Sick and Insane, to Which Is Appended a Report Relating to the Management of the Insane in Great Britain by H. B. Wilbur, M.D.* Albany: Weed, Parsons, 1876.

Andrews, Judson B. "Asylum Periodicals." *AJI* 33 (1876): 42–49.

———. "Case of Excessive Hypodermic Use of Morphia: Three Hundred Needles Removed from the Body of an Insane Woman." *AJI* 29 (1872): 13–20.

———. "Clinical Cases." *AJI* 25 (1869): 359–366.

———. "Early Indications of Insanity." *AJI* 35 (1879): 479–502.

———. "Exophthalmic Goitre with Insanity." *AJI* 27 (1870): 1–13.

———. "Memoirs of John Perdue Gray, M.D., L.L.D." *AJI* 44 (1887): 21–32.

———. "State *versus* County Care." *AJI* 45 (1889): 395–407.

"April-Day at the Asylum." *AJI* 2 (1852): 144.

Bibliography

"Apropos of Recent Insane Asylum Investigations." *Alienist and Neurologist* 4 (1880): 491–492.

"Annual Meeting of the AMSAII." *AJI* 19 (1862): 22–86; 20 (1863): 60–143.

"Asylum for Inebriates." *AJI* 20 (1864): 353–355.

"An Asylum for the Insane Should Be Near a Large City." *AJI* 22 (1865): 252–255.

"Asylum Life: or, The Advantages of a Disadvantage." *Opal* 3 (1853): 228.

"Asylum Mismanagement." *New York Medical Journal*, December 1883, 608.

"Asylum Reform in New York State." *AJI* 44 (1888): 407–408.

"Asylum Reform in New York State." *JNMD* 6 (1879): 530–536.

"Attack on an English Asylum Superintendent." *AJI* 41 (1885): 377.

Atwood, C. E. "Three Cases of Multiple Neuritis Associated with Insanity." *AJI* 45 (1888): 58–64.

"Audi Alteram Partem." *Opal* 3 (1853): 320.

B., C. A. "A Token of Remembrance." *AJI* 12 (1856): 73–87.

Bagg, M. M., ed. *Memorial History of Utica, New York, from Its Settlement to the Present Time*. Syracuse: D. Mason, 1892.

Bannister, N. M., and Moyer, H. N. "On Restraint and Seclusion in American Institutions for the Insane." *JNMD* 9 (1882): 457–478.

Beard, George. "Why We Need a National Association for the Protection of the Insane." In *Proceedings of the Seventh Annual Conference of Charities and Corrections, Held at Cleveland, June and July, 1880*, edited by F. B. Sanborn, 144–151. Boston: Williams, 1880.

Bell, Clark. "The Rights of the Insane and Their Enforcement." *American Psychological Journal* 1 (1883); 1–23.

Bennett, Alice. "Medical Restraints in the Treatment of the Insane." *Medico-Legal Journal* 1 (1884): 285–296.

"The Better Care of the Insane." *American Psychological Journal* 1 (1884): 436–438.

"Bibliographical." *AJI* 37 (1881): 470–471.

"Bibliographical Notice." *AJI* 25 (1869): 265–272.

Blumer, G. Alder. "A Half-Century of American Medico-Psychological Literature." *AJI* 51 (1895): 40–50.

Blumer, G. Alder, and Richardson, A. B., ed. *Commitment, Detention, Care and Treatment of the Insane, Being a Report of the Fourth Section of the International Congress of Charities, Correction and Philanthropy, Chicago, June, 1893*. Baltimore: Johns Hopkins Press, 1894.

Brigham, Amariah. "Asylums Exclusively for the Incurable Insane." *AJI* I (1844): 44–45.

———. *The Asylum Souvenir*. Utica: Asylum, 1849.

———. "Brief Notice of the New York State Lunatic Asylum, at Utica, and of the Appropriations by the State, for the Benefit of the Insane." *AJI* I (1844): 1–7.

———. "Cases of Insanity." *AJI* 1 (1844): 146–155.

———. "Cases of Insanity—Illustrating the Importance of Early Treatment in Preventing Suicide." *AJI* 1 (1845): 243–249.

———. "Definition of Insanity: Nature of the Disease." *AJI* 1 (1844): 97–116.

———. "Exemption of the Cherokee Indians and Africans from Insanity." *AJI* 1 (1845): 287–288.

———. "The Human Brain." *AJI* 1 (1844): 191–192.

————. "Influence of the Weather upon the Disposition and the Mental Faculties." *AJI* 1 (1845): 340–346.

————. *An Inquiry concerning the Diseases and Functions of the Brain, the Spinal Cord, and the Nerves.* New York: George Adlard, 1840.

————. "Insanity and Insane Hospitals." *North American Review* 44 (1837): 91–121.

————. "Insanity Illustrated by Cases, and by the Conversation and Manners of the Insane." *AJI* 1 (1884): 46–62.

————. *A Letter from Doctor Brigham to David M. Reese, M.D., Author of Phrenology Known by Its Fruits, Etc.* Hartford, Conn.: N.p., 1836.

————. "Long-continued Insanity, with Speechlessness, Etc." *AJI* 1 (1844): 148–155.

————. "The Medical Jurisprudence of Insanity." *AJI* 3 (1845): 258–274.

————. "The Medical Treatment of Insanity." *AJI* 3 (1847): 353–355.

————. "Millerism." *AJI* 1 (1845): 249–252.

————. "Money-making Mania." *AJI* 5 (1849): 327–343.

————. "The Moral Treatment of Insanity." *AJI* 4 (1847): 1–15.

————. "Noble on the Brain." *AJI* 2 (1847): 353–358.

————. *Observations on the Influence of Religion upon the Health and Physical Welfare of Mankind.* Boston: Marsh, Capen, & Lyon, 1835.

————. *Remarks on the Influence of Mental Cultivation and Mental Excitement upon Health.* 3d ed. Philadelphia: Blanchard & Lea, 1845.

————. "Schools in Lunatic Asylums." *AJI* 1 (1845): 326–340.

————. "Second Annual Fair at the New York State Lunatic Asylum." *AJI* 1 (1845): 347–352.

————. "Sleep: Its Importance in Preventing Insanity." *AJI* 1 (1845): 319–325.

"The Brown Case and the Buffalo Asylum." *AJI* 44 (1888): 407–408.

Brush, Edward N. "A Case of Cerebral Hyperaemia with Delirium Following Sudden Change of Temperature," *AJI* 39 (1882): 55–58.

————. "Obituary: John B. Chapin, M.D., L.L.D." *AJI* 74 (1918): 689–705.

————. "On the Employment of Women Physicians in Hospitals for the Insane." *AJI* 47 (1891): 323–330.

————. "Sarcoma of the Dura Mater: Report of a Case, with Illustrations." *AJI* 36 (1880): 342–348.

Bucknill, John Charles. "Notes on Asylums for the Insane in America." *AJI* 33 (1876): 21–41.

Bucknill, John Charles, and Tuke, Daniel Hake. *A Manual of Psychological Medicine: Containing the History, Nosology, Description, Statistics, Diagnosis, Pathology, and Treatment of Insanity.* Philadelphia: Blanchard & Lea, 1858.

Butler, John S. "The Individualized Treatment of the Insane." *Alienist and Neurologist* 7 (1886): 425–460.

Butolph, H. A. "The Relation between Phrenology and Insanity." *AJI* 6 (1849): 127–136.

————. "Remarks on the Organization and Management of Hospitals and Asylums for the Insane." *Alienist and Neurologist* 8 (1887): 471–482.

Campbell, J. A. "On Three Cases of Recovery after a Lengthened Duration of Insanity, with Remarks." *AJI* 45 (1888): 1–9.

"Cannabis Indica as a Narcotic." *AJI* 42 (1886): 357–358.

"Case of Mania with Delusions and Phenomena of Spiritualism." *AJI* 16 (1860): 321–340.

"Cases Illustrating the Pathology of Mental Disease." *AJI* 13 (1857): 231–248; 14 (1857): 159–171; 15 (1858): 366–376.

"Celebration of the Birthday of Pinel, at the State Lunatic Asylum, Utica, N.Y., April 11, 1846." *AJI* 3 (1846): 78–82.

Channing, Walter. "A Consideration of the Causes of Insanity." *Journal of Social Sciences* 18 (1883): 68–92.

Chapin, John B. "Cases Illustrating the Pathology of Mental Disease Arising from Syphilitic Infection." *AJI* 15 (1859): 249–258.

———. *A Compendium of Insanity.* Philadelphia: Saunders, 1898.

———. "Fifty Years in Psychiatry." *AJI* 61 (1905): 399–416.

———. "Insanity in the State of New York." *AJI* 13 (1856): 39–52.

———. "Lunatic Asylum Reform." *Medical Record,* December 31, 1881, 754.

———. "On Provision for the Chronic Insane Poor." *AJI* 24 (1867): 29–42.

———. "Public Complaints against Asylums for the Insane, and the Commitment of the Insane." *AJI* 40 (1883): 33–49.

———. "Report on Provision for the Chronic Insane." *Transactions of the American Medical Association* 19 (1868): 191–201.

Chase, Hiram. *Two Years and Four Months in a Lunatic Asylum, from August 20, 1863 to December 20, 1865.* Saratoga Springs, N.Y.: N.p., 1868.

Clark, A. Campbell. "The Special Training of Asylum Attendants." *AJI* 40 (1884): 326–343.

Clark, Daniel. "Wrinkles in Ancient Asylum Reports." *AJI* 46 (1890): 339–353.

Cleaves, M. Abbie. "The Medical and Moral Care of Female Patients." In *Proceedings of the Sixth Annual Conference of Charities, Held at Chicago, June, 1879,* edited by F. B. Sanborn, 73–83. Boston: Williams, 1879.

"Clinical Contributions to Melancholia." *AJI* 47 (1890): 71–72.

"Clitoridectomy in Insanity." *Alienist and Neurologist,* 16 (1895): 478–479.

"Code of Laws Relating to the Insane in the State of New York, Passed May 1, 1874." *AJI* 31 (1874): 81–89.

"The Commencement Exercises of the Training School for Attendants at the Buffalo Asylum." *AJI* 43 (1886): 120–126.

"The Commitment and Detention of the Insane." *AJI* 45 (1888): 177–178.

"Complaints by Insane Patients." *AJI* 39 (1882): 74.

"Concerning Asylum Reform." *Medical Record,* October 1, 1881, 380.

"Considerations in the Subject of Insanity." *Opal* 2 (1852): 41–43, 86–88, 104–105, 143–144, 167–168.

Cook, George. "Provision for the Insane Poor in the State of New York." *AJI* 23 (1866): 45–75.

"The County Superintendents of the Poor." *AJI* 15 (1858): 245–246.

Coventry, Charles B. "Amariah Brigham, M.D." *AJI* 6 (1849): 185–192.

———. "Physiology of the Brain." *AJI* 3 (1846): 193–207.

Cowles, Edward. "Progress in the Care and Treatment of the Insane during the Half-Century." In *Proceedings of the American Medico-Psychological Association, at the Fifteenth Annual Meeting, Held in Philadelphia, May 15–May 18, 1894,* 122–135. Utica: State Hospital Press, 1895.

Curwen, John. "On the Propositions of the AMSAII." *Alienist and Neurologist* 1 (1880): 1–17.

Dana, C. L. "The Asylum Superintendents on the Needs of the Insane, with Statistics of Insanity in the United States." *JNMD* 9 (1882): 241–257.

Danillo, S. "Female Diseases among the Insane." *Alienist and Neurologist* 4 (1884): 113–118.

Davis, Phoebe B. *Two Years and Three Months in the New York Lunatic Asylum at Utica: Together with the Outlines of Twenty Years' Peregrinations in Syracuse.* Syracuse, N.Y.: By the Author, 1855.

"Death of an Asylum Superintendent from a Bite." *AJI* 39 (1883): 390.

"Death of John B. Chapin." *AJI* 74 (1919): 481.

"The Debate on Insanity." In *Proceedings of the Eighth Annual Conference of Charities and Correction, Held at Boston, July 25–30, 1881,* edited by F. B. Sanborn, 26–28, 319–360. Boston: Williams, 1881.

Deecke, Theodore. "The Condition of the Brain in Insanity." *AJI* 37 (1881): 361–396.

———. "On Progressive Meningo-Cerebritis of the Insane." *AJI* 39 (1883): 391–410; 40 (1884): 379–403.

———. "On the Pathology of Heat-Stroke." *AJI* 40 (1883): 178–204.

———. "Retrospect of German." *AJI* 33 (1876): 78–91.

———. "The Structure of the Vessels of the Nervous Centers in Health, and Their Changes in Disease." *AJI* 36 (1880): 328–341, 422–440; 37 (1881): 273–294.

———. "Urea and Phosphoric Acid in the Urine in Anaemia." *AJI* 36 (1879): 50–73.

Dewey, Richard S. "Differentiation in Institutions for the Insane." *AJI* 39 (1882): 1–21.

———. "Present and Prospective Management of the Insane." *JNMD* 5 (1878): 60–94.

———. "Training-Schools for Attendants in Asylums for the Insane." In *Proceedings of the National Conference of Charities and Correction, at the Fourteenth Annual Session,* edited by Isabel C. Barrows, 221–228. Boston: Ellis, 1887.

"Dipsomania." *AJI* 19 (1862): 246–247.

"Discussion." In *Proceedings of the National Conference of Charities and Correction at the Twelfth Annual Session Held in Washington, D.C., June 4–10, 1885,* edited by Isabel C. Barrows, 435–444. Boston: Ellis, 1885.

"Discussion of the Papers on Insanity." In *Proceedings of the National Conference of Charities, Held in Connection with the General Meeting of the American Social Science Association, at Saratoga, September 1876,* 106–114. Albany: Munsell, 1876.

"Discussion on Provisions for the Insane." In *Proceedings of the National Conference of Charities and Correction, at the Fifteenth Annual Meeting,* edited by Isabel C. Barrows, 384–394. Boston: Ellis, 1888.

"The Dose of Bromide of Potassium." *AJI* 27 (1871): 502.

"Dr. Brigham and the Association of Medical Superintendents." *Opal* 3 (1853): 33–36.

"Dr. Ray on Moral Insanity." *AJI* 18 (1861): 183–188.

Earle, Pliny. *The Curability of Insanity: A Series of Studies*. Philadelphia: Lippin-cott, 1887.

Eaton, Dorman B. "Despotism in Lunatic Asylums." *North American Review* 132 (1881): 263–275.

"Editor's Table." *Opal* 1 (1851): 317; 2 (1852): 25–28, 59–64, 91–96, 121–128, 154–160, 187–192, 221–224, 251–256, 283–288, 316–320; 3 (1853): 26–31, 59–66, 115–120, 176–182, 207–214, 229–248, 272–280, 304–312, 337–344, 367–368; 4 (1854): 43–48, 67–72, 116–120, 137–144, 163–168, 193–200, 217–224, 242–248, 267–272; 6 (1856): 20–24, 93–96; 7 (1857): 161–168.

"Eighteenth Annual Meeting of the Association of Superintendents of Institutions for the Insane." *AJI* 21 (1864): 113–157.

Everts, Orpheus. "The American Style of Public Provision for the Insane, and Despotism in Lunatic Asylums." *AJI* 37 (1881): 113–139.

"Exactness in Psychological Nomenclature." *New York Medical Journal*, Decem-ber 12, 1885, 675.

Falret, J. "Dr. J. Falret on the Classification of Insanity." *AJI* 18 (1862): 355–384.

Farnham, Alice May. "Uterine Disease as a Factor in the Production of Insanity." *Alienist and Neurologist* 8 (1887): 532–547.

Farnham, Eliza W. "Case of Destitution of Moral Feelings." *AJI* 3 (1846): 129–135.

"Fatal Assault on Dr. Metcalf." *AJI* 42 (1885): 259–264.

"A Few Facts concerning a Patient, by Himself." *Opal* 7 (1857): 4–6.

"A Few Words by an Old Patient." *Opal* 3 (1853): 20–21.

Folsom, Charles. "The Jurisprudence of Insanity in New York." *Boston Medical and Surgical Journal* 96 (1877): 508–510.

Ford, Willis E. "Clinical Cases: Syphilitic Insanity." *AJI* 31 (1874): 73–80.

———. "Phosphorus in Insanity." *AJI* 30 (1874): 335–341.

"Fortieth Annual Report of the Managers of the State Lunatic Asylum, Utica, New York, for the Year 1882." *JNMD* 10 (1882): 110–120.

"Fourth Annual Meeting of the AMSAII." *AJI* 6 (1849), 52–60.

"Fourth of July at the Asylum." *AJI* 2 (1852): 201–209.

"The Frequency of Relapse in Insanity." *AJI* 19 (1862): 117–123.

Godding, W. W. "Progress in Provision for the Insane, 1844–1884." *AJI* 41 (1885): 129–141, 217–234.

———. "The State in Its Care of the Insane." In *Proceedings of the National Con-ference of Charities and Correction, at the Sixteenth Annual Session Held in San Francisco, California, September 11–18, 1889*, edited by Isabel C. Bar-rows, 63–82. Boston: Ellis, 1889.

Goodrich, Chauncey E. *Biographical Sketch of Amariah Brigham, M.D., Late Superintendent of the New York State Lunatic Asylum, Utica, New York*. Utica: McClure, 1858.

———. *A Sermon on the Death of Amariah Brigham, M.D., Superintendent of the New York State Lunatic Asylum, Who Died September 8, 1849, Delivered at the Asylum, October 8, 1849, and Again in the First Presbyterian Church, Utica, November 11, 1849*. New York: Trow, 1850.

Gray, John P. "Address on Mental Hygiene." Philadelphia: Collins, n.d.

———. *Annual Address before the Medical Society of the State of New York, Feb-ruary 5, 1868*. Utica: Roberts, Book, & Job, 1868.

————. "The Care of the Chronic Insane Poor of the State of New York." *AJI* 23 (1866): 252–260.

————. "Case of Pellagra of the Insane." *AJI* 21 (1864): 223–227.

————. "The Dependence of Insanity on Physical Disease." *AJI* 27 (1871): 377–408.

————. "General View of Insanity: Lecture Delivered before the Bellevue Hospital Medical College, Session of 1874–75." *AJI* 31 (1875): 443–465.

————. "Heredity." *AJI* 41 (1884): 10–21.

————. "Hints on the Prevention of Insanity." *AJI* 41 (1885): 295–304.

————. "Hyoscyamia in Insanity." *AJI* 36 (1880): 394–403.

————. "Insanity and Its Relation to Medicine." *AJI* 25 (1868): 145–172.

————. "Insanity: Its Frequency: and Some of Its Preventable Causes." *AJI* 42 (1885): 1–45.

————. *Introductory Address of the Course of 1883–1884, at the Albany Medical College, Delivered September 11, 1883.* Albany: Weed, Parsons, 1883.

————. "Moral Insanity." *AJI* (1858): 311–322.

————. "Pathological Researches." *AJI* 33 (1877): 331–351.

————. "Pathology of Insanity." *AJI* 30 (1874): 305–311; 31 (1874): 1–29; 31 (1875): 153–183.

————. "Reparation of Brain-Tissue after Injury." *AJI* 32 (1876): 488–501.

————. "Responsibility of the Insane: Homicide in Insanity." *AJI* 32 (1875): 153–183.

————. "Suicide." *AJI* 35 (1878): 37–73.

————. "Thoughts on the Causation of Insanity." *AJI* 29 (1872): 264–283.

Gray, Landon C. "Lunacy Reform." *Medical Record*, January 31, 1880, editorial page.

————. "Three Diagnostic Signs of Melancholia." *JNMD* 15 (1890): 1–9.

Green, Traill. "Functions of a Medical Staff of an Insane Asylum." *American Psychological Journal* 1 (1883): 225–233.

Grissom, Eugene. "Mechanical Protection for the Violent Insane." *AJI* 34 (1877): 27–58.

H. "Life at Asylumia." *Opal* 4 (1854): 347–348.

H., C. A. "A Token of Remembrance." *Opal* 6 (1856): 191–192.

"Habeas Corpus." *AJI* 29 (1872): 302–306.

Hallock, Winthrop B. "Accommodations for the Insane on the Cottage Plan." *New York Medical Journal* 29 (1874): 1–9.

Hammond, William A. "The Non-asylum Treatment of the Insane." In *Transactions of the Medical Society of the State of New York for the Year 1879*, 280–297. Syracuse: Truair, Smith, & Bruce, 1879.

————. "The Treatment of the Insane." *International Review* 8 (1880): 225–241.

"The Hospitalization of Asylums." *AJI* 47 (1890): 563–564.

"Hospital versus Asylum." *AJI* 47 (1890): 90–91.

Hotchkiss, William. *Five Months in the New-York State Lunatic Asylum.* Buffalo: Danforth, 1849.

"How the Jealous Public Protect the Insane." *Alienist and Neurologist* 4 (1883): 329.

"Humanity's Bonfire." *AJI* 16 (1858): 253.

Hun, Edward R. "Haematoma Uris." *AJI* 26 (1870): 13–28.
———. "The Pulse of the Insane." *AJI* 26 (1870): 324–336.
Hunt, E. K. *Biographical Sketch of Amariah Brigham, M.D., Late Superinten-dent of the New York State Lunatic Asylum, Utica, New York.* Utica: McClure, 1858.
———. "Memoir of Amariah Brigham." *AJI* 14 (1857): 1–29.
Hurd, Henry M. "The Minor Treatment of Insane Patients." *AJI* 40 (1883): 205–209.
———. "A Plea for Systematic Therapeutical, Clinical, and Statistical Study." *AJI* 38 (1881): 16–31.
"In Memoriam." *Alienist and Neurologist* 8 (1887): 152–154.
"Insanity: My Own Case." *AJI* 13 (1856): 25–36.
"Insanity *vs.* Devilment." *AJI* 45 (1889): 569–570.
"Investigation of Insane Asylum Methods." *Medical Record,* December 11, 1880, 669–670.
Jarvis, Edward. "Influence of Distance from and Nearness to an Insane Asylum on Its Use by the People." *AJI* 22 (1866): 361–406.
———. "Mechanical and Other Employments for Patients in the British Lunatic Asylums." *AJI* 29 (1862): 129–146.
———. "On the Comparative Liability of Males and Females to Insanity and Their Comparative Curability and Mortality When Insane." *AJI* 7 (1850): 142–171.
Jones, Pomroy. *Annals and Recollections of Oneida County.* Rome, N.Y.: By the Author, 1851.
"Judge Lawrence on the Release of Lunatics." *AJI* 40 (1884): 521.
"The July Days at Asylumia." *Opal* 8 (1858): 181–182.
Kellogg, A. O. "Consideration on the Reciprocal Influence of the Physical Orga-nism and Mental Manifestations." *AJI* 12 (1856): 366–376; 13 (1856): 1–13.
———. "Imbecility and Insanity." *AJI* 24 (1868): 280–287.
———. "Notes on a Visit to Some of the Principal Hospitals for the Insane in Great Britain, France, and Germany, with Observations on the Use of Me-chanical Restraint in the Treatment of the Insane." *AJI* 25 (1869): 281–308.
———. "On William Shakespeare as a Physiologist and Psychologist." *AJI* 16 (1859): 129–148; 17 (1860): 409–435.
Kempster, Walter. "Clinical Cases." *AJI* 25 (1868): 79–88.
Kiernan, James G. "Contributions to Psychiatry." *JNMD* 10 (1883): 26–35.
———. "School Training of the Insane." *Alienist and Neurologist* 7 (1886): 581–591.
Kitchen, Daniel H. "Conium in the Treatment of Insanity." *AJI* 29 (1873): 457–480.
———. "Ergot in the Treatment of Nervous Diseases." *AJI* 30 (1873): 83–96.
———. "Nitrate of Amyl in the Treatment of Spasmodic Asthma and Acute Bron-chitis." *AJI* 30 (1873): 250–255.
Knox, W. E. *A Sermon Delivered at the Dedication of the Chapel of the New York State Lunatic Asylum, October 27, 1858.* Utica: Curtiss & White, 1858.
Krauss, William C. "The Hypnotic State of Hysteria." *JNMD* 15 (1890): 526–533.
Lathrop, Clarissa. *The Secret Institution.* New York: Bryant, 1890.
Laws Relating to the Willard Asylum for the Insane and Rules and Regulations of

Said Asylum, Adopted July 1, 1869, Revised October 15, 1884. Buffalo: Baker, Jones, 1884.

Lee, Charles A. "Medico-Legal Suggestions on Insanity." In *Papers Read before the Medico-Legal Society*, 467–488. New York: Medico-Legal Association, 1889.

———. *On Provision for the Insane Poor of the State of New York and the Adaptation of the "Asylum and Cottage Plan" to Their Wants, As Illustrated by the History of the Colony of Fitz James, at Clermont, France*. Albany: Van Benthuysen, 1866.

Leonard, Clara. "Women as Hospital Physicians." In *Proceedings of the Eighth Annual Conference of Charities and Correction Held at Boston, July 25–30, 1881*, edited by F. B. Sanborn, 322–323. Boston: Williams, 1881.

"A Letter from an Old Patient." *Opal* 3 (1853): 109–110.

"A Letter from a Patient." *Opal* 2 (1852): 245–246.

"Life at Asylumia." *Opal* 5 (1855): 347.

"Life in the Asylum." *Opal* 5 (1855): 4–5.

"Life in the New York State Lunatic Asylum; or, Extracts from the Diary of an Inmate." *AJI* 5 (1849): 289–302.

Lindsay, W. Lauder. "Mechanical Restraint in English Asylums." *AJI* 35 (1879): 542–555.

———. "The Theory and Practice of Non-restraint in the Treatment of the Insane." *AJI* 35 (1878): 272–304.

"Lines on the Departure of Dr. George Cook for Europe." *Opal* 2 (1852): 182.

"The Lunacy Commission's Report of the State of New York." *JNMD* 15 (1890): 124–127.

"Lunatic Asylum Reform." *Medical Record*, December 31, 1881, 754–755.

"Lunatics at Large versus Sane Persons in Lunatic Asylums." *AJI* 39 (1883): 474–480.

Luther, Diller. "The Extent to Which the State Should Assume the Care of the Indigent Insane." In *Proceedings of the Fifth Annual Conference of Charities Held in Connection with the General Meeting of the American Social Science Association, at Cincinnati, May, 1878*, 90–97. Boston: Williams, 1878.

Mabon, William. "Clinical Cases: Chloralamid as a Hypnotic for the Insane." *AJI* 46 (1890): 492–503.

———. "Clinical Observations on the Action of Sulfonal in Insanity." *AJI* 45 (1889): 493–499.

MacDonald, A. E. "The Examination and Commitment of the Insane." *AJI* 32 (1876): 502–522.

MacDonald, Carlos F. "Hydrate of Chloral." *AJI* 34 (1878): 360–367.

MacFarland, Andrew. "Reminiscences of the Association and Reflections." *AJI* 34 (1878): 347–359.

Mann, Edward C. "Insanity in the Middle States." In *Proceedings of the National Conference of Charities, Held in Connection with the General Meeting of the American Social Science Association, at Saratoga, September, 1876*, 54–65. Albany: Munsell, 1876.

———. "A Plea for Lunacy Reform." *Medico-Legal Journal* 1 (1884): 159.

———. "A Plea for Medico-Legal Protection of Those Suffering from That Form of Mental Disease Known as Moral or Affective Insanity, Where the Affective

Bibliography

Instead of the Intellectual Faculties of the Mind Are Primarily and Principally Affected." *American Psychological Journal* 1 (1884): 81–85.

"Medical Experts in Cases of Suspected Insanity." *New York Times*, March 16, 1873.

"Medical Jurisprudence." *AJI* 45 (1856): 508–523.

"Medical Notes: New York." *Boston Medical and Surgical Journal* 104 (1881): 44–46.

"Memorial to the President." *Opal* 6 (1856): 289–290.

"Method of Calculating Statistical Results." *AJI* 21 (1865): 571–572.

"Minutes and Discussion." In *Proceedings of the National Conference of Charities and Correction, at the Thirteenth Annual Session*, edited by Isabel Barrows, 435–444. Boston: Ellis, 1887.

"Mismanagement of Public Institutions for the Insane." *American Psychological Journal* 1 (1853): 57–62.

Mitchell, S. Weir. "Address before the Fiftieth Annual Meeting of the American Medico-Psychological Association, Held in Philadelphia, May 16, 1894." *JNMD* 21 (1894): 413–437.

Nellis, A. "Case of Cerebral Atrophy with Subsequent Cystic Degeneration." *AJI* 44 (1887): 220–223.

"New Jersey Lunatic Asylum, *AJI* 3 (1847): 384.

"New York State Lunatic Asylum." *AJI* 6 (1850): 287.

"Notes and Comments." *AJI* 42 (1886): 550.

"On the Claims of the Insane to the Respect and Interest of Society." *Opal* 2 (1852): 242.

"On the Increase of Insanity in the State of New York Compared with the Increase of Population." *AJI* 39 (1883): 387–390.

Ordronaux, John. *Commentaries on the Lunacy Laws of New York, and on the Judicial Aspects of Insanity at Common Law and in Equity, including Procedure, as Expounded in England and the United States*. Albany: Parsons, 1878.

"Our Charitable and Humane Institution." *Opal* 3 (1853): 43.

"Our Fair." *Opal* 3 (1853): 57.

"Our Version of the Song of the Shirt." *Opal* 2 (1852): 150–151.

"Our Visit to Barnum's Panorama of the Crystal Palace." *Opal* 2 (1852): 368–369.

Packard, Mrs. E. P. W. *Marital Power Exemplified in Mrs. Packard's Trial, and Self-defence from the Charge of Insanity: or, Three Years Imprisonment for Religious Belief, by the Arbitrary Will of a Husband, with an Appeal to the Government to So Change the Laws as to Afford Legal Protection to Married Women*. Hartford, Conn.: Case, Lockwood, 1866.

———. *Modern Persecution, or Insane Asylums Unveiled, as Demonstrated by the Report of the Investigating Committee of the Legislature of Illinois*. 12th ed. Vol. 1. Hartford, Conn.: Case, Lockwood, & Brainard, 1891.

———. *The Mystic Key: or, The Asylum Secret Unlocked*. Hartford, Conn.: Case, Lockwood, & Brainard, 1886.

Paoli, G. C., and Kiernan, James G. "Female Physicians in Insane Hospitals: Their Advantages and Disadvantages." *Alienist and Neurologist* 8 (1887): 21–29.

Parigot, J. "General Medical Therapeutics." *AJI* 24 (1868): 381–405.

"People *ex. rel.* Norton v. N.Y. Hospital." *Abbott's New Cases* (1876): 252–273.

"Persons Discharged from Asylums as Not Insane." *New York Medical Journal* 41 (1885): 201.

"Physician in Chief of an Asylum." *AJI* 22 (1865): 261–266.

Pilgrim, Charles W. "Pyromania (So-Called), with Case." *AJI* 41 (1885): 463–465.

———. "Report of a Case of Epileptic Insanity, with the 'Echo Sign' Well Marked." *AJI* 40 (1884): 404–411.

———. "A Visit to Gheel." *AJI* 42 (1886): 317–327.

Plans and Elevations and a Historical Sketch of the Willard Asylum for the Insane, at Willard, on Seneca-Lake, New York. Ovid: Willard, 1887.

"Poisonous Dose of Chloral." *AJI* 27 (1871): 502–503.

"Practical Insanity: A Lecture." *Opal* 6 (1856): 289–290.

"Prejudice against Institutions for the Insane." *American Psychological Journal* 1 (1853): 153–160.

"The Prevention of Insanity." *New York Medical Journal*, September 4, 1886, 226.

Proceedings of the American Medico-Psychological Association, at the Fifty-first Annual Meeting Held in Denver, June 11–13, 1895. Utica: State Hospital Press, 1896.

"Proceedings of the AMSAII." *AJI* 23 (1866): 75–251.

"Proceedings of the Association." *AJI* 37 (1880): 1–164; 43 (1886): 135–220.

"Proceedings of the Association of Medical Superintendents." *AJI* 24 (1870): 129–224; 26 (1869): 147–202; 27 (1879): 129–223; 28 (1871): 201–342; 30 (1873): 161–249; 31 (1874): 129–240; 32 (1876): 266–404; 33 (1876): 161–323; 34 (1877): 160–381; 35 (1878): 74–181; 38 (1881): 155–262; 43 (1886): 156–178; 45 (1888): 65–162; 47 (1890): 166–186; 47 (1890): 166–240.

"Proceedings of the Association: Provision for the Chronic Insane." *AJI* 24 (1868): 288–336.

"Proceedings of the Eighth Annual Meeting of the Medical Superintendents of American Institutions for the Insane." *American Psychological Journal* 1 (1853): 97–117.

Proceedings of the Employees and Resident Officers of the Willard Asylum on the Occasion of Dr. John B. Chapin Severing His Official Connections with This Institution. Waterloo, N.Y.: News Office, 1884.

"Proceedings of the Fifteenth Annual Meeting of the AMSAII." *AJI* 17 (1860): 32–73.

"Proceedings of the Fourteenth Annual Meeting of the AMSAII," *AJI* 16 (1859): 42–96.

"Proceedings of the Thirteenth Annual Meeting of the AMSAII." *AJI* 15 (1858): 77–132.

"Proceedings of the Twenty-fourth Meeting of the AMSAII," *Alienist and Neurologist* 5 (1875): 210–223.

"The Proposed Law Submitted by the Committee of the Medico-Legal Society to the Legislature of the State of New York, Session of 1873." *Medico-Legal Journal* 1 (1884): 119–139.

"Proposed 'Reforms' in Pennsylvania." *AJI* 47 (1890): 85–88.

Prudden, Lewis. "A Few Facts Concerning a Patient." *Opal* 7 (1857): 4–6.

"Psychological Retrospect." *AJI* 36 (1880): 447–449; 37 (1880): 66–68.

"Puerperal Insanity." *AJI* 7 (1850): 374–375.

Bibliography

"Quarterly Summary: New Jersey." *AJI* 45 (1888): 329.

R., S. "Life in the N.Y. State Lunatic Asylum: or, Extracts from the Diary of an Inmate." *AJI* 4 (1849): 289–302.

Ray, Isaac. "American Hospitals for the Insane." *North American Review*, 79 (1854): 67–90.

———. "The Cost of Constructing Hospitals for the Insane." *JNMD* 5 (1878): 47–56.

———. "Popular Feeling towards Hospitals for the Insane." *AJI* 9 (1851): 36–65.

———. "Recoveries from Mental Diseases." *Alienist and Neurologist* 1 (1880): 131–143.

"Report of the Committee of the New York Neurological Society upon the Gallup Lunacy Bill." *JNMD* 15 (1890): 181–187.

"Report of the Committee to Investigate the Affairs and Management of the State Lunatic Asylum at Utica." *JNMD* 12 (1885): 377–382.

"Reports of American Asylums." *AJI* 16 (1859): 97–115, 200–241; 17 (1860): 73–90; 18 (1862): 263–286; 19 (1862–1863): 185–198, 366–376; 20 (1869): 474–519; 21 (1865): 544–570; 30 (1873–1874): 97–153, 362–381, 481–499; 36 (1879): 90–120.

"Restraint in British and American Asylums." *AJI* 34 (1878): 512–530.

"Review." *AJI* 42 (1886): 119.

"Review: Annual Report of the State Lunatic Asylum, Northampton." *AJI* 40 (1883): 89–91.

"Review: Lunacy Legislation." *AJI* 39 (1883): 494–508.

"Review: *Materialism in Its Relation to the Causes, Conditions, and Treatment of Insanity.*" *Journal of Psychological Medicine* 6 (1872): 29–61.

"Review of the *Second Annual Report of the State Commissioner in Lunacy, for the State of New York, for 1874,*" *AJI* 31 (1875): 466–470.

"Review of the *Tenth Annual Report of the State Commissioner in Lunacy, for the Year 1882.*" *AJI* 40 (1884): 475–503.

"Review: *Twenty-fifth Report of the State Lunatic Asylum at Northampton.*" *AJI* 37 (1881): 460–463.

"Rights of the Insane." *AJI* 39 (1883): 411–436.

"The Rights of the Insane." *American Psychological Journal* 1 (1884): 422–428.

Russell, James. "Asylum vs. Hospital." In *Proceedings of the American Medico-Psychological Association at the Fifty-Fourth Annual Meeting, Held in St. Louis, May 10–13, 1898*, 239–253. New York: American Medico-Psychological Association, 1898.

Seguin, E. C. "Lunacy Reform: I. Historical Considerations." *Archives of Medicine* 2 (1879): 184–198.

———. "Lunacy Reform: II. Insufficiency of the Medical Staff of Asylums." *Archives of Medicine* 2 (1879): 310–318.

Shaw, A. M. "Mechanical Restraint." *AJI* 35 (1879): 556–562.

Shaw, J. C. *The Practicability and Value of Non-restraint in Treating the Insane, a Paper Read at Cleveland, Ohio, July 1, 1880, before the Conference of Charities.* Boston: Tolman & White, 1880.

———. "The Progress of the Non-restraint System." *American Psychological Journal* 1 (1884): 376–380.

———. "A Second Year's Experience with Non-restraint in the Treatment of the

Insane." In *Papers and Proceedings of the National Association for the Protection of the Insane*, 44–55. New York: Putnam's, 1882.

Smith, Stephen. "Care of the Filthy Insane." In *Proceedings of the National Conference of Charities and Correction, at the Twelfth Annual Session Held in Washington, D.C., June 4–10, 1885*, edited by Isabel C. Barrows, 148–153. Boston: Ellis, 1885.

————. "Compensation of Insane Labor: Suggestions in Reference to the Better Organization of a System of Labor for the Chronic Insane." In *Eleventh Annual National Conference of Charities and Correction*, edited by Isabel C. Barrows, 222–228. Boston: Ellis, 1884.

————. "Remarks on the Lunacy Laws of the State of New York, as Regards Their Provisions for Commitment and Discharge of the Insane." *AJI* 40 (1883): 50–70.

Spitzka, E. C. "Merits and Motives of the Movement for Asylum Reform." *JNMD* 5 (1878): 694–714.

————. "Reform in the Scientific Study of Psychiatry." *JNMD* 5 (1878): 201–229.

Spurzheim, Johann Christoph. *Observations on the Deranged Manifestations of the Mind, or Insanity*. Appendix by Amariah Brigham. Boston: Marsh, Capon & Lyon, 1833.

"The State Commission in Lunacy." *AJI* 46 (1890): 566–569.

"State *versus* County Care." *AJI* 46 (1890): 504–534.

"Statistics of Insanity." *AJI* 18 (1861): 2–14.

Stribling, Francis T. "Qualifications and Duties of Attendants on the Insane." *AJI* 9 (1852): 97–102.

"Summary: On Separate Asylums for Curables and Incurables." *AJI* 22 (1865): 246–252.

"Summary: The Care of the Chronic Insane Poor of the State of New York." *AJI* 23 (1866): 252–260.

"To Dr. C—— by a Sick Patient." *Opal* 3 (1853): 58.

"To Dr. C——K." *Opal* 3 (1853): 109–110.

"To Dr. G——y." *Opal* 2 (1852): 346.

"To Dr. ————, on His Return from the Annual Meeting of Superintendents of Asylums." *Opal* 1 (1851): 54.

"To My Attendant." *Opal* 3 (1853): 4.

"To My Children at Home." *Opal* 2 (1852): 392.

"To My Mother." *Opal* 6 (1856): 185.

"To Our Apothecary." *Opal* 2 (1852): 275.

"To the Schoolmaster." *Opal* 3 (1853): 257.

Tourtellot, L. A. "Mechanical Restraint in the Treatment of the Insane." *AJI* 13 (1857): 281–290.

————. "The Senate Committee on the Insane Asylums of New York." *JNMD* 9 (1882): 349–358.

————. "Utica Asylum Investigation." *Amerian Psychological Journal* 2 (1884): 31–40.

"Training School for Attendants." *AJI* 42 (1885): 267–269.

Trull, William L. *An Inner View of the State Lunatic Asylum at Utica, or How Patients Are Treated in the Model (?) Mad House of New York*. Cohoes, N.Y.: Craig, 1881.

Bibliography

Tuke, Daniel Hake. *The Insane in the United States and Canada*. London: Lewis, 1885.

"Twentieth Annual Meeting of the Association of Medical Superintendents of American Institutions for the Insane." *AJI* 23 (1866): 79–251.

"Unlocked Doors in Asylums." *AJI* 37 (1880): 93–95.

"The Use of Sedatives in Insanity." *AJI* 43 (1887): 367–368.

Van Deusen, E. H. "Observations on a Form of Nervous Prostration (Neurasthenia), Culminating in Insanity." *AJI* 26 (1869): 446–461.

———. "Provision for the Care and Treatment of the Insane." *AJI* 28 (1872): 514–529.

"A Walk in the Woods: By Two Little Girls from No. 3." *Opal* 3 (1853): 161.

Wells, Francis. "Hospital Building." In *Proceedings of the Conference of Charities, Held in Connection with the General Meeting of the American Social Science Association*. 114–119. Albany: Munsell, 1876.

Wilbur, H. B. "Buildings for the Management and Treatment of the Insane." In *Proceedings of the Fourth Annual Conference of Charities*, edited by F. B. Sanborn, 134–158. Boston: Williams, 1877.

———. "Governmental Supervision of the Insane." In *Proceedings of the Third Annual Conference of Charities*, edited by F. B. Sanborn, 72–90. Boston: Williams, 1876.

———. *Materialism in Its Relation to the Causes, Conditions, and Treatment of Insanity*. New York: Appleton, 1872.

"The Willard Asylum Act and Provision for the Insane." *AJI* 22 (1865): 192–255.

Wines, Frederick H. "Hospital Building for the Insane." In *Proceedings of the Conference of Charities Held in Connection with the General Meeting of the American Social Science Association, at Saratoga, September 1877*, 143–150. Boston: Williams, 1877.

Wise, P. M. "The Barber Case: The Legal Responsibility for Epileptics." *AJI* 45 (1888): 360–373.

———. "The Care of the Chronic Insane." *AJI* 44 (1887): 170–175.

———. "Case of Sexual Perversion." *Alienist and Neurologist* 4 (1883): 87–91.

———. "Recovery of the Chronic Insane." *AJI* 42 (1886): 484–498.

———. " Vaginal Hernia and Uterine Fibroids, with Delusions of Pregnancy." *AJI* 46 (1889): 76–78.

Workman, Joseph. "Asylum Management." *AJI* 38 (1881): 1–15.

———. "Insanity of the Religious-Emotional Type, and Its Occasional Physical Relations." *AJI* 26 (1869): 33–48.

Wright, A. O. "The Increase of Insanity." In *Proceedings of the Eleventh Annual Session of the National Conference of Charities and Correction Held at St. Louis, October 13–17, 1884*, edited by Isabel C. Barrows, 229–236. Boston: Ellis, 1885.

"The Writ of Habeas Corpus and Insane Asylums." *AJI* 39 (1883): 301–317.

Secondary Sources: Articles and Books

Adams, Francis R. "From Association to Union: Professional Organization of Asylum Attendants, 1869–1919." *British Journal of Sociology* 20 (1969): 11–26.

Adelson, Pearle Yaruss. "The Back Ward Dilemma." *Amerian Journal of Nursing* 80 (1980): 422–425.

Atwater, Edward C. "The Medical Profession in a New Society, Rochester, New York (1811–1860)." *BHM* 47 (1973): 221–235.

Bachrach, Leona. "Asylum and Chronically Ill Psychiatric Patients." *American Journal of Psychiatry* 141 (1984): 975–978.

Bakan, David. "The Influence of Phrenology on American Psychology." *Journal of the History of Behavioral Sciences* 2 (1966): 200–220.

Bell, Leland V. *Treating the Mentally Ill: From Colonial Times to the Present.* New York: Praeger, 1980.

Blum, Alan F. "The Sociology of Mental Illness." In *Deviance and Respectability: The Social Construction of Moral Meanings,* edited by Jack D. Douglas, 52–53. New York: Basic Books, 1970.

Bluestein, Bonnie Ellen. "'A Hollow Square of Psychological Science': American Neurologists and Psychiatrists in Conflict." In *Madhouses, Mad-Doctors and Madmen,* edited by Andrew Scull, 241–270. Philadelphia: University of Pennsylvania Press, 1981.

––––––. "New York Neurologists and the Specialization of American Medicine." *BHM* 53 (1979): 170–183.

Bockoven, J. S. *Moral Treatment in American Psychiatry.* New York: Springer, 1963.

Braginsky, Benjamin M.; Braginsky, Dorothea D.; and Ring, Kenneth. *Methods of Madness: The Mental Hospital as a Last Resort.* New York: Holt, Rinehart & Winston, 1969.

Brenzel, Barbara M. *Daughters of the State: A Social Portrait of the First Reform School for Girls in North America, 1856–1905.* Cambridge: MIT Press, 1983.

Brock, William R. *Investigation and Responsibility: Public Responsibility in the United States, 1865–1900.* Cambridge: Cambridge University Press, 1984.

Brown, Edward M. "'What Shall We Do with the Inebriate?': Asylum Treatment and the Disease Concept of Alcoholism in the Late Nineteenth Century." *Journal of the History of the Behavioral Sciences* 21 (1985): 48–59.

Brown, George William. *Social Origins of Depression: A Study of Psychiatric Disorders in Women.* London: Tavistock, 1978.

Brown, Thomas E. "The Mental Hospital and Its Historians." *BHM* 56 (1982): 109–114.

Brumberg, Joan Jacobs. "'Ruined Girls': Changing Family and Community Responses to Illegitimacy in Upstate New York, 1890–1920," *Journal of Social History* 18 (1984): 247–272.

Bullough, Vern L., and Voght, Martha. "Homosexuality and Its Confusion with the 'Secret Sin' in Pre-Freudian America." *Journal of the History of Medicine and the Allied Sciences* 28 (1973): 143–155.

———. "Women, Menstruation, and Nineteenth-Century Medicine." *BHM* 47 (1973): 66–82.

Burnham, John C. "The Royal Derwent Hospital in Tasmania: Historical Perspectives on the Meaning of Community Psychiatry." *Australian and New Zealand Journal of Psychiatry* 9 (1975): 163–168.

Bynum, William. "Rationales for Therapy in British Psychiatry: 1780–1835." *Medical History* 18 (1964): 317–334.

Cancro, Robert, and Pruyser, Paul W. "A Historical Review of the Development of the Concept of Schizophrenia." *Bulletin of the Menninger Clinic* 34 (1970): 61–70.

Caplan, Ruth B., and Caplan, Gerald. *Psychiatry and the Community in Nineteenth-Century America*. New York: Basic Books, 1969.

Cardno, J. A. "The Aetiology of Insanity: Some Early American Views." *Journal of the History of the Behavioral Sciences* 4 (1968): 99–108.

Carlson, Eric T. "Amariah Brigham: I. Life and Works." *American Journal of Psychiatry* 112 (1956): 831–836.

———. "Amariah Brigham: II. Psychiatric Thought and Practice." *American Journal of Psychiatry* 113 (1957): 911–916.

———. "Cannabis Indica in Nineteenth-Century Psychiatry." *American Journal of Psychiatry* 131 (1974): 1004–1007.

———. "The Influence of Phrenology on Early American Psychiatric Thought." *American Journal of Psychiatry* 115 (1958): 535–538.

Carlson, Eric T., and Dain, Norman. "The Psychotherapy That Was Moral Treatment." *American Journal of Psychiatry* 117 (1960): 519–524.

Carlson, Eric T., and McFadden, R. Bruce. "Dr. William Cullen on Mania." *American Journal of Psychiatry* 117 (1960): 463–465.

Carlson, Eric T., and Simpson, Maribeth M. "Opium as a Tranquilizer." *American Journal of Psychiatry* 120 (1964): 112–117.

Carpenter, Mick. "Asylum Nursing before 1914." In *Rewriting Nursing History*, edited by Celia Davies, 123–146. London: Croom Helm, 1975.

Cassedy, James H. *American Medicine and Statistical Thinking, 1800–1860*. Cambridge: Harvard University Press, 1984.

Caudill, William. *The Psychiatric Hospital as a Small Society*. Cambridge: Harvard University Press, 1958.

Church, Olga Maranjian. "That Noble Reform: The Emergence of Psychiatric Nursing in the United States, 1882–1963." Ph.D. diss., University of Illinois at the Medical Center, 1982.

Clark, Lucy. *A Century of Progress at Utica State Hospital*. Utica: Hospital Alumnae Association, 1943.

Cohen, Patricia Cline. *A Calculating People: The Spread of Numeracy in America*. Chicago: University of Chicago Press, 1982.

Cohen, Stanley, and Scull, Andrew, eds. *Social Control and the State*. New York: St. Martin's, 1983.

Cooter, Roger. "Phrenology and British Alienists, ca. 1825–1845." In *Madhouses, Mad-Doctors and Madmen*, edited by Andrew Scull, 58–104. Philadelphia: University of Pennsylvania Press, 1971.

Courtwright, David T. "The Female Opiate Addict in Nineteenth-Century America." *Essays in Arts and Science* 10 (1982): 161–171.

———. "Opiate Addiction as a Consequence of the Civil War." *Civil War History* 24 (1978): 101–111.

Cressy, Donald. "Prison Organization." In *Handbook of Organizations*, edited by James Marsh, 1024. New York: Rand McNally, 1965.

Dain, Norman. *Concepts of Insanity in the United States, 1789–1865*. New Brunswick, N.J.: Rutgers University Press, 1964.

Dain, Norman, and Carlson, Eric T. "Moral Insanity in the United States, 1835–1866." *American Journal of Psychiatry.* 118 (1962): 795–801.

———. "Social Class and Psychological Medicine in the United States, 1789–1824." *BHM* 33 (1959): 454–465.

Davies, Celia, ed. *Rewriting Nursing History*. London: Croom Helm, 1980.

Degler, Carl M. "What Ought to Be and What Was: Women's Sexuality in the Nineteenth Century." *American Historical Review* 79 (1974): 1467–1490.

De Guistino, David. *Conquest of Mind: Phrenology and Victorian Sociological Thought*. London: Croom Helm, 1975.

Deutsch, Albert. *The Mentally Ill in America: A History of Their Care and Treatment from Colonial Times*. Garden City, N.Y.: Doubleday, Doran, 1937.

Digby, Anne. *Madness, Morality, and Medicine: A Study of the York Retreat 1796–1914*. Cambridge: Cambridge University Press, 1985.

Dohrenwend, Barbara; Dohrenwend, Bruce P.; Dodson, Margaret; and Shrout, Patrick. "Symptoms, Hassles, Social Supports, and Life Events: Problems of Confounded Measures." *Journal of Abnormal Psychology* 93 (1984): 222–230.

Dohrenwend, Bruce P., and Dohrenwend, Barbara Scull. "Sex Differences and Psychiatric Disorder." *American Journal of Sociology* 81 (1976): 1447–1454.

Doran, Robert E. "History of the Willard Asylum for the Insane and the Willard State Hospital." Willard: N.p., 1978.

Douglas, Jack D., ed. *Deviance and Respectability: The Social Construction of Moral Meanings*. New York: Basic Books, 1970.

Dudden, Faye E. *Serving Women: Household Service in Nineteenth-Century America*. Middletown, Conn.: Wesleyan University Press, 1983.

Duffy, John. "Masturbation and Clitoridectomy: A Nineteenth Century View." *Journal of the American Medical Association* 186 (1963): 246–248.

Dunham, H. Warren, and Weinberg, S. Kirson. *The Culture of the State Mental Hospital*. Detroit: Wayne University Press, 1960.

Dwyer, Ellen. "A Historical Perspective." In *Sex Roles and Psychopathology*, edited by Cathy S. Wilson, 19–48. New York: Plenum, 1984.

———. "The Weaker Vessel: The Law versus Social Realities in the Commitment of Women to Nineteenth-Century New York Asylums." In *Women and the Law*, vol. 1, edited by Kelly Weisberg, 85–106. Cambridge: Schenkman, 1983.

Eaton, Leonard. "Eli Todd and the Hartford Retreat." *New England Quarterly* 26 (1953): 435–453.

Ewalt, Donald H., Jr., "Patients, Politics, and Physicians: The Struggle for Control of State Lunatic Asylum Number 1, Fulton, Missouri." *Missouri Historical Review* 78 (1983): 170–188.

Finnane, Mark. *Insanity and the Insane in Post-Famine Ireland*. London: Croom Helm, 1981.

Forster, Robert, and Ranum, Orest, eds. *Deviants and the Abandoned in French Society*. Baltimore: Johns Hopkins University Press, 1978.

Bibliography

Foucault, Michel. *Madness and Civilization: A History of Insanity in the Age of Reason.* New York: Random House, 1965.

Fox, Richard. *"So Far Disordered in Mind": Insanity in California, 1870–1930.* Berkeley and Los Angeles: University of California Press, 1978.

Freedberger, Mark. "The Decision to Institutionalize: Families with Exceptional Children in 1900." *Journal of Family History* 6 (1981): 396–409.

Freedman, Estelle B. *Their Sister's Keepers: Women's Prison Reform in America, 1831–1930.* Ann Arbor: University of Michigan Press, 1981.

Friedman, Lawrence J. "The Demise of the Asylum." *Reviews in American History* 12 (1984): 241–247.

Fullinwider, S. P. "Insanity as the Loss of Self: The Moral Insanity Controversy Revisited." *BHM* 49 (1975): 87–101.

Gaines, Atwood D. "Definitions and Diagnoses: Cultural Implications of Psychiatric Help-seeking and Psychiatrists' Definition of the Situation in Psychiatric Emergencies." *Culture, Medicine, and Psychiatry* 3–4 (1979): 386–387.

Gardinier, Walter R., Jr. "Pauperism and Insanity: Aspects of Social Welfare in Nineteenth Century Chautauqua County." M.A. thesis, State University College at Fredonia, 1978.

Garfinkel, Harold. "Conditions of Successful Degradation Ceremonies." *American Journal of Sociology* 61 (1856): 420–424.

Goffman, Erving. *Asylums: Essays on the Social Situation of Mental Patients and Other Inmates.* Garden City, N.Y.: Doubleday, Anchor, 1961.

———. *Interaction Ritual: Essays on Face-to-Face Behavior.* Garden City, N.Y.: Doubleday, 1967.

———. *Relations in Public: Microstudies of the Public Order.* New York: Harper & Row, 1971.

Golden, Janet, and Schneider, Eric C. "Custody and Control: the Rhode Island State Hospital for Mental Diseases, 1870–1970." *Rhode Island History* 41 (1982): 113–125.

Goldhammer, Herbert, and Marshall, Andrew W. *Psychosis and Civilization: Two Studies in the Frequency of Mental Disease.* Glencoe, Ill.: Free Press, 1949.

Goldstein, Michael S. "The Sociology of Mental Health and Illness." *Annual Review of Sociology* 5 (1979): 381–409.

Gove, Walter R., ed. *Deviance and Mental Illness.* Beverly Hills, Calif.: Sage, 1982.

Grob, Gerald N. "Abuse in American Mental Hospitals in Historical Perspective: Myth and Reality." *International Journal of Law and Psychiatry* 3 (1980): 295–310.

———. "Class, Ethnicity, and Race in American Mental Hospitals." *Journal of the History of Medicine and Allied Sciences* 28 (1973): 207–229.

———. *Mental Illness and American Society, 1875–1940.* Princeton, N.J.: Princeton University Press, 1983.

———. *Mental Institutions in America: Social Policy to 1875.* New York: Macmillan, 1973.

———. "The Origins of American Psychiatric Epidemiology." *American Journal of Public Health* 75 (1985): 229–236.

———. "The Political System and Social Policy in the Nineteenth Century: Legacy of the Revolution." *Mid-America* 56 (1976): 5–19.

————. "Public Policy-making and Social Policy." In *Policy Studies Review Annual*, vol. 15, edited by Irving Louis Horowitz, 703–730. Beverly Hills, Calif.: Sage, 1981.

————. "Rediscovering Asylums: The Unhistorical History of the Mental Hospital." *Hastings Center Report* 7 (1977): 33–41.

————. "Reflections on the History of Social Policy in America." *Reviews in American History* 7 (1979): 293–306.

————. *The State and the Mentally Ill: A History of Worcester State Hospital in Massachusetts, 1830–1920.* Chapel Hill: University of North Carolina Press, 1966.

Gunn, L. Ray, "The Decline of Authority: Public Policy in New York, 1837–1860." Ph.D. diss., Rutgers University, 1957.

————. "The New York State Legislature: A Developmental Perspective, 1777–1846." *Social Science History* 4 (1980): 277–280.

Hahn, Nicolas F. "Too Dumb to Know Better: Cacogenic Family Studies and the Criminology of Women." *Criminology* 18 (1980): 3–25.

Hall, J. K. et al. *One Hundred Years of American Psychiatry.* New York: Columbia University Press, 1944.

Hannon, Joan. "Poverty in the Antebellum Northeast: The View from New York State's Poor Relief Rolls." *Journal of Economic History* 44 (1984): 1007–1032.

Henderson, S.; Duncan-Jones, P.; McAuley, H.; and Ritchie, K. "The Patient's Primary Group." In *Psychosocial Disorders in General Practice*, edited by P. Williams and A. Clare, 109–130. London: Academic, 1979.

Herrmann, Frederick M. *Dorothea L. Dix and the Politics of Institutional Reform.* Trenton: New Jersey Historical Commission, 1981.

Himmelhoch, Myra S., and Shaffer, Arthur H. "Elizabeth Packard: Nineteenth Century Crusader for the Rights of Mental Patients." *Journal of American Studies* 13 (1979): 343–376.

Hoch, Paul. "History of the Department of Mental Hygiene." Albany: State of New York, 1955.

Hollander, Russell. "Life at the Washington Asylum for the Insane, 1871–1880." *Historian* 44 (1982): 229–241.

Horwitz, Allan V. *The Social Control of Mental Illness.* New York: Academic, 1982.

Hunter, Richard, and Macalpine, Ida. *Psychiatry for the Poor, 1851 Colony Hatch Asylum-Friern Hospital 1973: A Medical and Social History.* Kent: Dawson, 1974.

Hurd, Henry M., ed. *The Institutional Care of the Insane in the United States and Canada.* 4 vols. Baltimore: Johns Hopkins Press, 1916–1917.

Ignatieff, Michael. *A Just Measure of Pain: The Penitentiary in the Industrial Revolution.* New York: Pantheon, 1978.

————. *The Needs of Strangers.* New York: Viking, 1984.

————. "State, Civil Society and Total Institutions: A Critique of Recent Social Histories of Punishment." In *Legality, Ideology and the State*, edited by David Sugarman, 183–211. New York: Academic, 1983.

Jackson, Stanley W. "Melancholia and Mechanical Explanation in Eighteenth-Century Medicine." *Journal of the History of Medicine and Allied Sciences* 38 (1983): 298–314.

Bibliography

————. "Melancholia and Partial Insanity." *Journal of the History of the Behavioral Sciences* 19 (1983): 173–184.

Jacobs, James. *New Perspectives on Prisons and Imprisonment.* Ithaca, N.Y.: Cornell University Press, 1983.

Jacyna, L. S. "Somatic Theories of Mind and the Interests of Medicine in Britain, 1840–1879." *Medical History* 26 (1982): 233–258.

Jones, Colin. "The Treatment of the Insane in Eighteenth- and Early Nineteenth-Century Montpellier." *Medical History* 24 (1980): 371–390.

Jones, Robert E. "Correspondence of the American Psychiatric Association Founders." *American Journal of Psychiatry* 119 (1963): 1121–1134.

Katz, Michael B. "Origins of the Institutional State." *Marxist Perspective* 1 (1978): 6–22.

————. *Poverty and Policy in American History.* New York: Academic, 1983.

Katz, Michael B., Doucet, Michael J., and Stern, Mark J. *The Social Organization of Early Industrial Capitalism.* Cambridge: Harvard University Press, 1982.

Katzman, David. *Seven Days a Week: Women and Domestic Service in Industrializing America.* New York: Oxford University Press, 1978.

Kempe, Ruth S., and Kempe, Henry C. *Child Abuse.* Cambridge: Harvard University Press, 1978.

Kessler, Ronald C.; Brown, Roger L.; and Broman, Clifford L. "Sex Differences in Psychiatric Help-keeping: Evidence from Four Large-Scale Studies." *Journal of Health and Social Behavior* 22 (1979): 49–64.

Klein, Stanley B. "A Study of Social Legislation Affecting Prisons and Institutions for the Mentally Ill in New York State, 1822–1846." Ph.D. diss., New York University, 1956.

Kolko, Gabriel. *The Triumph of the Conservatives: A Re-interpretation of American History, 1900–1916.* New York: Free Press, 1963.

Krasnick, Cheryl L. "'In Charge of the Loons': A Portrait of the London, Ontario, Asylum for the Insane in the Nineteenth Century." *Ontario Quarterly* 74 (1982): 138–184.

Laing, R. D. *The Politics of the Family and Other Essays.* New York: Random House, Vintage, 1972.

————. *Sanity, Madness and the Family.* London: Tavistock, 1964.

Lamb, H. Richard, ed. *The Homeless Mentally Ill.* Washington, D.C.: American Psychiatric Association, 1984.

Lasch, Christopher. *A Haven in a Heartless World.* New York: Basic Books, 1977.

————. *The World of Nations: Reflection on American History, Politics, and Culture.* New York: Knopf, 1973.

Leavitt, Judith Walzer, and Numbers, Ronald L., eds. *Sickness and Health in America: Readings in the History of Medicine and Public Health.* Madison: University of Wisconsin Press, 1978.

Leiby, James. *A History of Social Welfare and Social Work in the United States.* New York: Columbia University Press, 1978.

Lewis, W. David. *From Newgate to Dannemora: The Rise of the Penitentiary in New York, 1796–1848.* Ithaca, N.Y.: Cornell University Press, 1965.

Lincoln, Charles A., ed. *Messages from the Governor.* Vols. 3–5. Albany: J. B. Lyon, 1907.

Lively, Carrie E. "Reminiscences of a State Mental Hospital Attendant." *Indiana Medical History Quarterly* 9 (1983): 13–22.

Longo, Lawrence D. "The Rise and Fall of Battey's Operation: A Fashion in Surgery." *BHM* 53 (1979): 244–267.

McCandless, Peter. "'Build! Build!': The Controversy over the Care of the Chronically Insane in England, 1855–1870." *BHM* 53 (1979): 553–594.

————. "Liberty and Lunacy: The Victorians and Wrongful Confinement." *Journal of Social History* 11 (1978): 366–386.

MacDonald, Michael. *Mystical Bedlam: Madness, Anxiety, and Healing in Seventeenth-Century England.* Cambridge: Cambridge University Press, 1981.

McGovern, Constance M. "Doctors or Ladies? Women Physicians in Psychiatric Institutions, 1872–1900." *BHM* 55 (1980): 88–109.

McKelvey, Blake. *American Prisons: A History of Good Intentions.* Montclair, N.J.: Patterson Smith, 1977.

McPeak, William. "Family Interactions as Etiological Factors in Mental Disorders: An Analysis of the *American Journal of Insanity*, 1844–1848." *American Journal of Psychiatry* 132 (1975): 1327–1329.

Marshall, James R., and Dowdell, George W. "Employment and Mental Hospitalization: The Case of Buffalo, New York, 1914–1955." *Social Forces* 60 (1982): 843–853.

Mellett, D. J. "Bureaucracy and Mental Illness: The Commissioners in Lunacy, 1845–1890." *Medicla History* 25 (1981): 221–250.

Midelfort, H. C. Erik. "Madness and the Problems of Psychological History in the Sixteenth Century." *Sixteenth Century Journal* 12 (1981): 5–12.

Mitchinson, Wendy. "Gender and Insanity: A Nineteenth Century Case." Paper presented at the Social Science History Association Annual Meeting, 1985.

————. "Gynecological Operations on Insane Women: London, Ontario, 1895–1901." *Journal of Social History* 15 (1982): 467–484.

Monkkonen, Eric H. "A Disorderly People? Urban Order in the Nineteenth and Twentieth Centuries." *Journal of American History* 68 (1981): 539–559.

Mora, George. "The Historiography of Psychiatry and Its Development: A Reevaluation." *Journal of the History of the Behavioral Sciences* 1 (1965): 43–52.

Mora, George, and Brand, Jeanne L., eds. *Psychiatry and Its History: Methodological Problems in Research.* Springfield, Ill.: Thomas, 1970.

Morgan, Norman C., and Johnson, Nelson A. "Failures in Psychiatry: The Chronic Hospital Patient." *American Journal of Psychiatry* 113 (1957): 824–830.

Morrissey, Joseph P.; Goldman H.; Klerman, L.; and associates. *The Enduring Asylum: Cycles of Institutional Reform at Worcester State Hospital.* New York: Grune & Stratton, 1980.

Neugebauer, Richard. "Treatment of the Mentally Ill in Medieval and Early Modern England: A Reappraisal." *Journal of the History of the Behavioral Sciences* 14 (1978): 158–169.

Numbers, Ronald L., and Numbers, Janet S. "Millerism and Madness: A Study of 'Religious Insanity' in Nineteenth-Century America." *Bulletin of the Menninger Foundation* 49 (1985): 289–320.

Parkerson, Donald H. "The Structure of New York Society: Basic Theories in Nineteenth-Century Social History." *New York History* 65 (1984): 159–187.

Paykel, E. S. "Life Stress in Psychiatric Disorders: Applications of the Clinical Approach." In *Stressful Life Events: Their Nature and Effects*, edited by B. S. Dohrenwend and B. P. Dohrenwend, 135–139. New York: Wiley, 1974.

Pickett, Robert S. *Houses of Refuge: Origins of Juvenile Reform in New York State, 1815–1857.* Syracuse: Syracuse University Press, 1969.

Pitts, John A. "The Association of Medical Superintendents of American Institutions for the Insane, 1844–1892: A Case Study of Specialism in American Medicine." Ph.D. diss., University of Pennsylvania, 1979.

Pollack, Horatio M. "The Development and Extension of the Parole System in New York State." *Psychiatric Quarterly* 1 (1927): 53–56.

Polsky, Howard W., Claster, Daniel S., and Goldberg, Carl, eds. *Social System Perspectives in Residential Institutions.* East Lansing: Michigan State University, 1970.

Quen, Jacques. "Asylum Psychiatry, Neurology, Social Work, and Mental Hygiene: An Explanatory Study in Interprofessional History." *Journal of the History of the Behavioral Sciences* 13 (1977): 3–11.

———. "Early Nineteenth-Century Observations on the Insane in the Boston Almshouse. *Journal of the History of Medicine and the Allied Sciences* 23 (1968): 80–85.

Rafter, Nicole Hahn. *Partial Justice: Women in State Prisons, 1800–1935.* Boston: Northeastern University Press, 1985.

Reverby, Susan. "The Search for the Hospital Yardstick: Nursing and the Rationalization of Hospital Work." In *Health Care in America: Essays in Social History*, edited by Susan Reverby and David Rosner, 206–225. Philadelphia: Temple University Press, 1979.

Reverby, Susan, and Rosner, David, eds. *Health Care in America: Essays in Social History.* Philadelphia: Temple University Press, 1979.

Riese, William. "History and Principles of Classification of Nervous Disease." *BHM* 18 (1945): 465–512.

Risse, Guenter B. "Epidemics and Medicine: The Influence of Disease on Medical Thought and Practice." *BHM* 53 (1979): 505–519.

Rosen, George. "Historical Trends and Future Prospects in Public Health." In *Medical History and Medical Care: A Symposium of Perspectives*, edited by Gordon McLachlan and Thomas McKeown, 57–81. London: Oxford University Press, 1971.

———. *Madness in Society: Chapters in the Historical Sociology of Mental Illness.* Chicago: University of Chicago Press, 1958.

———. "Problems in the Application of Statistical Analysis to Questions of Health, 1700–1880." *BHM* 29 (1955): 27–45.

———. "Social Stress and Mental Disease from the Eighteenth Century to the Present: Some Origins of Social Psychiatry." *Milbank Memorial Fund Quarterly* 37 (1959): 5–32.

Rosenberg, Charles E. "And Heal the Sick: The Hospital and the Patient in Nineteenth Century America." *Journal of Social History* 10 (1977): 428–447.

———. "Inward Vision and Outward Glance: The Shaping of the American Hospital, 1880–1914." *BHM* 53 (1979): 346–391.

———. "The Practice of Medicine in New York a Century Ago." *BHM* 41 (1967): 223–253.

———. *The Trial of the Assassin Guiteau: Psychiatry and the Law in the Gilded Age.* Chicago: University of Chicago Press, 1968.

Rosenfield, Sarah. "Sex Differences in Depression: Do Women Always Have Higher Rates?" *Journal of Health and Social Behavior* 21 (1980): 33–42.

Rosenham, David. "The Contextual Nature of Psychiatric Diagnoses." *Journal of Abnormal Psychology* 84 (1975): 462–467.

Rosenkrantz, Barbara G., and Vinovskis, Maris A. "Caring for the Insane in Ante-Bellum Massachusetts: Family, Community, and State Participation." In *Kin and Communities: Families in America,* edited by Allan J. Lichtman and Joan R. Challinor, 187–218. Washington: Smithsonian Institution Press, 1979.

———. "The Invisible Lunatics: Old Age and Insanity in Mid-nineteenth Century Massachusetts." In *Aging and the Elderly: Humanistic Perspectives in Gerontology,* edited by Stuart F. Spicker, Kathleen M. Woodward, and David Van Tassel, 95–125. Atlantic Highlands, N.J.: Humanities, 1978.

———. "Sustaining the 'Flickering Flame of Life.'" In *Health Care in America,* edited by Susan Reverby and David Rosner, 154–182. Philadelphia: Temple University Press, 1979.

Rosner, David. *A Once Charitable Enterprise: Hospitals and Health Care in Brooklyn and New York, 1885–1915.* Cambridge: Cambridge University Press, 1982.

Rothman, David. *Conscience and Convenience: The Asylum and Its Alternatives in Progressive America.* Boston: Little, Brown, 1980.

———. *The Discovery of the Asylum: Social Order and Disorder in the Early Republic.* Boston: Little, Brown, 1971.

Rubin, Julius H. "Mental Illness in Early Nineteenth Century New England and the Beginnings of Institutional Psychiatry as Revealed in a Sociological Study of the Hartford Retreat 1824–1843." Ph.D. diss., New School for Social Research, 1979.

Russell, William L. *The New York Hospital: A History of the Psychiatric Service, 1771–1936.* New York: Columbia University, 1945.

Ryan, Mary P. *Cradle of the Middle Class: The Family in Oneida County, New York, 1790–1865.* Cambridge: Cambridge University Press, 1981.

Santos, Elvin H., and Stainbrook, Edward. "A History of Psychiatric Nursing in the Nineteenth Century." *Journal of the History of Medicine and Allied Sciences* 4 (1949): 48–74.

Savino, Michael E., and Mills, Alden B. "The Rise and Fall of Moral Treatment in California Psychiatry: 1852–1870." *Journal of the History of the Behavioral Sciences* 3 (1967): 359–369.

Scheff, Thomas J. *Being Mentally Ill: A Sociological Theory.* Chicago: Aldine, 1966.

———. "Control over Policy by Attendants in a Mental Hospital." *Journal of Health and Human Behavior* 2 (1961): 93–105.

———. "The Labeling Theory of Mental Illness." *American Sociological Review* 39 (1974): 44–52.

Schlossman, Steven L. *Love and the American Delinquent: The Theory and Practice of "Progressive" Juvenile Justice, 1825–1920.* Chicago: University of Chicago Press, 1977.

Bibliography

Schneider, David M. *The History of Public Welfare in New York State, 1609–1866.* Chicago: University of Chicago: 1938.

Schneider, David M., and Deutsch, Albert. *The History of Public Welfare in New York State, 1867–1940.* Chicago: University of Chicago Press, 1941.

Schwartz, David B. "Asylum: Late Nineteenth Century View." *Hospital and Community Psychiatry* 27 (1976): 485–489.

Schwartz, Joel. "Women and the Mental Hospital in Nineteenth Century America: The Case of the Trenton State Asylum." Paper presented at the Newberry Conference on Women's History and Quantitative Methodology, July 1979.

Scull, Andrew. *Decarceration: Community Treatment and the Deviant—a Radical View.* Englewood Cliffs, N.J.: Prentice-Hall, 1977.

——. "The Domestication of Madness." *Medical History* 27 (1983): 233–248.

——. "From Madness to Mental Illness: Medical Men as Moral Entrepreneurs." *Archives Européennes de Sociologie* 16 (1975): 218–259.

——. "Mad-Doctors and Magistrates: English Psychiatry's Struggle for Professional Autonomy in the Nineteenth Century." *Archives Européennes de Sociologie* 17 (1976): 279–305.

——. *Museums of Madness: The Social Organization of Insanity in Nineteenth Century England.* New York: St. Martin's, 1979.

——, ed. *Madhouses, Mad-Doctors, and Madmen: The Social History of Psychiatry in the Victorian Era.* Philadelphia: University of Pennsylvania Press, 1981.

Sederer, Lloyd. "Moral Therapy and the Problem of Morale." *American Journal of Psychiatry* 134 (1977): 267–272.

Showalter, Elaine. *The Female Malady: Woman, Madness, and English Culture, 1830–1980.* New York: Pantheon, 1985.

——. "Victorian Women and Insanity." *Victorian Studies* 23 (1980): 157–181.

Shryock, Richard Harrison. *Medicine and Society in America: 1660–1860.* Ithaca, N.Y.: Cornell University Press, 1980.

Sicherman, Barbara. "The Paradox of Prudence: Mental Health in the Gilded Age." *Journal of American History* 52 (1976): 890–912.

——. *The Quest for Mental Health in America, 1880–1917.* New York: Arno, 1980.

Skultans, Vieda. *English Madness, Ideas on Insanity, 1580–1890.* London: Routledge & Kegan Paul, 1979.

Smith, Roger. *Trial by Medicine: Insanity and Responsibility in Victorian Trials.* Edinburgh: Edinburgh University Press, 1981.

Smith-Rosenberg, Carroll. "The Cycle of Femininity: Puberty and Menopause in Nineteenth Century America." *Feminist Studies* 1 (1973): 58–72.

Spitzer, Stephan, and Denzin, Norman, eds. *The Mental Patient: Studies in the Sociology of Deviance.* New York: McGraw-Hill, 1968.

Starr, Paul. "Medicine, Economy, and Society in Nineteenth-Century America." *Journal of Social History* 10 (1979): 588–607.

Straus, Murray A.; Gelles, Richard J.; and Steinmetz, Suzanne K. *Behind Closed Doors: Violence in the American Family.* New York: Doubleday, 1980.

Sykes, Gresham M. *The Society of Captives: A Study of a Maximum Security Prison.* Princeton, N.J.: Princeton University Press, 1958.

Szasz, Thomas S. *Ideology and Insanity: Essays on the Psychiatric Dehumaniza- tion of Man*. Garden City, N.Y.: Doubleday, Anchor, 1970.

———. *The Myth of Mental Illness*. New York: Harper & Row, 1961.

Taylor, Laurie. "Vocabularies, Rhetoric and Grammar: Problems in the Sociology of Motivation." In *Deviant Interpretations: Problems in Criminological Theory*, edited by David Downes and Paul Rock, 145–162. New York: Harper & Row, 1979.

Tomes, Nancy. "The Domesticated Madman: Changing Concepts of Insanity at the Pennsylvania Hospital, 1780–1830." *Pennsylvania Magazine of History and Bi- ography* 56 (1982): 271–286.

———. *A Generous Confidence: Thomas Story Kirkbride and the Art of Asylum- keeping, 1840–1883*. New York: Cambridge University Press, 1984.

———. "A Generous Confidence: Thomas Story Kirkbride's Philosophy of Asy- lum Construction and Management." In *Madhouses, Mad-Doctors, and Mad- men*, edited by Andrew Scull, 121–143. Philadelphia: University of Pennsyl- vania Press, 1981.

Tourney, Garfield. "A History of Therapeutic Fashions in Psychiatry, 1800–1966." *American Journal of Psychiatry* 124 (1967): 92–104.

Tyor, Peter L. "'Denied the Power to Choose the Good': Sexuality and Mental Defect in American Medical Practice, 1850–1920." *Journal of Social History* 10 (1977): 472–489.

Tyor, Peter L., and Bell, Leland V. *Caring for the Retarded in America: A History*. Westport, Conn.: Greenwood, 1984.

Tyor, Peter L., and Zainaldin, Jamil S. "Asylum and Society: An Approach to In- stitutional Change." *Journal of Social History* 13 (1979): 23–46.

Vogel, Morris J. *The Invention of the Modern Hospital: Boston, 1870–1930*. Chi- cago: University of Chicago Press, 1980.

Vogel, Morris J., and Rosenberg, Charles E., eds. *The Therapeutic Revolution: Essays in the Social History of American Medicine*. Philadelphia: University of Pennsylvania Press, 1979.

Waldinger, Robert J. "Sleep of Reason: John P. Gray and the Challenge of Moral Insanity." *Journal of the History of Medicine and Allied Sciences* 34 (1979): 163–179.

Walk, Alexander. "The History of Mental Nursing." *Journal of Mental Science* (1961): 1–17.

Walton, John K. "Lunacy in the Industrial Revolution: A Study of Asylum Admis- sions in Lancashire, 1848–1850." *Journal of Social History* 13 (1979): 1–22.

———. "The Treatment of Pauper Lunatics in Victorian England: The Case of the Lancaster Asylum." In *Madhouses, Mad-Doctors, and Madmen*, edited by An- drew Scull, 166–197. Philadelphia: University of Pennsylvania Press, 1981.

Weinstein, Raymond M. "The Mental Hospital from the Patient's Point of View." In *Deviance and Mental Illness*, edited by Walter R. Gove, 121–146. Beverly Hills, Calif.: Sage, 1982.

Wender, Paul H. "Dementia Praecox: The Development of the Concept." *Ameri- can Journal of Psychiatry* 119 (1963): 1143–1151.

Werman, D. S. "True and False Experts: A Second Look." *American Journal of Psychiatry* 130 (1973): 1351–1354.

Bibliography

Wexler, David B. "The Structure of Civil Commitment: Patterns, Presures and Interaction in Mental Health Legislation." *Law and Human Behavior*, 7 (1983): 1–15.

Wiebe, Robert. *The Search for Order, 1877–1920*. New York: Hill & Wang, 1967.

Yarrow, Marion Radke; Schwartz, Charlotte Green; Murphy, Harriet S.; and Deasy, Leila Calhoun. "The Psychological Meaning of Mental Illness in the Family." *Journal of Social Issues* 11 (1955): 12–24.

Index

abuse, 14–16, 22–23, 129–130, 176–178, 180–183, 201–208. *See also* attendants; restraints

addiction, drug, 92, 103, 122–123, 153, 267

admission procedures, 117–119, 224

AJI, 20, 23, 46–47, 64, 68, 70, 74, 119, 234, 254

alcoholism, 69, 92, 96, 153

AMSAII, 46–47, 49, 67, 70, 71–72, 193, 254

Apgar Report, 193–195, 203, 205

assistant physicians, 14–15, 61, 70–71; daily lives, 83–84; duties, 76, 82; female, 78–80, 147–148, 207, 241–242, 267; leaves, 81–82; qualifications, 77–80; and ratio to patients, 19; and relations with patients, 14, 19–21, 226

attendants, 128, 130, 132, 138–139, 157–158, 224, 225, 226–227, 263, 264–265, 268; and abuse, 176, 177–179, 180–183, 201–206, 265, 267–268; as domestic servants, 163, 178; drinking problems, 17–18, 168–169; duties, 15, 16–18, 164–167; as part of asylum family, 163–164, 176–177, 178, 183–184; qualifications, 170–172, 261, 262; ratio to patients, 24; resignations or firings, 17–18, 165, 169, 260, 263, 265; salaries, 174–175, 264; training schools, 179–180, 266; uniforms, 175–177, 268; at Utica, 172; at Willard, 167–169, 172–175

Ayers vs. Russell, 113

Beard, George M., 195–196

Benedict, Nathan: background, 65; relations with John Gray, 66–67; as superintendent, 20, 65–67, 125, 149

Blumer, George Alder, 20, 26, 56–57, 74–75, 81, 167, 176, 179

Brigham, Amariah: and attendants, 88, 154, 178, 264–265; early life of, 58–60, 236; as editor of the *AJI*, 64; at Hartford Retreat, 61; on insanity, 59–63, 106; on phrenology, 60–61; and record keeping, 88–89; and relations with patients, 11, 149; on religion, 59; as superintendent, 11, 19, 38, 40, 56, 57, 63; on treatment, 60–61, 62–65, 119–120, 158

Butolph, H. A., 38, 61

casebook records, xiii, 5–6, 86–89, 117, 119–120, 213–214

Chapin, John, 49, 201; as assistant physician, 72, 167; and attendants, 167–168, 177–178; on care of the chronic insane, 131–136; and conflicts with John Gray, 43–50; early life of, 71–72; and female physicians, 78; on the function of the asylum, 81–82; as superintendent, 23, 43–49, 56–57, 72–73

Chase, Hiram, 26

chronically insane, 45–47, 54, 131, 132, 139–140, 143, 210

classification, 12–15, 118–119, 157, 167, 224, 249; as punishment, 14, 124, 137–140, 224 commissioner in lunacy, 23, 136, 157–158, 178, 186, 189, 190–193, 203, 208, 209. *See also* Ordronaux, John; Smith, Stephen

commission in lunacy, 186, 208

commitment, 10–12, 22, 85–98, 117, 243; laws, 86, 109–115, 117, 190–193. *See also* families

Cook, George, 45–48, 65, 132, 254

county care, 30–31, 34, 39–41, 44–45, 50–51, 86, 93, 134, 153, 155, 159, 187–193, 209, 211

county superintendent of the poor, 30–31, 40–41, 85–86, 209–210, 299

Coventry, C. B., 31, 44

Davis, Phoebe, 129

dementia, 5, 92, 117–118, 134, 139–140, 145, 150, 158

diagnosis, 5, 117–118, 158, 249

discharge, 6, 54, 94–95, 106, 111, 114–115, 127, 149–157, 257, 258; as "not insane," 94, 114, 117, 153. *See also* patients

Dix, Dorothea, 38–42, 189

Downing, A. J., 222

entertainments, 120, 124, 141–143, 167–168, 247, 251, 261

epilepsy, 91, 92, 93, 98, 100, 123, 133, 138, 144–145, 154

escapes, 155–156, 225

families, 3, 28, 104, 114–115; and the asylum, 116; asylum as surrogate for, 4–5, 28, 57, 125–127, 142, 148, 163–164, 178–179, 183–185, 214–215; and commitment, 3, 86–98; distance from patients, 28

Farnham, Alice, 80

Foucault, Michel, xii

Goffman, Erving, xii, 7, 182

Gray, John, 26, 40, 49, 56–57, 67–68, 72, 73, 90, 92, 111, 125, 130, 149–152, 192; and attendants, 18, 165–166, 171, 175, 176, 177, 205; background of, 68; and conflicts with Nathan Benedict, 66–67, 239; and conflicts with staff, 43–49, 67–68, 77, 82, 196; criticisms of, 70–71, 73, 192–208, 272; death of, 71; and defense of Utica Asylum, 21–23; as editor of the *AJI*, 20, 23, 46–47, 68; at Guiteau trial, 69; on insanity, 68–70, 90, 98–104; and political skills, 77; on treatment, 120–125, 158–159

Grob, Gerald, 161, 188, 208, 230

habeas corpus, writs of, 112–113, 114, 154

Hammond, William, 126, 135, 192, 195–196

heredity, 70, 72–73, 94, 98, 100

Hotchkiss, William, 10–12, 128–129

Hoyt, Charles, 189

Hughes, Evan, 201–206

Ignatieff, Michael, 217

imbecility, 118

insane asylums: architecture of, 72; critics of, 161–162, 170, 176–177, 179, 186–212; history and historiography of, xi–xii, 106, 217; images of, 1, 57; multiple functions of, xii–xiii, 1–5; New York State system of, 28, 30–34, 49–50; and relations with public, 6–9, 17, 26–28; and

social control, xii, 1, 83; and visitors, 26–28. *See also* New York State Lunatic Asylum; patients; Willard Asylum for the Chronic Insane
insanity, xi, 4, 61–62, 69–70, 72–73, 85, 98–104, 112, 114, 215, 244; conceptions of, 32–33, 61–62; diagnosis of, 5, 65, 117–118, 158, 249; duration of, 247; and gynecological abnormalities, 80, 81; and heredity, 70, 72–73; and menstruation, 120; moral, 98; and poverty, 3 (*see also* patients, and class); and religion, 70; and sex differences, 98, 104 (*see also* women, and mental illness); and sexual deviance, 102–103
insanity defense, 69

Jarvis, Edward., 43, 77

legislature, 29–36, 52, 53, 187, 192–208, 202–203, 230–231, 232
Lynds, Elam, 35–36

mania, 5, 92, 118, 150, 152
Marcy, William, 33
matron, 38, 170, 264
melancholia, 5, 96, 118, 150, 251
mental hospitals. *See* insane asylums
mental illness. *See* insanity
Mitchell, S. Weir, 24–25, 73
Monkkonen, Eric, 97

National Association for the Protection of the Insane and the Prevention of Insanity (NIAPIPI), 186, 193
National Conference of Charities and Corrections, 193

New York Neurological Society, 190, 195, 199
New York State Lunatic Asylum: board of managers of, 27, 37–38, 55, 175; budget of, 12–54; daily routines of, 13–16; discharge policies of, 149–150, 152–153; early history of, 2, 29–38; injury books of, 22–23; investigations of, 22–23, 24, 192–208; setting of, 8, 13–14, 35–36, 222; superintendents of (*see* Blumer, George Alder; Brigham, Amariah; Gray, John). *See also* patients; treatment

Oneida County Medical Society, 31–34
Opal, 13, 19–20, 25, 26–27, 126, 127–128, 156
Ordronaux, John, 73–74, 111–113, 191–193, 196–200, 270, 271

parole, 16–17, 155, 225
patients: age, 93, 104–105; arrival at asylum of, 10–12; and class, 2–3, 24–25, 85–86, 92, 97, 104–109, 114, 148, 153, 225, 243, 269; and community, 6, 10–11; costs of care of, 86–87, 92–93, 110–111, 131–132 (*see also* treatment); criminal, 94–95; daily routines of, 27; discharge of, 114–115, 116; duration of illness of, 247; eccentricity of, 95–98; escapes of, 17, 65–66, 139, 161; ethnicity of, 5, 6, 105, 246, 262; and families, 85–98, 126–127, 154 (*see also* families); forced feeding of, 182–183; marital status of, 106; parole of, 16–17, 155, 225; private, 85, 110–111; race

patients (*continued*)
of, 106–108; and relations with doctors, 19–20; and relations with each other, 21–45; and sex, 5, 6, 25–26, 106–108; and transfers to Willard, 115; views of treatment of, 3, 12–13, 127–130, 148; and violence, 21–23, 90–91, 128, 138–139, 161, 227–228
Pilgrim, Charles, 81
Pratt, Daniel, 191–192
Prudden, Lewis, 113–114
pyromania, 91

recovery rates, 150–152, 154–155
restraints, 22–24, 124, 140–141, 156, 196, 197, 207, 214, 223, 224, 228; abolition of, 74, 140–141; in Utica crib, 93, 124, 196, 207

Scull, Andrew, xii
senility, 101, 103
sexual disorders, 146–148
Silkman, James B., 112–113
Smith, Stephen, 13, 135, 152, 167, 199–200, 203, 224, 225, 271–272
Spitzka, E. C., 193, 195
State Board of Charities, 186, 188–189, 190, 192–193, 195, 196–198, 199–200, 205, 207
State Care Act, 108, 188, 208–212, 215
State Charities Aid Association, 189, 190, 209, 269
suicide, 98, 118
superintendents, 3, 6, 8, 19, 53–56, 73, 83, 235. *See also* Blumer, George Alder; Brigham, Amariah;

Chapin, John; Gray, John; Wise, P. M.
syphilis, 92, 93, 98, 101, 123, 144–145
Szasz, Thomas, xi, xii

Thropp, Enos, 31–33
Tourtellot, Louis, 82, 196
treatment: acute versus chronic, 131–132, 157–162; of the chronic, 131–132; drug, 80, 120–122, 129–130, 144–145, 146, 149, 250–251; and economic considerations, 85–86, 110, 131, 146, 153, 157–158, 194–195, 213, 231, 232, 253; heroic, 62–63, 74–75, 136, 252, 255, 256; moral, 4, 14–15, 119–120, 128, 137–143 (*see also* entertainments); and punishment, 15–16; and recovery, 150–152, 154–155; routines, 14–16; of sexual disorders, 146–148; at Utica, 118–131; at Willard, 53–54; and work, 4, 13, 27–28, 75, 131–136, 160
tuberculosis, 144

Wilbur, Hervey B., 192–193, 196
Wilkins, Theoda, 78
Willard, Sylvester, 44–45, 189
Willard Asylum for the Chronic Insane: budget of, 51–54; classification of, 137–141; daily routines of, 16–17; detached cottages at, 9, 48, 137; discharge policies of, 150–151, 154–157; early history of, 2, 43–49, 147, 209; infirmary at, 139–140; mechanical restraints at, 140–141; medical care at, 143–148, 160–161; mechanical restraints at, 140–141;

medical care at, 143–148, 160–161; moral treatment at, 137–143; physical setting of, 8–9, 12, 45–46. *See also* Chapin, John; Wise, P. M.

Wise, P. M., 56–57, 69, 75, 81, 136

women: and domestic violence, 94, 107, 114; and mental illness, 3–4, 18, 102, 104, 106–108, 116, 121, 146–148, 256; and treatment, 4, 133

Woodward, Samuel, 57